THIRD EDITION

Population Health

Creating a Culture of Wellness

David B. Nash, MD, MBA
Founding Dean Emeritus
Jefferson College of Population Health
Thomas Jefferson University
Philadelphia, PA

Alexis Skoufalos, EdD, MS
Associate Dean, Strategic Development
Jefferson College of Population Health
Thomas Jefferson University
Philadelphia, PA

Raymond J. Fabius, MD, FACPE
Co-Founder and President
HealthNEXT
Philadelphia, PA

Willie H. Oglesby, PhD, MBA, MSPH, FACHE
Interim Dean
Jefferson College of Population Health
Thomas Jefferson University
Philadelphia, PA

JONES & BARTLETT
LEARNING

World Headquarters
Jones & Bartlett Learning
5 Wall Street
Burlington, MA 01803
978-443-5000
info@jblearning.com
www.jblearning.com

Jones & Bartlett Learning books and products are available through most bookstores and online booksellers. To contact Jones & Bartlett Learning directly, call 800-832-0034, fax 978-443-8000, or visit our website, www.jblearning.com.

Production Credits
VP, Product Management: Amanda Martin
Director of Product Management: Laura Pagluica
Product Manager: Sophie Fleck Teague
Product Specialist: Sara Bempkins
Senior Project Specialist: Dan Stone
Senior Marketing Manager: Susanne Walker
Manufacturing and Inventory Control Supervisor: Amy Bacus
Composition: codeMantra U.S. LLC
Cover Design: Michael O'Donnell
Rights & Media Specialist: Rebecca Damon
Media Development Editor: Troy Liston (TBD)
Cover Image (Title Page, Part Opener, Chapter Opener):
    © chomplearn/Shutterstock
Printing and Binding: LSC Communications

18847-9

Library of Congress Cataloging-in-Publication Data
Library of Congress Cataloging-in-Publication Data unavailable at time of printing
Library of Congress Control Number: 2019913111

6048

Printed in the United States of America
22   10 9 8 7 6 5 4

Brief Contents

Contents

**Chapter 7   Developing the Workforce
to Enhance Population
Health 137**

Robert Sachs, Alexis Skoufalos

PART III   Creating Culture Change   155

**Chapter 8   Health Promotion and
Health Behavior 157**

Amy Leader, Preethi Selvan

Foreword to the Third Edition

Population health was first defined by Kindig and Stoddard in 2003 as "the health outcomes of a group of individuals, including the distribution of such outcomes within the group."[1] The Institute of Medicine (IOM, now the National Academy of Medicine) built on this definition: in 2011, the IOM Roundtable on Population Health Improvement developed its working definition, in which "population health outcomes are the product of multiple determinants of health, including medical care, public health, genetics, behaviors, social factors, and environmental factors."[2] Indeed, population health involves the consideration of a broader array of determinants of health beyond health care or public health. Importantly, achieving population health requires the convergence of multiple sectors and disciplines.

Population health has never been more important. In the United States (U.S.), we are facing challenges achieving the triple aim (simultaneously improving the health of the population, enhancing the experience and outcomes of care, at a lower per capita cost).[3] Healthcare spending has been rising and is widely considered unsustainable; it already accounts for nearly 18% of the nation's gross domestic product.[4] Furthermore, such high rates of spending have not translated to better outcomes. U.S. health outcomes lag behind almost every other industrialized nation despite higher spending on health care.[5] For example, the U.S. lags behind similarly developed countries in terms of rates of all-cause mortality, premature death, thirty-day mortality following hospital admission, and hospital-acquired conditions. Furthermore, many groups in the U.S. face significant disparities across racial and ethnic lines and income levels. For example, the differences in life expectancy that Murray and colleagues (2006)[6] noted in their study "Eight Americas" suggest that we are living in different countries rather than different counties. Murray et al. found a difference of nearly 21 years between the healthiest of the epidemiologically clustered groups of Americans and the least healthy groups. To improve the health of the population, nationally or locally, we must overcome these disparities and focus on improving outcomes while also providing high-value care. It will take a collective effort to address the social determinants and ensure the integration of public health and primary care (IOM 2011,[7] IOM 2012[8]).

At the same time as we are facing all these healthcare challenges, the U.S. health policy landscape is evolving, offering new opportunities for population health. In particular, the passage of the Patient Protection and Affordable Care Act (ACA) in 2010 was a major step toward the reform necessary to improve the health of the nation. An orientation toward population health is a strong theme throughout the ACA. Many provisions of the ACA enacted reforms to the health insurance market. The ACA expanded Medicaid and established health insurance exchanges for individuals and small businesses to buy health insurance. However, under the current U.S. administration and Congress, the future of the ACA has become uncertain. Nevertheless, the Trump administration has indicated that value-based care will continue to be a priority. In a March 2018 speech to the Federation of American Hospitals, the Department of Health and Human Services (HHS) Secretary Alex Azar noted, *"There is no turning back to an unsustainable system that pays for procedures rather than value. In fact, the only option is to charge forward—for HHS to take bolder action, and for providers and payers to join with us."*[94] However, much work remains. Fee-for-service is still the dominant form of healthcare payment, health care and social services continue to be separate, and too many Americans lack access to the social and environmental conditions necessary to achieve good health.

In light of these conditions, how can we make progress toward population health?

This textbook serves as an important roadmap to achieving population health. Across 14 chapters divided into three discrete sections, it presents an overview of the current state of health in the U.S. and discusses the population health ecosystem, which encompasses the healthcare delivery and payment models, legal and regulatory landscape, and more, that provide the backdrop to all population health efforts. It places population health squarely in the context of multiple determinants of health. Importantly, it calls for a widespread culture change. Achieving population health will not be possible without a sustained focus on prevention and health promotion, accountability for outcomes, development of new payment and care delivery models, cross-sector collaboration, and a focus on health in all policies. The rise of new tools and technologies also presents an important opportunity. New sources of data combined with advances in informatics, analytics, and data science will allow for better prediction and management of risk. Consumer-facing technologies, such as wearables and apps, will provide patients with new opportunities to be engaged in their care.

As discussed in this book, all of these changes will require the engagement of multiple sectors, accompanied by the development of a skilled healthcare workforce with training across many different disciplines. In a recent paper, my coauthor and I have called for a new science and practice of convergence in population health. Convergence science has been defined as "an approach to problem solving that integrates expertise from life sciences with physical, mathematical, and computational sciences as well as engineering to form comprehensive frameworks that merge areas of knowledge from multiple fields to address specific challenges."[10] In our opinion, "in addition to harnessing advances in health care and biomedical research, population health requires the engagement of social, behavioral, economic, data, legal, and political science sectors and must involve policy decisions and practice in all sectors. Improving the health of populations requires the collective participation of all stakeholders to converge on research, policy, and implementation that can influence health outcomes. ***Accordingly, population health needs to be reconceived as a new science and practice of convergence.***"[11]

Universities and academic health sciences centers have an important role to play in advancing population health as a convergence science. They must create the culture, ecosystem, and incentives to bring relevant sectors together and establish frameworks that integrate knowledge from many disciplines and implement the new convergence science of population health. Institutions, such as the Jefferson College of Population Health, are leading the way by working to "prepare leaders with global vision to examine the social determinants of health and to evaluate, develop and implement health policies and systems that will improve the health of populations and thereby enhance the quality of life."[12] However, more work is needed.

Fortunately, we are at a turning point for making progress toward population health. The healthcare landscape is evolving: overall, we are seeing a shift from volume to value and a growing emphasis on prevention and health promotion, recognition of the importance of the social determinants of health, and the engagement of non-health sciences and sectors. Indeed, population health must be reimagined as convergence science and practice. Advances in technology and the entry of new stakeholders into the healthcare field, such as Uber, Amazon, JP Morgan, and Berkshire Hathaway's new healthcare partnership, further signal the growing recognition of the important role of population health. For these reasons, we are optimistic about the future health of citizens in the U.S.

Victor Dzau, MD
President, National Academy of Medicine

▶ References

1. Kindig D, and Stoddart, G. What is population health? *American J Public Health*. 2003;93(3):380–383.
2. Roundtable on Population Health Improvement. Available at: http://nationalacademies.org/HMD/Activities/PublicHealth/PopulationHealth ImprovementRT.aspx. Accessed December 2, 2018.
3. What is the Triple Aim? Available at: http://www.ihi.org/Topics/TripleAim/Pages/Overview.aspx
4. Martin AB, Hartman M, Washington B, Catlin A, and The National Health Expenditure Accounts Team. National Health Care Spending in 2017: Growth Slows to Post–Great Recession Rates; Share of GDP Stabilizes. *Health Affairs*. 2019;38(1):96–106.
5. OECD (2017), Health at a Glance 2017: OECD Indicators, OECD Publishing, Paris. http://dx.doi.org/10.1787/health_glance-2017-en
6. Murray, CJ, Kulkarni, SC, Michaud, C, Tomijima, N, Bulzacchelli, MT, Iandiorio, TJ, and Ezzati M. 2012. Eight Americas: Investigating mortality disparities across races, counties, and race-counties in the United States. *PLoS Medicine*. 2012;3(9):e260.
7. Institute of Medicine. For the public's health: revitalizing law and policy to meet new challenges. Washington, DC: The National Academies Press, 2011.
8. Institute of Medicine. 2012. Primary Care and Public Health: Exploring Integration to Improve Population Health. Washington, DC: The National Academies Press. https://doi.org/10.17226/13381
9. Remarks on Value-Based Transformation to the Federation of American Hospitals. Available at: https://www.hhs.gov/about/leadership/secretary/speeches/2018-speeches/remarks-on-value-based-transformation-to-the-federation-of-american-hospitals.html
10. Massachusetts Institute of Technology. Convergence: the future of health. Cambridge, MA: Massachusetts Institute of Technology, 2016. Available at: http://www.convergencerevolution.net/2016-report/
11. Dzau VJ and Balatbat CA. Reimagining population health as convergence science. *Lancet*. 2018 (August 4);392 (10145):367–368.
12. Jefferson College of Population Health. About Us. Available at: https://www.jefferson.edu/university/population-health/about.html

Preface

As I write this preface to the third edition of *Population Health: Creating a Culture of Wellness,* the Jefferson College of Population Health (JCPH) is celebrating a major milestone: our 10th birthday. In July 2008, the Board of Trustees of Thomas Jefferson University in Philadelphia, PA, voted unanimously to approve the creation of the nation's first College of Population Health.

The creation of our college was an integral part of the university's critical public commitment to improving the health of our citizens and an important step toward its goal of becoming a national leader in health sciences education. As the country's first college of population health, we felt then—and we reaffirm now—our particular and unique responsibility and burden. Our challenge is to train leaders for the future from across the healthcare stakeholder spectrum who will go forward and improve the health of the population. Ours was the first college to build the bridge between health and health care. This book provides a strong foundation for this bridge, and helps us to meet the challenge of creating tomorrow's leaders today.

A number of important questions still need to be addressed as the national population health agenda matures. Among these questions are, "What exactly is population health? How does it differ from public health?"

David Kindig's breakthrough paper, published in 2003, is the one that most thought leaders call out as having provided the best working definition of population health—namely, "the distribution of health outcomes within a population, the health determinants that influence distribution and the policies and interventions that impact the determinants."[1]

Kindig also provided us with the view that population health could be "the aggregate health outcome of health adjusted life expectancy of a group of individuals in an economic framework that balances relative marginal returns from the multiple determinants of health. This definition proposes a specific unit of measure of population health, and considers the relative cost-effectiveness of resource allocation to multiple determinants."[1]

There are five essential goals to consider when applying the population health concept across the continuum of care: 1) keeping healthy those who are well; 2) reducing health risks; 3) providing quick access to care for acute illness so that health does not deteriorate; 4) managing chronic illness to prevent complications, and 5) treating those with complex or catastrophic illnesses at centers of excellence where they can receive high-quality, high-value care. To accomplish these goals effectively, we will need to draw from sister areas of emphasis, such as health informatics, organizational design and construction, and human factors engineering. We recognize now that collaboration is required to accomplish these goals effectively, and progress must be regularly assessed across the spectrum of care.

As we take the next steps forward, the leadership of Jefferson Health (our $5.2 billion delivery system) and the faculty of our college are beginning to coalesce around the differences between population health and public health. We strongly believe that population health connects prevention, wellness, and behavioral health science with healthcare quality and safety, disease prevention and management, and economic issues of value and risks, all in the service of specific populations. Like public health, population health builds on the science of epidemiology and biostatistics, but population health takes these disciplines in a new direction by means of applied metrics and analytics.

Historically, the U.S. healthcare system rewarded reactive care rather than proactive care and financially encouraged doctors to focus on treating acute episodes of illness and disease rather than managing those illnesses or diseases to avert future crises. In most cases, doctors were paid for piecework. That is, they were paid more for providing a higher volume and higher intensity of acute-care services. At the same time, doctors were underpaid, or not paid at all, to coordinate effective preventive health care to keep their patients out of the hospital. We must learn to focus our efforts (and incentives) upstream on prevention rather than working to fix problems after people become ill. To address obesity and its risks to health, instead of building yet another bariatric surgical operating room, we need to offer nutritional counseling and improve the quality of school lunches. Rather than building another cardiac catheterization laboratory, we need to focus on prevention as the core strategy to reduce the burden of coronary artery disease. If we want to make progress, it's more efficient and effective to "shut off the faucet" rather than constantly "mop up the floor."

It has been nearly 10 years since the passage of the Affordable Care Act, and there is value in examining the key trends that have emerged. The financial realities of the traditional payment system, prior to systemic reform, generated terrible conflicts of interests and pernicious incentives. If hospitals could be incentivized to succeed in their mission of truly improving health rather than merely filling beds, then patients and society would benefit. We believe, and we reaffirm with the third edition, that population health represents just such a paradigm shift and that it has already begun to tackle the transformation of our system now readily described as moving from volume to value. In fact, we believe that a good part of population health management could be readily described by the phrase "no outcome, no income."

Accumulating national evidence supports the central thesis of this third edition and is best exemplified by Dr. Victor Dzau's authorship of the Foreword of this book. In his leadership role at the National Academy of Medicine (NAM), Dr. Dzau impaneled the leading experts in the industry to reaffirm the idea that we must learn to "shut off the faucet" instead of always "mopping up the floor." In the watershed publication, *Vital Signs for the Nation*, the NAM made it explicitly clear that population health would be the lever to move 18% of the GDP in the right direction, and that practicing population health would eventually help move our nation from #17 in the world with regard to the health of our population, to at least into the top 10, given the fact that we now spend nearly $3 trillion dollars a year, or $10,000 per person annually, including children.

I strongly believe that a "no outcome, no income" system must be characterized by the following: 1) practicing medicine based on the best available evidence and tying payments to those outcomes, 2) reducing unexplained clinical variation, 3) continually measuring and closing the feedback loop between physicians and the supply chain that supports them, 4) trading professional autonomy for clinical collaboration, and 5) engaging with patients across the continuum, especially capitalizing on advances in modern technology.

In addition to the NAM, other major groups, including the American College of Physicians (ACP) and the American Medical Association (AMA), have also endorsed population health. Indeed, the AMA has led a consortium of 30 medical schools through a process to completely revamp undergraduate medical education and align it with the tenets of population health. As of this writing, the 2nd edition has been deployed in more than 80 graduate programs nationwide and in schools of medicine, nursing, pharmacy, public health, and related health sciences. A decade ago, I found myself explaining the nomenclature regarding our field, and indeed our college, to virtually every colleague, on nearly a daily basis. As I traveled across the country, people were unfamiliar with the terminology of population health. Ten years later, the JCPH is at the forefront of a national movement to become more responsible stewards of the vast public resources for which we are accountable to our citizens. Perhaps our nation will become a world leader in providing a healthcare system characterized by the original Institute of Medicine's (now the NAM's) six domains of safety, effectiveness, efficiency, patient-centeredness, timeliness, and equity. Instead of a set of a half-dozen lofty and seemingly unattainable goals, population health has emerged as the roadmap for successfully closing the quality chasm and achieving improvement in health.

▶ How Is This Book Organized?

This 3rd edition is focused on the expanding role of population health and its importance in bringing about a nationwide culture of wellness. The text has been completely revised and updated to incorporate considerable changes in the delivery system, and it recognizes the powerful role that new technology will continue to play in improving the health of the population.

This book is organized into 15 chapters, divided into three discrete sections. We have instituted one consistent definition of population health throughout the book, agnostic to whatever approach the nation continues to take to implement health reform. In Part Three, each chapter includes closing vignettes that help to illustrate the key take-home messages.

Part One, "**Population Health in the United States,**" lays the groundwork with a thorough review of the scholarship in the field. It helps to define the impact of the social determinants of health and takes a closer look at the impact of disparities on health.

Part Two, "**The Population Health Ecosystem**," takes population health and analyzes the structures, systems, stakeholders, and the regulatory environment within the ecosystem itself. It ends with a serious discussion on workforce development to support improvement in the health of the population. This is a critical component of the long-range goals of our college, and is certainly consistent with the goals as elucidated by *Vital Directions* from the NAM.

The third section of the book, "**Creating Culture Change**," recognizes that we must give our readers tools that will help them to leverage change. These include a better understanding of the science of prevention and health promotion and the use of technology to support consumer engagement. Of course, culture change continues to be an important tool in our toolbox.

The third edition concludes with a special section by Dr. Stephen K. Klasko, the visionary President and CEO of our health system. Dr. Klasko has stimulated a national discussion on the future of academic medicine and its role in promoting the health of the population.

▶ Who Should Read This Book?

My co-editors and I are grateful for the participation of a large number of nationally recognized experts, and our own faculty, who helped to conceptualize and execute this third edition. While we, of course, believe every section contains important information for anyone who cares about how we might more effectively improve the health of the country, we recognize that for many, this may be their first exposure to the field. As a result, the book appeals to a broad spectrum of learners, including undergraduates in colleges and universities across the country, and professional schools of medicine, public health, health administration, nursing, and the pharmaceutical sciences.

Many dedicated people have played an important role in the genesis of this third edition. I would particularly like to thank our amazing university President and CEO Stephen K. Klasko, MD, MBA, for his continued visionary leadership and his ongoing and unwavering support of the Jefferson College of Population Health and me as the Senior Editor. I want to also recognize the steadfast support of our school from the Provost, Dr. Mark Tykocinski. With the recent merger of Thomas Jefferson University and Philadelphia University, Dr. Tykocinski now has ten deans reporting to him, with a student body of nearly 8,000. Selfishly speaking, I am proud that the College of Population Health is widely viewed as the innovation engine within the academic pillar that supports the entire Jefferson Health System.

As the Senior Editor, I continue to be very appreciative of the hard work of my co-editors Drs. Alexis Skoufalos, Willie H. Oglesby, and Ray Fabius. We are strongly supported by Ms. Sonja Sherritze, an accomplished medical editor. Sonja is deeply connected to our college in her role as Editor of *Pharmacy and Therapeutics*, a peer-reviewed journal for which I have had the privilege of being the Editor-in-Chief for nearly 20 years.

I am particularly grateful to the faculty and staff of the Jefferson College of Population Health who have boldly travelled this unmarked path with us in the successful launch and early growth of our college. I am especially grateful to our relatively new colleague, Willie H. Oglesby, who helped conceptualize this third edition and was central in organizing the three-part strcture, and providing us with deep insight about the language surrounding the ecosystem of population health. Finally, we would also like to mention our gratitude to friends and family who have supported us as we pursued our passion for improving the health and well-being of the population.

At this important 10th anniversary, we are truly grateful to our current and future students who challenge us with their complex questions and whose quest for solutions will bring about much-needed improvements in population health in the future. It has been an incredible privilege for me, as the founding Dean, to lead this talented team, and I am confident that our students will go forth and make a world of difference. We will continue to build the bridge between health and health care.

As all good editors know, we take full responsibility for any errors of omission or commission. Most importantly, we greatly value feedback from our readers and fellow pioneers in population health. We are particularly interested in the value of the text as a pedagogic tool as well.

I have always felt strongly that one of the tenets of good leadership is to help prepare those who will take the mantle tomorrow. I am supremely confident that this third edition of *Population Health: Creating a Culture of Wellness,* will provide just such a foundation for training the future healthcare leaders that our nation so desperately needs today to help nurture a healthier, happier, and more productive nation tomorrow.

David B. Nash, MD, MBA
Summer 2019

▶ Reference

1. Kindig D, Stoddart, G. What is population health? *Am J of Public Health.* 2003;93(3):380–383.

The Optimistic Future for HealthCare: Population Health from Philosophy to Practice

Stephen K. Klasko, MD, MBA

David Nash has led the fight for the transformation of American health care—long before he founded Jefferson's College of Population Health more than 10 years ago. He stands at the most critical intersection of our time: across public health, personalized health, and the huge ecosystem that has created an overpriced and inequitable healthcare delivery system. I believe it is this intersection that will determine our future. And David has a favorite catch phrase that perfectly captures that future: "No outcome, no income."

But the disconnects that challenge an optimistic future remain strong, all the way from our popsicle-stick-and-glue federal policies to the way we select and license clinicians to our inability to coordinate and deliver complex care to the "superutilizers," the 5% of patients who account for 50% of the total cost.[1]

American healthcare delivery remains fragmented, unfriendly, often unsafe, and deeply inequitable. It is an industry that takes Star Trek–level medicine and grafts it onto a Fred Flintstone delivery system. We are all the worse for it.

The key is this: we know a lot about the social determinants of health. We know that 80% of what determines our health takes place outside the health delivery system. But we knew that 20 years ago. We knew it 10 years ago. We still don't know how to bring that knowledge home—to ensure that the billions of dollars we spend bolsters an individual's physical health, mental health, and indeed social health. We need to look outside the delivery system and work hand in hand with community partners, government, and industry to develop solutions to these complex problems.

It is time to stop talking about population health and, instead, make it happen throughout America's massive healthcare enterprise. This book describes the different structures and stakeholders in the healthcare ecosystem, explains how they connect and complement one another, and offers all of us a clear resource to construct meaningful population health interventions. The next step is to embrace disruption, find creative partners, and seek the radical transformation that will build the optimistic future we all fight for.

Reading this book, and listening to David Nash speak, is like taking a series of golf lessons. The book can guide us to position ourselves to care for an entire population; tell us what club to use to overcome inequities in food, education, and housing; and give us a feeling of where the fairways of success and sandtraps of the old model lie. But it is time for the leaders of healthcare organizations in all areas to actually solve these problems and deal with the rough across all sectors of the healthcare ecosystem—providers, hospitals, pharma, insurers, PBMs, and especially consumers themselves.

▶ The Iron Triangle Lives

William Kissick outlined the famous Iron Triangle of Healthcare in the 1990s, based on his work on Medicaid in the 1960s. It remains true: there is an iron triangle of access, quality, and cost containment. Increasing or decreasing any side of that triangle changes at least one other side. [2] But we cannot kid ourselves—disruption is painful.

The Patient Protection and Affordable Care Act (ACA) did not escape Kissick's Iron Triangle. The ACA did exactly what it was supposed to do—it increased access to our broken delivery system and then hoped we would transform ourselves. Quite to the contrary, we have seen instead a debate in which everyone continues the game of pointing fingers at each other.

Incremental change will not be sufficient to break the Iron Triangle. Healthcare transformation requires disruption. Part of disruption involves creative collaboration. And some of it will lead to parts of the industry failing, especially if they cannot show outcomes that make sense to payers, but also to the new boss: patients.

▶ Disruption Can Be Creative

I had the honor of taking part in a panel on the future of hospitals at the World Economic Forum in Davos, Switzerland, in January 2019. It gave me the opportunity to talk with people from multiple nations, with many different delivery systems and needs.

The experience reinforced my belief that health care must become global—we have to learn by "thinking globally," more than we like to admit in the United States. The global problem is stark: the World Economic Forum estimates that 100 million people a year are forced into poverty because they cannot afford to pay for health care, and far too many people simply do not have access to a basic package of health care. [3] That is as true in my hometown of Philadelphia, which hosts a prestigious array of academic health institutions, as it is in Johannesburg or Durban. In fact, Philadelphia has the dubious lead among major U.S. cities when it comes to the greatest disparity in average life expectancy—20 years between our richest and poorest zip codes.

That means it's time to embrace disruption. In my 2016 book, *We Can Fix Healthcare*, [4] I laid out 12 disruptors that could have been embraced by both political parties and become the basis for a new delivery system in the United States. I still believe we can do it, and in Davos, I advocated for several disruptors.

While disruption is painful, it can also be optimistic, creative, exciting, and good for the people involved. It can be especially great for the people at the center—patients, their families, and their communities.

▶ Health Care with No Address

We need to use technology to create "health care with no address." As I said at the World Economic Forum, I cannot wait for a future Davos when we talk less about self-driving cars and more about self-healing humans. That future is closer than we think. Nor is the vision of phones and watches and clothes that monitor our health limited to the rich: cell phones have spread further than anyone anticipated. But if we don't shift our thinking, we cannot keep up. Shobana Kamineni of Apollo Hospitals in India was on the Davos panel and said: "In India, we cannot build enough hospitals. The mobile phone is the disruptive technology, and that is where the hospital will move."

To be clear: The iPhone will never be your primary care physician. Artificial intelligence (AI) is not a magic panacea. But we need to get to the point where most health care happens at home. That means we need to stop talking about "telehealth"—it's just health.

▶ Is There an Avatar in the House? The Clinician in the Age of AI

In an age in which augmented intelligence will take over the tasks of memorization and robotics, we need clinicians who are selected and trained in ways that enhance their innate human qualities: to help them to be creative, communicative, and empathetic. I always begin with the DNA of the clinical system—the selection and licensing of clinicians. We still select clinicians, especially physicians, on the basis of biochemistry grades and memorization tests. Then we're surprised that doctors aren't more empathetic team builders. But when we attempt to select medical students with empathy, emotional intelligence, and leadership—the kids who built free clinics instead of studying biochemistry—those students face board exams that force them to compete with each other for residency slots based on memorization skills. Medical education has a lot that it needs to change.

Regardless of discipline, the clinician must be trained and licensed to be the human being in the room, even if that room is virtual. As Alibaba founder Jack Ma said at the World Economic Forum, "When we invented cars, we didn't teach our kids to run faster. When we invented planes, we didn't teach our kids to fly." Computers will replace our ability to crunch numbers and remember data, but they will never be as wise as we are. We need to produce clinicians who understand the human question, "What does this mean?"

I saw this firsthand as an obstetrician, after a baby was born with unanticipated Down syndrome. The first question the parents often ask is some form of "What does this mean?" I've seen good obstetricians answer by describing the genetic basis for Down syndrome. I've seen great ones answer by saying, "It means you've delivered a beautiful baby who will love you very much. And we will connect you with other parents who have delivered beautiful babies like yours so you can find out more, and share experiences."

There's no question that in the near future, there will be a robot/AI/he/she/it next to me when I deliver a baby. And there is no question that he/she/it will be better than we humans are at immediately naming whatever anomaly exists. But it will never understand what is going through the minds of the mother and father and what they need emotionally and spiritually. Technology will replace a good part of what doctors must do today, but the next generation of nurses and doctors will be greater teammates to patients when we stop trying to make clinicians better robots than the robots themselves.

▶ The Crisis of Complex Care

At Jefferson, we have been pioneers in teaching "hot-spotting," with support from the Robert Wood Johnson Foundation; we are one of four national hubs for interprofessional education targeting "super-utilizers." This is critical because our globe has a crisis in what's called complex care—helping people who have multiple, frequently chronic illnesses combined with mental health challenges and complex social needs. The Jefferson Center for Interprofessional Education has trained teams of students to meet people who are caught in a cycle of emergency-room visits—for example, to repeatedly change a colostomy bag. That small pilot program showed cuts in cost, increases in empathy and self-efficacy for the students, and increases in optimism for the faculty mentors. The data are being readied for publication, but the bottom line is that it showed a significant reduction in emergency room visits and a notable reduction in length of stay in the hospital and in 30-day readmissions.

If we want self-healing humans, we need a platform of technology that makes it possible for interdisciplinary teams to deliver the simple human solutions that people need.

▶ Equity Matters

We need a far more diverse group of clinicians. We must excite young women and men from all backgrounds about the profession of health care, give them the confidence to pursue it, and then accept them into our schools. I would rather see the kid who volunteered to build a free clinic get accepted to medical school than the kid who spent his or her time taking multiple MCAT prep courses while sitting at home studying biochemistry. We did this with the SELECT program at the University of South Florida, and it works: set a minimum bar of grades and/or MCAT scores, and then select students based on emotional intelligence and leadership. In Jefferson's JeffDESIGN curriculum, we eliminated the MCATs. It can be done.

To think globally and act locally demands that we create a truly global healthcare system. It is ridiculous that a well-trained clinical professional from another country must start over in the United States. That's why Thomas Jefferson University has created the first joint-MD program between the United States and the European Union. Based at Cattolica University in Italy, Italian students will be able to earn both Italian and American medical degrees that will allow them to practice on either continent.

Building on the global clinician, we further need an understanding of integrative medicine that does not sneer at holistic health developed in other countries. When I accidentally hurt myself in India, I was offered solutions related to movement and diet, not pain pills. Global health care is not an "either/or" (either "Western" or "Eastern") but a "both/and." Given our poor track record with chronic and non-communicable disease prevention, we need to embrace all forms of diagnosis, prevention, and treatment that have been shown to be effective, regardless of their place of origin.

These new professionals—the empathetic, creative, and communicative clinicians of the future—are the ones who will tackle health disparities; who will understand the integration of mental and physical health; and who will find solutions for social health, working with teams we haven't yet defined. We know health depends on employment, education, and opportunity—it's time we made zip code no longer the primary predictor of a person's destiny.

▶ Yes, It Is About Health

We use a variety of words to describe the "movements" we need in healthcare delivery. But to me, combining integrative medicine, personalized medicine, and population health is possible. It means we have to think of "health" as physical, mental, and social. Once we do that, we can better serve individuals, their families, communities, and populations. That would be a true goal for an optimistic future.

There is plenty of pessimism about our ability to make these changes. One conference I sat through reminded me of the old quotation: "We're a crossroads. One road leads to total destruction, the other to utter despair. Let's hope we choose the right one." But that's not the future I see.

What I see is a future where the Iron Triangle is replaced by a diamond of consumer-centric care in which everyone has the ability to connect, and form human relationships; the ability to easily navigate the system on patients' own terms; and the ability to understand what they need to do. We need to replace the "winter is coming" rhetoric of the old healthcare delivery system with a new mantra of reimagining health care to create unparalleled value.

(Stephen K. Klasko, MD, MBA is President of Thomas Jefferson University and CEO of Jefferson Health.)

▶ References

1. Mitchell EM. *Concentration of Health Expenditures in the U.S. Civilian Noninstitutionalized Population, 2014.* November 2016, AHRQ Statistical Brief #497. Available at: https://meps.ahrq.gov/data_files/publications/st497/stat497.pdf
2. Kissick WL. Medicine's Dilemmas: Infinite Needs Versus Finite Resources. New Haven: Yale University Press; 1994.
3. Klasko SK. Dispatch from Davos. *STATNews First Opinion*, January 26, 2019. Available at: https://www.statnews.com/2019/01/26/dispatch-from-davos-future-hospitals/
4. Klasko SK, Shea GP, Hoad MJ. We Can Fix Healthcare: The 12 Disruptors That Will Create Transformation. Mary Ann Liebert Inc.; 2016.

Contributors List

Jillian Baker, DrPH, EdM
Medical Scholarship Director
Rowan University School of Osteopathic
  Medicine
Stratford, NJ

Justin Beaupre, EdD, MHA, LAT, ATC
Postdoctoral Research Fellow
Main Line Health Center for Population
  Health Research etc
Main Line Health Center for
  Population Health Research
  at Lankenau Institute for
  Medical Research
Wynnewood, PA

Janice L. Clarke, RN, BBA
Project Director
Jefferson College of
  Population Health
Thomas Jefferson University,
Philadelphia, PA

Joe Coughlin, PhD
Director
MIT AgeLab
Massachusetts Institute of Technology
Cambridge, MA

Myles Dworkin, MD (c), MPH (c)
Thomas Jefferson University
Philadelphia, PA

Victor J. Dzau, MD
President
National Academy of Medicine
Washington, DC

Adam Felts, MFA
Technical Associate
MIT AgeLab
Massachusetts Institute of Technology
Cambridge, MA

Rosemary Frasso, PhD, MSc, MSc, CPH
Program Director
Public Health
Jefferson College of Population Health
Thomas Jefferson University
Philadelphia, PA

Livia Frasso Jaramillo, MSPH
Public Health Analyst
The Innovation Center (CMMI)
Centers for Medicare and Medicaid Services
Washington, DC

Stephen K. Klasko, MD, MBA
President
Thomas Jefferson University
Chief Executive Officer
Jefferson Health
Philadelphia, PA

Michael Kobernick, MD, MS-HSA, MS-PopH, FAAFP
Senior Medical Director
Health Plan Business
Blue Cross Blue Shield of Michigan
Detroit, MI

Amy Leader, DrPH, MPH
Associate Professor
Jefferson College of Population Health
Thomas Jefferson University
Philadelphia, PA

Y. Brian Lee, JD, MPH
Senior Associate
Alston and Bird, LLP
Washington DC

John McAna, PhD, MA
Associate Professor
Jefferson College of Population Health
Thomas Jefferson University
Philadelphia, PA

Russell K. McIntire, PhD, MPH
Assistant Professor
Jefferson College of Population Health
Thomas Jefferson University
Philadelphia, PA

Michael H. Park, JD, MPH
Partner
Alston and Bird, LLP
Washington, DC

Jennifer Puzziferro, DNP, RN-BC, CCM
Vice President of Case Management
RWJ Barnabas Health
Oceanport, NJ

Jennifer Ravelli, MPH
Assistant Dean for Student Affairs
Jefferson College of Population Health
Thomas Jefferson University
Philadelphia, PA

Martha Romney, MS, JD, MPH
Assistant Professor
Jefferson College of Population Health
Thomas Jefferson University
Philadelphia, PA

Robert Sachs, PhD
Sachs Talent Advisors
Benicia, CA

Somava Saha, MD, MS
Vice President
IHI
Lexington, MA

Harm J. Scherpbier, MD, MS
Chief Medical Information Officer
Health Share Exchange
Philadelphia, PA

Katherine A. Schneider, MD , MPhil, FAAFP
President
Delaware Valley ACO
Radnor, PA

Preethi Selvan, BS, MPH
Associate Professor
Clinical Study Coordinator
Sidney Kimmel Cancer Center
Jefferson Health
Philadelphia, PA

Vicki Shepard, ACSW, MPA
Vice President
Tivity Health
Franklin, Tennessee

Matthew Stiefel, MPA, MS
Senior Director
Center for Population Health
Kaiser Permanente
Care Management Institute
Oakland, CA

Karen Walsh, MS, MBA
Program Director
Population Health Intelligence
Jefferson College of Population Health
Thomas Jefferson University
Philadelphia, PA

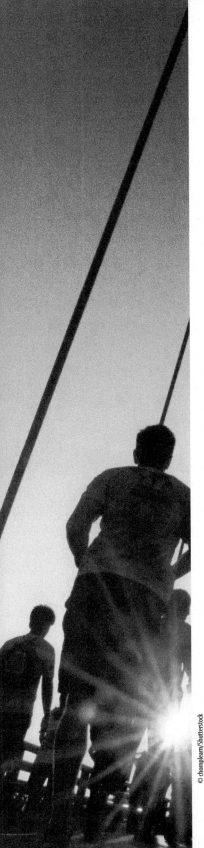

© champleam/Shutterstock

PART I

Population Health in the United States

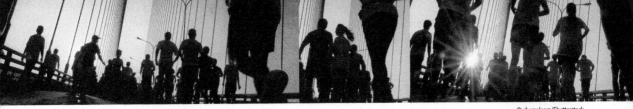

CHAPTER 1

The Population Health Promise

Raymond J. Fabius*

EXECUTIVE SUMMARY

The population health promise is to promote health and prevent disease; the strategy is to create a culture of health and wellness.

The Patient Protection and Affordable Care Act (ACA) of 2010 codified and set in motion an array of programs and initiatives aimed at improving the health of the U.S. population. Although considerable progress is being made on many fronts—from making health insurance accessible to more Americans to increasing accountability for and quality of healthcare delivery and services—the need for population health management continues to be urgent.[1]

Population health refers broadly to the distribution of health outcomes within a population, the health determinants that influence distribution, and the policies and interventions that affect those determinants.[2,3] Accordingly, population health is holistic in that it seeks to reveal patterns and connections within and among multiple systems and to develop approaches that respond to the needs of populations. Population health tactics include rigorous analysis of outcomes. Understanding population-based patterns of outcomes distribution is a critical antecedent to addressing population needs in communities (i.e., patterns inform the selection of effective population health management strategies to diminish problems and develop approaches to prevent reoccurrence in the future).

Convened by the National Quality Forum in 2008, the **National Priorities Partnership** addressed four major healthcare challenges that affect all Americans: eliminating harm, eradicating disparities, reducing disease burden, and removing waste.[4] One of the priorities identified to address these challenges is *improving the health of the population*. While ambitious, this goal is fundamental to health care and healthcare reform. Improving the health of the population will require improved efforts to provide health insurance coverage, promote healthy behaviors, and prevent illness. The "silos" in healthcare delivery must be dismantled, and providers must work cooperatively to

---

* This chapter includes contributions made in the first and second editions by Valerie Pracilio, David B. Nash, Janice L. Clarke, and JoAnne Reifsnyder.

advance seamless, coordinated care that traverses settings, health conditions, and reimbursement mechanisms. Interdisciplinary teams of healthcare providers committed to diligent management of chronic conditions and providing safe, high-quality care will play a central role. The emergence of a preventive health focus within primary care will be required. The pattern of infrequent health checkups supplemented by more frequent visits for treatment of illness must become more balanced. Policy makers will be called upon to craft policies that support illness prevention, health promotion, and public health, and healthcare professionals must continue their efforts to enforce recommendations in communities. All of these efforts must align to promote health and wellness and to advance a new population health agenda. Population health is no longer a mere strategy—it is the solution that holds the greatest promise for creating *a culture of health and wellness*.

LEARNING OBJECTIVES

By the end of this chapter, the reader will be able to:

1. Explain the concept of population health.
2. Recognize the need for a population health approach to healthcare education, delivery, and policy.
3. Discuss the integration of the four pillars of population health.
4. Use this text as a resource for further population health study and practice.

KEY TERMS

Chronic care management
Compression of morbidity
Health determinants
Health policy

Healthcare quality
National Priorities Partnership
Patient safety
Population health

Population health
  management
Public health

▶ Introduction

Although the term **population health** is not new, there is still no clear consensus on a single definition. In the evolving U.S. healthcare environment, where the need for positive change is evident and ongoing, population health is viewed across constituencies as a promising solution for closing key gaps in healthcare delivery. In the context of this text, population health is defined as the distribution of health outcomes within a population, the health determinants that influence distribution, and the

policies and interventions that affect the determinants.[2,3]

Population health embraces a comprehensive agenda that addresses the healthy and unhealthy, the acutely ill and chronically ill, the clinical delivery system, and the public sector and private sector. While there are many determinants that affect the health of populations, the ultimate goal for healthcare providers, public health professionals, employers, payers, and policy makers is the same: healthy people comprising healthy populations that create productive workforces and thriving communities.

Population health is both a concept of health and a field of study.[2] Populations can be defined by geography or grouped according to some common element (e.g., employer, ethnicity, medical condition, provider organization). As the name implies, population health is inclusive of every individual and group, comprising a heterogeneous population that wears many labels. For example, a man of Mexican descent who works for a contractor and belongs to a carpenters' union may be a member of three different populations: the community of Mexican descent, his employer's organization, and the carpenters' union. To address needs at the population level, all of these associations must be considered.

As a field of study, attention must be given to multiple determinants of health outcomes, including medical care, public health interventions, and the social environment, as well as the physical environment and individual behaviors, and the patterns among each of these domains.[5] The purpose of this chapter is to promote an understanding of population health, to encourage discussions and engagement of key stakeholders (healthcare providers, public health professionals, payers/health plans, employers, and policy makers), and to foster the development and dissemination of strategies aimed at improving population health.

▶ The Current State of Population Health

Health care in the United States is complex, and many would argue that its method of delivery bears little resemblance to a true system. Considering the characteristics of systems (e.g., interactivity of independent elements to form a complex whole, harmonious or orderly interaction, and coordinated methods or procedures), U.S. health care may well represent the antithesis of a system.

Despite devoting nearly 18% of its gross domestic product (GDP) to health care (projected to approach 20% by 2025),[6] the United States performs lower on five dimensions of performance (quality, access, efficiency, equity, and healthy lives) compared to similar developed countries, including Australia, Canada, Germany, the Netherlands, New Zealand, and the United Kingdom. The common element among the aforementioned nations is a universal healthcare delivery system, and some argue that the absence of universal health care in the United States explains the access disparities, inequity, and poor outcomes in addition to the exorbitant and uncontrolled costs.[7]

Unfortunately, the health status of the U.S. population does not reflect the high level of spending on health care. For example:

- One-third (33%) of U.S. adults went without recommended care, did not see a doctor when sick, or failed to fill a prescription because of costs in 2016.[8]
- Major disparities exist based on socioeconomic status. Roughly 28.5 million[9] Americans were still uninsured as of 2017, and 133 million Americans (almost half of the U.S. population, 45%) suffer from at least one chronic condition.[10]
- **Healthcare quality** is suboptimal, and **patient safety** is lagging.[8,11]
- The public health system continues to be egregiously underfunded.[12]

The passing of the ACA and the subsequent phased implementation of a broad range of regulations and initiatives aimed at improving the health of the U.S. population have brought about some positive change; however, it will take many years before the benefits are realized on a population scale,[1] and the need for **population health management** remains urgent. Recent governmental limitations placed on the ACA, including the December 2017 repeal of the individual mandate, have resulted in a steady increase in the number uninsured (13.7%, the highest rate since 2016).[13]

Because important advances in science and technology have contributed to increases in life expectancy in the 20th century, unprecedented growth in the population of older adults has introduced new pressures on healthcare providers, payers, and communities. Roughly two-thirds of Medicare recipients contend with two or more chronic conditions, and 16% deal with six or more. In 2015, 55% of Medicare fee-for-service beneficiaries had hypertension, 27% had ischemic heart disease, and 27% were diabetic.[14] Chronic conditions require frequent monitoring and evaluation, which places a strain on the healthcare system and makes the need for care coordination imperative. Perhaps most disturbing is the recent announcement from the Centers for Disease Control and Prevention (CDC) that the average life expectancy for Americans is declining.[15] Traditionally, the United States has supported a "sick care" system bolstered by payment policies that reward both consumers and providers for health care that is sought primarily when acute illness strikes or in an emergency. While caring for the sick will always be an integral

part of health care, true population health can be achieved only by placing an equal emphasis on health promotion and disease prevention.

▶ Population Health Defined

Population health is the distribution of health outcomes within a population, the determinants that influence distribution, and the policies and interventions that affect the determinants.[2,3] These three key components—health outcomes, **health determinants**, and health policies—serve as the foundation for this chapter.

Health determinants, the varied factors that affect the health of individuals, range from aspects of the social and economic environment to the physical environment and individual characteristics or behaviors.[16] Although some of these factors can be affected by individuals, some are external to an individual's locus of control. For example, individuals may be coached to adopt healthier lifestyles, thereby reducing their risk for lifestyle-related diseases (e.g., hypertension, diabetes, and smoking-related illnesses). The same individuals may be genetically predisposed to cardiovascular disease or may reside in geographic locations where exercise outdoors is unsafe or air quality is extremely poor—these health determinants are outside of their control.

Health determinants are a core component of the ecological model used in **public health** to describe the interaction between behavior and health.[16] The model assumes that overall health and well-being are influenced by interaction among the determinants of health.[17] Relationships with peers, family, and friends influence behavior at the interpersonal level. At the community level, there are institutional factors (e.g., rules, regulations) that influence social networks. At the public level, policies and laws regulate certain behaviors.[13] These variables have a cumulative effect on health and the ability of individuals and populations to stay well in the communities where they live, work, and play.

Interaction among the determinants of health leads to outcomes, the second component of the population health definition. Population- and individual-level disparities and risk factors exert significant influence on health-related outcomes. General health outcomes could be improved by assuring access to quality health care for all populations, regardless of insurance status, with a primary focus on health maintenance and prevention to decrease health risks. Policy development is one mechanism used to support population health management and improvement. Support and guidance for these efforts is provided by policies at local, state, and federal levels. Laws that have promoted use of seat belts and infant care seats have had a profound impact on population health.[18]

Population health is not synonymous with public health. In fact, public health is a core element of population health that focuses on determinants of health in communities, preventive care, interventions and education, and individual and collective health advocacy and policies. The principal characteristic that differentiates population health from public health is its focus on a *broad set of concerns* rather than on just these specific activities.[2] Population health efforts generate information to inform public health strategies that can

be deployed in communities. The combination of information gathered to define problems and build awareness and the strategies to address needs comprises population health management.

Consider Wendy McDonald, a hypothetical community member whose situation illustrates the importance of considering multiple factors when using a population health approach. Wendy is obese and lives in a lower-income community where healthy food is not readily available. Safe neighborhood parks and recreation centers are lacking, making physical activity a challenge. Inadequate health insurance restricts her ability to receive primary medical care or guidance from a healthcare provider on how to manage her weight, and she is unaware of the increased risk factors for disease it presents. On a positive note, she regularly attends a place of worship where she receives spiritual enrichment and social support. Additionally, she works as a waitress at the local diner. The population health conceptual model suggests effective approaches to care delivery in such situations. A primary care practice in communities such as Wendy's could be reengineered as a patient-centered medical home that applies a comprehensive, integrated approach to disease and **chronic care management** and supports health promotion and disease prevention, which would lead to better short- and long-term health outcomes. A community-based population health approach to address Wendy's challenges might include adding green space for recreation and supporting healthy food options through tax credits to food stores that offer them. The church she attends could organize farmers' markets, health risk assessments, and 5K walk/run events. The diner she works at could provide health insurance. Underlying both of these approaches are policies that support community improvements, make health a priority that leads to better health outcomes, and may be shared with public health initiatives.

Donald Berwick, MD, President Emeritus and former CEO of the Institute for Healthcare Improvement (IHI), once remarked that health care has no inherent value, but health does. The population health promise requires a broader focus—one that encompasses health promotion and disease prevention as well as caring for the sick. Under the traditional healthcare model, individuals seek care to restore health when it is compromised and seek prevention primarily when they are fearful about potential loss of health. Under an aspirational model of health and wellness promotion, individuals would value their health and seek preventive care as a means to optimize it. Ultimately, the intrinsic reward of feeling well should be a major driver of population health in a true "culture of wellness."

▶ Foundations of Population Health

The Care Continuum

Nearly all of us spend our lives striving to be well, mitigating actual and potential health risks, seeking treatment when acutely ill, managing chronic illness and recovering from catastrophic health events. The promise of population health is to allow more and more people the opportunity to live healthily and well for the vast majority of their lives—limiting illness and suffering. Research is now clear that the longer you can maintain your health, the shorter the period of significant illness before one dies. This is known as the **compression of morbidity**. We all hear about vital people who live well into their 90s and die in their sleep. It must be the goal of population health to markedly increase this experience within communities.

The Science

Health is a state of well-being; population health provides a conceptual framework for the study of well-being and variability among populations.[19] In the United States, the delivery of healthcare services receives the lion's share of health-related resources and attention, and yet it is only one of many contributors to and drivers of a population's overall health (e.g., the business and political communities). There is substantial, yet unrealized, opportunity to advance the population health agenda and to improve health through efforts focusing on personal behavior and health promotion within each of these spheres.[20]

The expectation that healthcare providers must care for their own patients in their own practice settings is rapidly changing as new models for affecting outcomes at the population level are introduced. Treatment of populations aims to increase recommended prevention and screening practices and improve adherence to recommended treatment in accordance with evidence-based, nationally recognized guidelines. These aims can be achieved only with teams of healthcare providers cooperating within and across settings. While one-at-a-time treatment has been the traditional approach to patient care, population-level interventions that integrate a set of common aims and standards are needed to support significant and sustainable health improvements in the

United States. This effort has been aided by the adoption of electronic medical records and the promotion and incentivizing their meaningful use to improve accessibility of actionable health information.[21]

Keeping well people well is a key priority in population health. The notion that health professionals should only see their patients on an annual basis (or less often) unless they are ill must give way to a clinical relationship based on maximizing health and preventing illness. Periodic and dedicated preventative health visits should be completed with the intent of delivering all evidence-based preventive care, from biometric health screening to health risk assessments and immunizations. Reducing health risks is also a key priority in population health. Once identified unhealthy behaviors like smoking, excessive alcohol consumption, and sedentary lifestyles must be aggressively addressed and changed using our advancing understanding of behavior change. Management of chronic disease is another key priority in population health. The fact that nearly half of all Americans have one or more chronic diseases is only partly explained by population growth and increases in longevity. The present and predicted burden of chronic disease is the strongest signal that current strategies for helping people get well, and stay well, are ineffective. The burgeoning population, and the prevalence of chronic illness that accompanies it, drives both cost and utilization of healthcare services and now threatens Americans' progress in life expectancy.

There is ample evidence to inform population health improvement strategies, but processes remain poorly defined and success is variable. Although numerous national goals for population health have been proposed and targeted outcomes have been defined, translating best practices into action is a daunting challenge. The Chronic Care Model (**FIGURE 1-1**) is a

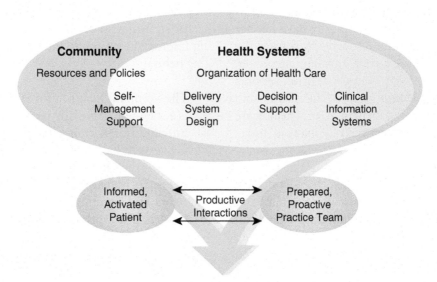

Improved Outcomes

FIGURE 1-1 The Chronic Care Model.

well-regarded conceptual model for guiding the development of effective programs to provide better chronic care to patients; it is comprised of Patient Care and Practice Improvement Organization, Clinical Information Systems, Delivery System Design, Decision Support, Self-Management, and Community Resources. The devil is, of course, in the details: the emerging understanding of what is required to build "cultures of health" will be of value, as will the recognition of complementary activities in support of an improved delivery process (e.g., social and environmental factors).[22]

The greatest contributor to premature death from preventable chronic illness is patient behavior. Of the six model components, the degree to which patients are informed and activated is critical to improved patient outcomes. Informed, activated patients are more likely to learn self-management strategies and to adopt healthy behaviors. Providers need an array of tools to effectively help patients manage their health risks and chronic conditions. Because they typically have neither the time nor the resources to consult the evidence base during a patient encounter, they need robust clinical decision support tools at the point of care. The relationship between the patient and the healthcare provider can be greatly enhanced today through the use of technology. Many avenues of communication need to be leveraged—such as text messaging via secure patient portals, phone calls, and video chat, and incorporating data from wearables and other remote monitoring devices into medical records. These can provide helpful feedback, help to track compliance and adherence, and alert clinicians through an early warning system

when health starts to deteriorate. Further, providers need a reimbursement model that rewards performance and outcomes while supporting the needed investment of time and money into appropriate interdisciplinary communication, collaboration, and follow-up, as well as access to interoperable technologies that permit data sharing in real time. All of these components must be supported by clinical information systems that track progress in the management of chronic conditions. These practice-based components, combined with community efforts (e.g., community-wide screenings, in-home support for elderly persons, nutritious school lunch programs) and active participation of patients who productively interact with healthcare providers, will support effective, quality chronic care management while reducing health risks and costs.[23]

One of the greatest challenges to improving the population's health is translating evidence into practice. Two state initiatives provide examples of population health strategies in action—one generating improvements, while the other is lagging behind:

- The Vermont Blueprint for Health is a state-led, nationally recognized initiative transforming healthcare delivery. At its foundation is the local Transformation Network, a network of Project Managers, Practice Facilitators, and Community Health Team Leaders who work with Patient-Centered Medical Homes (PCMHs), Community Health Teams (CHTs), and local health and human services leaders. This local network allows for rapid response to Vermont's health priorities through statewide implementation of new initiatives. Their 2017 Annual Report highlights progress in reducing health and pharmacy expenditures, increasing investment into focused social services, near comprehensive engagement of the state's primary care providers, greater training in self-care of its citizen and improved data and analytics.[24] Vermont remains among the healthiest states in the United States.[25]

In Wisconsin, David Kindig, a key thought leader in population health, is driving efforts to earn the designation of "healthiest state." For three decades, Wisconsin's *Healthiest Wisconsin 2020: Everyone Living Better, Longer* initiative of statewide community health improvement planning has targeted improving the health of all Wisconsin residents and communities. This plan's two key goals are to (1) improve health across the life span and (2) achieve health equity by eliminating health disparities among various segments of the population. Its mission is to ensure that Wisconsin's populace lives in healthy, safe, and resilient families and communities. *Healthiest Wisconsin 2020* fulfills Wisconsin Statutes section 250.07(1)(a), requiring the Department of Public Health to develop a public health agenda for the people of Wisconsin at least every decade. The initiative is both a state health plan and an ongoing process based in science, quality improvement, partnerships, and large-scale community engagement. Despite these efforts, Wisconsin has fallen from 11th in 2006 to 20th in the widely publicized America's Health State Rankings in 2016.[26,27]

Both the Vermont and Wisconsin initiatives demonstrate that population health extends beyond health care. Achieving health and well-being at the individual, population, state, and national levels requires the collective efforts of healthcare providers, public health professionals, payers and health plans, employers, and policy makers. That is why achieving success is difficult and can be elusive.

The Effect on and Response by the Marketplace

There is a shared responsibility for population health. Although the cost burden of health care is shared among all constituents, the distribution of costs is not always proportionate. With more than 60% of Americans obtaining health insurance coverage through their employers, businesses have a substantial stake in their employees' health.[28] As healthcare costs continue to escalate much faster than general inflation, businesses are searching for strategies to moderate their healthcare cost trend without compromising quality.

The health of its employees influences the economic health of a business—a healthy employee is more productive on the job and misses fewer days of work. The bottom line is that prevention and condition management programs generate a positive return on investment for employers. Studies have calculated returns as high as 6:1 and as low as 1.5:1.[29-31] In this scenario, everyone benefits—employees are healthier, businesses can operate more cost effectively through improved employee performance and reduced health benefits costs, and health plans reduce outlays for preventable morbidity. In some cases, the productivity gains exceed the healthcare cost savings for employers.[32] Moreover, there is increasing evidence that companies focusing on the health and safety of their workforces produce greater returns for their shareholders.[33-35] Worksites are an ideal venue for promoting health and wellness because many consumers spend the majority of their time at work.

While the business case for promoting wellness is becoming increasingly clear, competing priorities present a challenge in many organizations. Corporate cultures, investment costs, incentives for participation in the initiative, and employees' underlying health behaviors are potential barriers to implementing a successful workplace wellness program. However, workplace programs may be effective in three major domains of health: promoting behavior change to prevent illness, supporting employees to self-manage existing chronic conditions, and assisting in the navigation of a complex and fragmented healthcare system.

Forty percent of premature deaths can be attributed to behavior. In fact, behavior is a key contributor to two of the leading causes of preventable death: obesity and smoking.[28] The healthcare costs alone attributable to smoking topped $170 billion a year in 2012.[36] Workplace smoking cessation programs have been effective in mitigating risk for the health effects of smoking. Employer involvement in health plan–supported disease management efforts or health advocacy programs provides employees with access to education and tools to properly manage their health risks and conditions as well as seek the most appropriate care. The best available evidence concerning employer sponsorship of health and wellness programs supports the premise that employees who are well provide the greatest benefit to their organization.[37-39] Many enlightened employers realize that health care is not a cost but rather an investment into their most precious resource—their workforce.

The Politics

Prevention, health, and wellness efforts must be supported by policy and regulation to advance the population health agenda. Building awareness is the first step toward making lasting change, followed by identifying population health needs and recognizing the importance of data and measurements on which causal inferences are based and actions are taken. Two examples, current rates of smoking and obesity in the United States, represent needs that must be addressed through population-based initiatives. The rate of adult smoking has yielded to successful public health improvement efforts, falling from 42% to 14% prevalence over the past 50 years,[40] while obesity has proven more resistant to positive change. Policies that drive population health efforts must be created at the local, state, and national levels to serve as the foundation of the population health infrastructure. Because implementation of population health improvement policies often requires significant resources, stakeholders face difficult decisions about priorities. Federal monies made health improvement initiatives possible in Vermont and Wisconsin initially.[24-26]

The healthcare workforce that will provide high-quality population-based health care in the future must be trained now, and education reform is under way to ensure the competency of future leaders and practitioners in health care, public health, business, and **health policy**. Finally, research is needed to inform strategies to address population health approaches. Similar to the potential benefits of disease management and wellness initiatives realized by employers, policies that support health and wellness will also contribute to the wealth of the nation.

▶ Frameworks for Innovation

A few key initiatives provide a framework for innovation that aspires to make population health efforts the norm rather than the exception. As in all industries, common goals and objectives and guidelines and standards in health care provide an understanding of expectations and drive efforts to provide safe quality care.

Healthy People 2020

Since 1979, the U.S. Department of Health and Human Services (HHS) has been leading efforts to promote health and prevent disease through identification of threats and implementation of mechanisms to reduce threats. *Healthy People* sets national health objectives for a 10-year period based on broad consensus and founded on scientific evidence.[41] *Healthy People 2020* contains 38 focus areas and four overarching goals:

1. Attaining high-quality, longer lives free of preventable disease, disability, injury, and premature death
2. Achieving health equity, eliminating disparities, and improving the health of all groups
3. Creating social and physical environments that promote good health for all
4. Promoting quality of life, healthy development, and healthy behaviors across all life stages[42]

Public health professionals use the *Healthy People* objectives to drive community efforts based on defined needs. Containing both clinical and nonclinical measures, *Healthy People* also serves as a guide for population health efforts and a road map for interdisciplinary collaboration that leads to shared responsibility for health and wellness. Also important, it introduces the concept of cultural transformation and the benefits of leveraging social and physical environmental influences to elevate the health status of populations.

The development of objectives and priorities for *Healthy People 2030* is under way. The fifth edition of *Healthy People*, will aim at new challenges and build on lessons learned from its first four decades.[43]

Triple Aim

In 2007, the IHI launched the Triple Aim, providing an agenda for optimizing performance on three dimensions of care: the health of a defined population, the experience of care for individuals in the population, and the cost per capita for providing care for this population.[44] "Population" is defined by enrollment or inclusion in a registry. Groups of individuals defined by geography, condition, or other attributes can be considered a population if data are available to track them over time. At the core of this initiative are efforts to optimize value. A number of integrators across the United States are working to implement strategies to achieve the Triple Aim. At the macro level, integrators pool resources and make sure the system structure and processes support the needs of the population. At the micro level, integrators ensure that the most appropriate care is provided to patients with respect to overuse, underuse, and misuse.[45] To successfully achieve the Triple Aim, healthcare institutions and delivery systems must reduce hospitalizations, apply resources to patient care that are commensurate with their needs, and build sustained relationships that are mindful of patient needs.[45] While a great deal of work remains to achieve optimal performance on the three objectives, the Triple Aim has built awareness and offers a framework for population health management.

Practical National Priorities and Goals—The CDC 6/18 Initiative

The U.S. Centers for Disease Control and Prevention (CDC) has identified six common and costly health conditions with 18 proven interventions. It is collaborating with partners, including healthcare providers, public health workers, insurers, and employers who purchase insurance, to improve health and control healthcare costs by:

- Giving partners rigorous evidence about high-burden health conditions and related interventions

- Highlighting disease prevention interventions to increase their coverage, use, and quality
- Aligning proven preventive practices with value-based ways of paying for healthcare

With this information, partners can make decisions that improve people's health and help control costs.

It calls for the following actions:

1. Reduce tobacco use
2. Control high blood pressure
3. Prevent unintended pregnancy
4. Control asthma
5. Improve antibiotic use
6. Prevent type 2 diabetes

This a ground-breaking effort because it calls for the collaboration of many of the constituents of health care to attach prevalent health risks and conditions where there are known effective interventions.[46]

In 2015, the Agency for Healthcare Research and Quality developed six National Quality Strategy (NQS) priorities. These areas of focus address much of the population health continuum while also focusing on the equally germane issues of health equity and patient safety[47]:

1. **Patient Safety:** Making care safer by reducing harm caused in the delivery of care
2. **Person- and Family-Centered Care:** Ensuring that each person and family is engaged as partners in their care
3. **Care Coordination:** Promoting effective communication and coordination of care
4. **Effective Prevention and Treatment:** Promoting the most effective prevention and

treatment practices for the leading causes of mortality, starting with cardiovascular disease

5. **Healthy Living:** Working with communities to promote wide use of best practices to enable healthy living

6. **Care Affordability:** Making quality care more afford-able for individuals, families, employers, and governments by developing and spreading new health care delivery models

Achieving these national priorities requires health care and wellness to be fostered at the community level through a partnership between public health agencies, healthcare purchasers, and healthcare systems. The goal is to promote preventive services, healthy lifestyle behaviors, and high-quality, affordable healthcare. These priorities and projects will continue to spur action and innovation and serve as a model for population health improvement.

▶ **Preventive Strategies and Pillars of Population Health**

To achieve the ambitious goal of improving the U.S. healthcare system, we must be prepared to broaden our current focus beyond acute, episodic health care. This implies a collective commitment to incorporating population-based primordial, primary, and secondary prevention strategies—as citizens and as healthcare providers—as well as better coordinating care for those suffering from chronic

illnesses to mitigate complications, also known as tertiary prevention.

Preventive Strategies

National experts and policy analysts agree that focusing on primordial and primary prevention strategies (e.g., healthy environments, healthy cultures, health promotion, and wellness activities) will ultimately improve the overall health of citizens and decrease the costs associated with overmedicalization. Three lifestyle modifications—eliminating and reducing tobacco use, eating healthy foods with portion control, and increasing regular physical activity—are consistently identified in population-based epidemiologic research as most likely to reduce the prevalence of chronic conditions. Utilizing secondary preventive services (e.g., cancer screenings, blood pressure and cholesterol monitoring, health counseling) promotes early detection of disease. Secondary prevention strategies seek to reduce barriers to early treatment or completion of therapy, thereby improving treatment outcomes and reducing disease chronicity. For example, detecting an early-stage breast cancer during mammography and initiating treatment may prevent the need for mastectomy or indeed be lifesaving.

Tertiary prevention focuses on minimizing disease complications and comorbidities through appropriate, evidence-based treatment and—critical to reducing healthcare costs—by coordinating and providing continuity of care for chronic conditions. This is best accomplished by incorporating the Chronic Care Model into healthcare systems and monitoring disease-specific indicators to ensure quality care and maximize quality of life for patients and their families. Prevention and disease management are integral to maintaining population health and encouraging wellness. All healthcare professionals have a role to play.

The Four Pillars

Population health rests on four pillars[48] (FIGURE 1-2):

- Care Management
- Quality and Safety
- Public Health
- Health Policy

The interaction among each of these pillars in education and practice lays the foundation for achieving population health goals and strategies (FIGURE 1-3). National statistics show that only 55% of U.S. adults receive recommended preventive care, acute care, and care for chronic conditions, such as hypertension (high blood pressure) and diabetes.[11] Successful execution of these four pillars will markedly improve upon this metric, allowing many more people to receive evidence-based care and health-related services.

Care Management

When only slightly more than half of Americans receive care that they could benefit from, there is a need for collective efforts (involving patients, providers, public health, employers, health plans, and policy makers) to improve health and wellness. Given the large proportion of the population suffering from chronic conditions, it is clear that care coordination must be improved across the many settings where care is delivered and that

evidence-based clinical management and effective self-management must be actively promoted. Behavior and prevention play important roles in chronic care management. Access to screening and counseling for chronic conditions is integral to successful treatment. Education is another key component in chronic care management because treatment decisions need to be made jointly by the patient and the provider. Patients' understanding of their diseases and treatment options is essential for well-informed healthcare decisions and adherence to treatment. In combination, these efforts support quality of life and function, contribute to the health of populations, and reduce the use of costly acute care for preventable problems arising from poorly managed chronic illness.

Quality and Safety

Quality and safety improvement rely on "activated" patients and provider teams that are motivated to examine the structure and organization of healthcare delivery and rectify the processes or workflows that lead to errors. In the two decades since the 1999 National Academy of Medicine report, *To Err Is Human*, a number of national and professional organizations have identified best practices and made recommendations on how to design systems and processes to make healthcare safer.[49] Synergy across these groups will be integral to achieving gains in quality and safety. Local, state, and national public health efforts must support and complement the work being done in local healthcare institutions. The resulting public attention and awareness of quality and safety goals can serve to activate consumers.

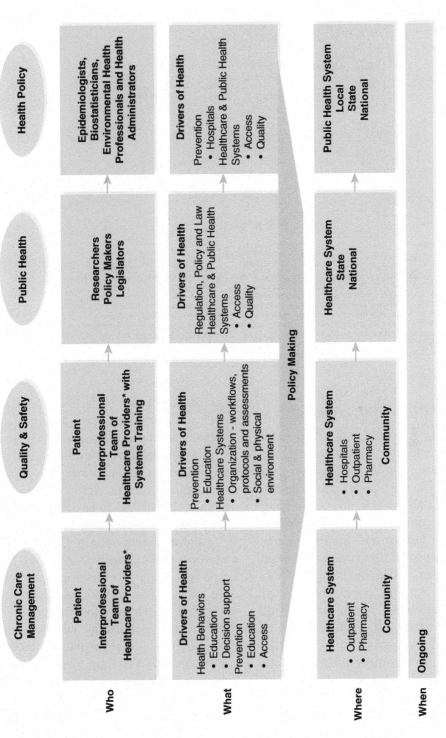

FIGURE 1-2 The Four Pillars of Population Health.

Data from Booske BC, Kindig DA, Nelson H, Remington PL. What Works? Policies and Programs for a Healthier Wisconsin–Draft. University of Wisconsin Population Health Institute, January 2009.

* An interprofessional team of healthcare providers includes both clinical (physicians, nurses, pharmacists, allied health professionals, dentists, radiologists) and nonclinical (healthcare administrators, quality, safety, and public health professionals) professionals.

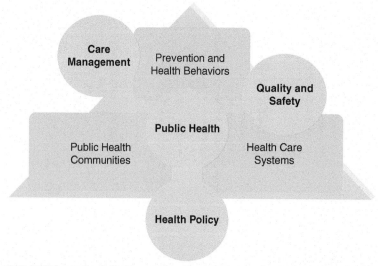

Public health communities and healthcare systems serve as the foundation on which the population health infrastructure rests. Healthcare providers, researchers, policy makers, legislators, and public health professionals who work in the public health communities and healthcare systems partner with patients to focus on prevention and healthy behaviors. Professionals in chronic care management, quality and safety, public health, and health policy must work together to develop a framework to prevent conditions that burden the population both physically and economically. Interdisciplinary collaboration will strengthen the foundation of the population health infrastructure and lead to improved population health management.

FIGURE 1-3 An Interdisciplinary Model for Population Health.

Public Health and Health Policy

Through interaction with communities and healthcare institutions, public health professionals serve as educators and advocates. The third pillar, public health, provides a framework for identifying health determinants, health disparities, and disease burden and for implementing strategies to address community-wide health concerns. As the fourth pillar, policy efforts support population-focused care management, quality and safety, and public health (e.g., policy support in pay-for-performance initiatives that drive adoption of community-wide quality and safety standards). Taken a step further, making comparison data available for other healthcare constituents and consumers (i.e., transparency) creates a sense of accountability for performance and an impetus for improvement. Future policy changes supporting transparency and public accountability for health and wellness will be necessary to meet the population health promise. Activated patients are seeking out guidance in both cost and quality when choosing between provider and treatment options. Commercial and non-profit enterprises, including the Leapfrog Group,[50] are developing promising websites and apps to assist consumers in their search for information. Taken together, the population health goals, strategies, and implementation tactics associated with the four pillars of care management, quality and safety, public health, and health policy will drive population health efforts to achieve health and wellness.

▶ Conclusion

The United States is faced with many challenges in health care, and the strategies used to address both existing and emerging issues will determine the future health status of our nation. To improve the health of the nation, our focus must shift from health care that is reactive to health care that is proactive and promotes health and wellness. Although population needs have been identified in current literature, a reproducible, population health action plan has yet to be established to address them. In the words of Goethe, "Knowing is not enough; we must apply. Willing is not enough; we must do."[51] It will require the collective efforts of many to truly create transformational change. This chapter is intended to prime readers for further exploration of population health efforts to promote health and wellness. In effect, it is a statement of population health's promise as well as a call to action.

Study and Discussion Questions

1. What is population health?
2. Why is a population health approach needed to promote health and wellness?
3. How do the four pillars of population health work together to improve population health?
4. What does the concept called "compression of morbidity" mean?
5. What do the four levels of prevention (primordial, primary, secondary and tertiary) represent?
6. What is your role in population health?

Suggested Readings and Websites

Readings

Agency for Healthcare Research and Quality. Priorities of the National Quality Strategy. Rockville, MD: Author. Available at http://www.ahrq.gov/research/findings/nhqrdr/nhqdr15/priorities.html (accessed May 5, 2019).

Centers for Disease Control and Prevention (CDC). CDC's 6/18 Initiative: Accelerating Evidence Into Action. Available at https://www.cdc.gov/sixeighteen/docs/6-18-factsheet.pdf (accessed May 5, 2019).

Dzau VJ, McClellan M, Burke S, Coye MJ, Daschle TA, Diaz A, et al. Vital Directions for Health and Health Care: Priorities from a National Academy of Medicine Initiative. Discussion Paper, National Academy of Medicine, Washington, DC. *NAM Perspectives* 2017; doi: 10.31478/201703e.

Maeshiro R (ed.) Responding to the challenge: Population health education for physicians. *Academic Med.* 2008;83(4):319–421. Population health education theme issue, available at https://journals.lww.com/academicmedicine/toc/2008/04000.

Kindig DA. Understanding population health terminology. *Milbank Q.* 2007;85:139–361.

Kindig D, Stoddart G. What is population health? *Am J Public Health.* 2003;93:380–383.

National Academy of Medicine (formerly the Institute of Medicine). *Crossing the Quality Chasm: A New Health System for the 21st Century.* Washington, DC: National Academy Press; 2001.

National Academy of Medicine (formerly the Institute of Medicine). *To Err Is Human: Building a Safer Health System.* Washington, DC: National Academy Press; 2000.

Websites

County Health Rankings: http://www.countyhealth
rankings.org/

Dartmouth Atlas of Health Care: http://www.dart
mouthatlas.org/

The Population Health Alliance: http://www
.populationhealthalliance.org/

Institute for Healthcare Improvement: http://www
.ihi.org/ihi

Partnership to Fight Chronic Disease: http://www
.fightchronicdisease.org/

Triple Aim: http://www.ihi.org/Engage/Initiatives
/TripleAim/pages/default.aspx

References

1. Centers for Disease Control and Prevention.
National Center for Chronic Disease Prevention
and Health Promotion (NCCDPHP): About
Chronic Diseases. Available at https://www
.cdc.gov/chronicdisease/about/index.htm
(accessed March 21, 2019).

2. Kindig D, Stoddart G. What is population
health? *Am J Public Health*. 2003;93:380–383.

3. Kindig DA. Understanding population health
terminology. *Milbank Q*. 2007;85:139–161.

4. Agency for Healthcare Research and Quality. Priorities of the National Quality Strategy.
Rockville, MD: Author. Available at http://www
.ahrq.gov/research/findings/nhqrdr/nhqdr15
/priorities.html (accessed March 21, 2019).

5. Kindig DA, Asada Y, Booske B. A population
health framework for setting national and state
health goals. *JAMA*. 2008;299:2081–2083.

6. Centers for Medicare and Medicaid Services.
National Health Expenditure Projections
2015-2025. Available at https://www.cms.gov
/Research-Statistics-Data-and-Systems/Statistics
-Trends-and-Reports/NationalHealth
ExpendData/Downloads/Proj2015.pdf (accessed
March 21, 2019).

7. Schneider EC, Sarnak DO, Squires D, Shah A,
Doty MM. *Mirror, mirror 2017: international
comparison reflects flaws and opportunities
for better U.S. health care*. New York: The
Commonwealth Fund; July 14, 2017. Available at
https://www.commonwealthfund.org/publications
/fund-reports/2017/jul/mirror-mirror-2017-
international-comparison-reflects-flaws-and
(accessed March 21, 2019).

8. Osborn R, Squires D, Doty MM, Sarnak DO,
Schneider EC. In new survey of 11 countries,
US adults still struggle with access to and
affordability of health care. New York: The
Commonwealth Fund; November 16, 2016.
Available at https://www.commonwealthfund
.org/publications/journal-article/2016/nov
/new-survey-11-countries-us-adults-still
-struggle-access-and-affordability-of-health
-care (accessed March 21, 2019).

9. Berchick ER, Hood E, Barnes JC. Health
insurance coverage in the United States: 2017.
United States Census Bureau, US Department
of Commerce Economics and Statistics
Administration. Sept 2018. Available at https://
www.census.gov/content/dam/Census/library
/publications/2018/demo/p60-264.pdf
(accessed March 21, 2019).

10. Raghupathi W, Raghupathi V. An empirical study
of chronic diseases in the United States: a visual
analytics approach to public health. *Int J Environ
Res Public Health*. 2018;15(3):431; doi: 10.3390
/ijerph15030431. Available at www.mdpi.com
/journal/ijerph (accessed March 21, 2019).

11. McGlynn EA, Asch SM, Adams J, Keesey J,
Hicks J, DeCristofaro A, Kerr EA. The quality
of healthcare delivered to adults in the United
States. *N Engl J Med*. 2003;348:2635–2645.

12. Christopher GC, McGhee HC, Gracia JN.
Creating Change through Leadership: Two
Extraordinary Leaders, a Mother and Daugh-
ter, Share Their Experiences Promoting Racial
Equity. Trust for America's Health Web Forum
Series—Taking Action to Promote Health
Equity. November 1, 2018. Available at http://
dialogue4health.org/web-forums/detail
/creating-change-through-leadership (accessed
March 28, 2019).

13. Witters D. US uninsured rate rises to four-year
high. *Gallup News*. January 23, 2019. Available at
https://news.gallup.com/poll/246134/uninsured
-rate-rises-four-year-high.aspx (accessed March
21, 2019).

14. Centers for Medicare and Medicaid Services.
Medicare Chronic Conditions Dashboard:
Region Level. Available at https://www.cms

.gov/Research-Statistics-Data-and-Systems /Statistics-Trends-and-Reports/Dashboard /chronic-conditions-region/cc_region _dashboard.html (accessed March 21, 2019).

15. Centers for Disease Control and Prevention. Life expectancy at birth, by sex, United States: 2006-2016. Available at https://www.cdc.gov /nchs/index.htm (accessed March 21, 2019).

16. World Health Organization. The determinants of health. Available at http://www.who.int/hia /evidence/doh/en/ (accessed March 21, 2019).

17. U.S. Department of Health & Human Services, National Institutes of Health, National Cancer Institute. *Theory at a glance: a guide for health promotion practice.* Bethesda, MD: Authors. 2005. Available at http://www .sbccimplementationkits.org/demandrmnch /wp-content/uploads/2014/02/Theory-at -a-Glance-A-Guide-For-Health-Promotion -Practice.pdf (accessed March 21, 2019).

18. U.S. Dept of Transportation, National Highway Safety Administration. Traffic safety facts: research note. January 2019. Available at https://crashstats.nhtsa.dot.gov/Api/Public /ViewPublication/812662 (accessed March 21, 2019).

19. Gebbie K, Rosenstock L, Hernandez LM, eds. *Who will keep the public healthy? Educating public health professionals for the 21st century.* Washington, DC: Institute of Medicine of the National Academies; 2003. Available at https://www.ncbi .nlm.nih.gov/books/NBK221695/ (accessed May 5, 2019).

20. Dzau VJ, McClellan M, Burke S, Coye MK, Daschle TA, Diaz A, et al. Vital Directions for Health and Health Care: Priorities from a National Academy of Medicine Initiative. Discussion Paper, National Academy of Medicine, Washington, DC. *NAM Perspectives* 2017; doi: 10.31478/201703e.

21. Office of the National Coordinator for Health Information Technology. MACRA and meaningful use. Available at https://www.healthit.gov /topic/meaningful-use-and-macra/meaningful -use-and-macra (accessed March 21, 2019).

22. Cigna. Creating a culture of health. Available at https://www.cigna.com/assets/docs/improving -health-and-productivity/837897 _CultureOfHealthWP_v5.pdf (accessed March 21, 2019).

23. Institute for Healthcare Improvement. Changes to improve chronic care. Available at http://www.ihi.org/resources/Pages/Changes /ChangestoImproveChronicCare.aspx/ (accessed March 21, 2019).

24. State of Vermont, Department of Vermont Health Access. *Blueprint for Health in 2017 Annual Report.* Waterbury, VT: Author. Available at http://blueprintforhealth.vermont.gov/sites/bfh /files/Vermont-Blueprint-for-Health-Annual -Report-2017.pdf (accessed March 21, 2019).

25. United Health Foundation. America's Health Rankings 2017 Annual Report. Minneapolis, MN. Available at https://www .americashealthrankings.org/learn/reports /2017-annual-report/findings-state-rankings (accessed March 28, 2019).

26. Wisconsin Department of Health Services. Healthiest Wisconsin 2020. Available at https:// www.dhs.wisconsin.gov/hw2020/index.htm (accessed March 21, 2019).

27. University of Wisconsin Population Health Institute. Health of Wisconsin report card 2016. Available at https://uwphi.pophealth .wisc.edu/health-of-wisconsin-report -card-2016-2/ (accessed March 21, 2019).

28. Baicker K, Cutler D, Song Z. Workplace wellness programs can generate savings. *Health Aff.* 2010;29(2):304–311.

29. Health Enhancement Research Organization and Population Health Alliance. *Program Measurement and Evaluation Guide: Core Metrics for Employee Health Management.* 2015. Alexandria, VA: Society for Human Resource Management. Available at https://www.shrm .org/ResourcesAndTools/hr-topics/benefits /Documents/HERO-PHA-Metrics-Guide -FINAL.pdf (accessed March 21, 2019).

30. Mattke S, Liu H, Caloyeras JP, Huang CY, Van Busum KR, Khodyakov D, Shier V, Exum E, and Broderick M. Do workplace wellness programs save employers money? Santa Monica, CA: RAND Corporation, RB-9744-DOL, 2014. Available at https://www.rand.org/pubs/research_briefs /RB9744.html (accessed March 28, 2019).

31. Walton J. Wellness programs generate a 6:1 ROI. *Work Design Magazine*, January 31, 2018. Available at https://workdesign.com/2018/01 /wellness-programs-for-healthy-workplace/ (accessed March 28, 2019).

32. Fabius R, Thayer RD, Konicki DL, Yarborough CM, Peterson KW, Isaac F, et al. The link between workforce health and safety and the health of the bottom line: tracking market performance of companies that nurture a "culture of health." *J Occup Environ Med*. 2013;55(9):993–1000.

33. Fabius R, Loeppke R, Hohn T, Fabius D, Eisenberg B, Konicki DL, Larson P. Tracking the market performance of companies that integrate a culture of health and safety: an assessment of Corporate Health Achievement Award applicants. *J Occup Environ Med*. 2016;58(1):3–8.

34. Goetzel RZ, Fabius R, Fabius D, Roemer EC, Thornton N, Kelly RK, Pelletier KR. The stock performance of C. Everett Koop Award winners compared with the Standard & Poor 500 Index. *J Occup Environ Med*. 2016;58(1):9–15.

35. Grossmeier J, Fabius R, Flynn JP, Noeldner SP, Fabius D, Goetzel RZ, Anderson DR. Linking workplace health promotion best practices and organizational financial performance. *J Occup Environ Med*. 2016;58(1):16–23.

36. Xu X, Bishop EE, Kennedy SM, Simpson SA, Pechacek TF. Annual healthcare spending attributable to cigarette smoking: an update. *Am J Prev Med*. 2015 Mar; 48(3):326–333. Available at doi: 10.1016/j.amepre.2014.10.012 (accessed March 21, 2019).

37. Society of Human Resource Management. Why employee well-being matters to your bottom line. Available at http://www.shrm.org/about /foundation/products/documents/6-11%20 promoting%20well%20being%20epg-%20final .pdf (accessed March 21, 2019).

38. Robert Walters. The value of promoting employee health and well-being. Available at https://www.robertwalters.com/content/dam /robert-walters/corporate/news-and-pr/files /whitepapers/health-and-wellbeing-white paper-aus.pdf (accessed March 21, 2019).

39. White M. The cost-benefit of well employees. *Harv Bus Rev*. December 2005. Available at http://hbr.org/2005/12/the-cost-benefit-of- well-employees/ar/1 (accessed March 21, 2019).

40. Centers for Disease Control and Prevention. Smoking is down, but almost 38 million American adults still smoke. [Press release.] January 18, 2018. Available at https://www .cdc.gov/media/releases/2018/p0118-smoking -rates-declining.html (accessed March 21, 2019).

41. U.S. Department of Health and Human Services Office of Disease Prevention and Health Promotion. *Healthy People 2020: History and development of Healthy People*. Available at http://healthypeople.gov/2020/about/history. aspx (accessed March 21, 2019).

42. U.S. Department of Health and Human Services Office of Disease Prevention and Health Promotion. *Healthy People 2020: Leading health indicators development and framework*. Available at https://www.healthypeople.gov/2020/leading -health-indicators/Leading-Health-Indicators -Development-and-Framework (accessed March 21, 2019).

43. U.S. Department of Health and Human Services Office of Disease Prevention and Health Promotion. *Healthy People 2030: Development of the national health promotion and disease prevention objectives for 2030*. Available at https:// www.healthypeople.gov/2020/About-Healthy -People/Development-Healthy-People-2030 (accessed March 21, 2019).

44. Institute for Healthcare Improvement. An overview of the IHI Triple Aim. Available at http://www.ihi.org/Engage/Initiatives/TripleAim /pages/default.aspx (accessed March 21, 2019).

45. Dentzer S. The "Triple Aim" goes global, and not a minute too soon. *Health Aff*. 2013;32(4):638.

46. Centers for Disease Control and Prevention. The 6/18 initiative: accelerating evidence into action. Available at https://www.cdc.gov/sixeighteen /index.html (accessed March 28, 2019).

47. Agency for Healthcare Research and Quality. Priorities in Focus. January 2017. Rockville, MD: Author. Available at http://www.ahrq.gov /workingforquality/reports/priorities-in-focus .html (accessed March 28, 2019).

48. Nash DB. Population health mandate: a broader approach to healthcare delivery. Boardroom Press, Feb. 2012. San Diego, CA: The Governance Institute.

49. National Academy of Medicine (formerly the Institute of Medicine). *To Err Is Human: Building a Safer Health System*. Washington, DC: National Academy Press; 2000.

50. The Leapfrog Group. Health care choices. Available at http://www.leapfroggroup.org/ (accessed March 21, 2019).

51. Internet Encyclopedia of Philosophy. Johann Wolfgang von Goethe. Available at http://www .iep.utm.edu/goethe/ (accessed March 21, 2019).

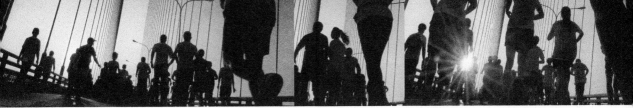

CHAPTER 2
Epidemiology

Russell McIntire
John McAna
Willie H. Oglesby

EXECUTIVE SUMMARY

This chapter provides a broad overview of the field of epidemiology and basic epidemiologic methods. Epidemiology works to measure the burden and search for the causes of disease among populations. Population health practitioners use epidemiologic methods to gather the scientific evidence for planning, implementing, and evaluating interventions to improve the health of populations. Descriptive epidemiology measures the burden of disease by generating morbidity and mortality rates to describe the extent of disease and death among groups. Analytic epidemiology uses experimental and observational study designs to uncover and understand the factors that cause disease. The application of epidemiologic principles and methods has become increasingly important in population health due to emerging infectious and chronic diseases, changing technologies, and shift in focus of health systems toward population-based health outcomes.

LEARNING OBJECTIVES

By the end of this chapter, the reader will be able to:

1. State the major objectives of epidemiology.
2. Define characteristics of descriptive and analytic epidemiology.
3. Discuss distinctions between epidemiology and medicine.
4. List sources of epidemiologic data.
5. Describe methods used in applied epidemiology.

▶ Introduction

Population health improvement efforts are informed by data from a variety of sources, including electronic medical records, population-based surveys, birth and death records, claims data, community input, expert opinion, and many others. Population health practitioners use these data to highlight health issues that should be addressed, identify sub-populations disproportionately affected, monitor and evaluate intervention efforts, and uncover factors contributing to disease and death.

Public health interventions, such as vaccination campaigns, seat belt use laws, workplace safety, and inspections to ensure safe food supplies have contributed to the dramatic increases in length and quality of life among people in the United States in the past century.[1] However, the aging population, economic instability, changes in technology, and emerging areas of concern such as obesity and the opioid epidemic are creating serious challenges that population health practitioners need to address in order to maintain the progress we have made.

▶ Leading Causes of Death in the United States

Currently, chronic diseases represent the majority of the causes of death in the United States. Of the 10 leading causes of death among U.S. residents in 2015, 7 were chronic diseases, 2 were behavioral (unintentional injuries and suicide), and only 1 was caused by infectious disease (influenza and pneumonia).[2] Heart disease and cancer have remained the top 2 causes of death in the United States for the past 40 years (**FIGURE 2-1**).

Determinants of Causes of Death and Disease in the United States

It is important to identify the major causes of death and disease among populations, but natural questions emerge: Why do people get sick? How do they acquire the diseases that lead to disability and death? What are the societal conditions, genetic factors, health behaviors, and environmental exposures that cause disease? A **determinant** is a definable entity that causes, is associated with, or induces a health outcome,[3] such as death or disease. Determinants might be easily recognizable factors such as biological agents that cause infection (such as viruses, bacteria, parasites), carcinogens (such as cigarette smoke, asbestos), or physical injuries (accidents, violence) that cause disease. Alternatively, determinants may be less specific factors, such as stress, physical inactivity, eating unhealthy foods, or sleep deprivation. Determinants are not

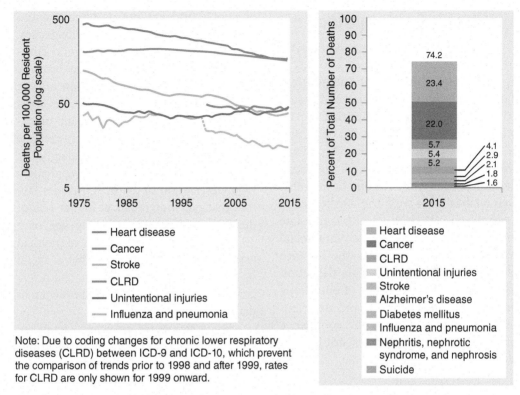

FIGURE 2-1 Leading Causes of Death.

Data from National Vital Statistics System. NCHS, Health United States, 2016.

just the things that make people sick; they can also be the things that make people healthy, such as wearing a condom during sex, getting immunizations, or seeking other preventative medical services.

Distributions and Health Disparities

The frequency of disease and mortality from disease vary among different population subgroups. For example, the 2008–2012 mortality rate from prostate cancer was higher among African Americans compared to non-Hispanic whites, Hispanics, Asian and Pacific Islanders, and American Indian and Alaska Natives in the United States.[4] These variations show how disease in populations has different **distributions** depending upon demographic, social, or behavioral characteristics of people. Demographic subgroups that have higher occurrence of disease compared to other groups are defined as having **health disparities**. Eliminating health disparities is a major priority of public health interventions and governmental planning initiatives, such as the Healthy People initiatives, by the U.S. Department of Health and Human Services.[5,6]

What Is Epidemiology and Why Is It Important?

Epidemiologists produce the scientific evidence about the determinants and distribution of major health issues that impact our lives. Before we discuss the definition and functions of the field of epidemiology, we must define health. There are many definitions of health, but one of the most well established is from the World Health Organization (WHO): "Health is the state of complete physical, mental, and social well-being and not merely the absence of disease or infirmity."[7] This definition focuses not just on the state of one's body but also on mental health and describes health in active terms as the confluence of physical and mental states, not just the lack of disease diagnosis.

Population Medicine

Epidemiology is often referred to as "population medicine" due to its focus on the health of groups of people. This is a major distinction from the field of medicine, where the primary focus is on individual patients. In epidemiology, the "patient" is the group, which in epidemiology parlance is called a cohort. A **cohort** is a group of people assembled or observed by researchers in order to learn about the extent or causes of health problems. Cohorts have similar demographic, risk factor, or health outcome characteristics. They may be a particular demographic group, neighborhood, or even a group organized by time, such as those born during a certain calendar year in a geographic location.

Epidemiologists explore the distribution and causes of disease among groups of people and are not as often focused on individual people's clinical diagnoses. As a result, the epidemiologic and clinical descriptions of a disease may be quite different. The clinical description of type 2 diabetes would include specific signs and symptoms such as frequent urination, weight loss, blurry vision, numbness in the extremities, and other diagnostic patient characteristics. The epidemiologic description of diabetes includes factors that put individuals at higher risk of developing diabetes, including age over 45, overweight or obesity, lack of physical activity, family history of diabetes, racial or ethnic minority, and other characteristics associated with higher frequency of diabetes in populations.

Epidemiology collects, analyzes, and interprets data regarding the distribution and determinants of disease among populations. This information is used to plan interventions to reduce the population burden of disease. Epidemiologic studies fall into two major categories, *descriptive* and *analytic*. **Descriptive epidemiology** focuses on summarizing the impact and extent of health-related events among particular groups. **Analytic epidemiology** focuses on searching for the determinants of diseases.

When patients present with bloody stool and kidney failure at a hospital, medical professionals and lab technicians collect and analyze the stool samples to determine the presence of the pathogen responsible, such as *E. coli*. Epidemiologists are the professionals who aggregate case reports and search for patterns among cases to determine the source of the infectious agent. If the epidemiologic investigation shows commonalities among cases that point to a potential source of the infection, epidemiologists make a plan for preventing further transmission of the disease. For example, if everyone who was sick consumed food from the same restaurant, epidemiologists might recommend temporarily closing down the restaurant to remove the source of the pathogen. Identification of the causes or determinants of disease is essential to take actions to prevent future cases and reduce the burden of the disease among populations.

"What Is Upon the People"

The word *epidemiology* is composed of the Greek words, *epi*, which means "upon," *demos*, which means "people," and *logy* which means "the study of." In essence, epidemiology is the study of "what is upon the people." This definition makes sense, as population health practitioners use epidemiology to identify what diseases are affecting populations. Identifying the causes of health among populations is the first major function of epidemiology. The second function is to use this knowledge to intervene to reduce the burden of disease among populations.[8] Epidemiology is an action-oriented science because it is focused on the end result of improved health among populations. Epidemiologists do not characterize the distribution and determinants of disease for actuarial purposes or for rote record keeping. The ultimate goal of all epidemiologic investigations is to inform interventions that will reduce the impact of disease on populations.

Objectives of Epidemiology

To that end, the objectives of the discipline of epidemiology that are used to achieve this goal include the following[9]:

1. **To determine the burden of disease among populations:** This objective is achieved through descriptive studies that generate rates of disease among groups of people in order to identify and compare distributions of disease. Interventions to improve health should then be focused on geographic areas or demographic subgroups with the highest burden of disease. This objective is critical for health planners and policymakers when choosing how to distribute resources or create priorities for disease prevention and treatment services.

2. **To determine the causes or etiology of disease:** Individual epidemiologic studies of different design combine to form the evidence base for the causes of disease. No one epidemiologic study, regardless of the strength of the study design or analysis, is sufficient by itself to determine that a risk factor, or exposure, causes disease. Determining causation is a slow process that improves and develops over time as new research is released through the peer-review process.

3. **To study the natural history and progression of disease:** Not all diseases have the same burden among populations. Some diseases, such as rabies, are lethal and have a high fatality rate yet affect a small percentage of people in populations. Some diseases, such as arthritis, are not fatal yet affect

a large percentage of people and are linked to genetics, behavior, and demographic characteristics such as age. Measuring the characteristics of diseases as they manifest, progress, and affect people during different life stages is important to identify and evaluate interventions to reduce the population impact of disease.

4.   **To evaluate health care services and interventions:** This objective aligns with the discipline of outcomes research. Researchers use epidemiologic methods to compare outcomes between groups that received healthcare or programmatic services versus those that did not receive services.

5.   **To provide a knowledge base:** Epidemiologic studies produce the body of literature used by population health decision makers to implement the most efficient and effective population health programs, interventions, and policies. Decision makers need to take actions to improve the health of populations after considering the full context of the breadth of knowledge about specific health topics.

▶ History of Epidemiology

Epidemiology is as old as the discipline of medicine. The Greek physician Hippocrates wrote extensively around 400 B.C. about his medical observations. In one

of Hippocrates' most famous treatises, he discussed the importance of the physical, environmental, and social environment on the development of disease.

> Whoever wishes to investigate medicine properly, should proceed thus: in the first place to consider the seasons of the year, and what effects each of them produces, for they are not at all alike, but differ much from themselves in regard to their changes. Then the winds, the hot and the cold, especially such as are common to all countries, and then such as are peculiar to each locality. We must also consider the qualities of the waters … which the inhabitants use, whether they be marshy and soft, or hard, and running from elevated and rocky situations, and then if saltish and unfit for cooking; and the ground, whether it be naked and deficient in water, or wooded and well-watered, and whether it lies in a hollow, confined situation, or is elevated and cold; and the mode in which the inhabitants live, and what are their pursuits, whether they are fond of drinking and eating to excess, and given to indolence, or are fond of exercise and labor, and not given to excess in eating and drinking.[10]

This line of thinking represented a rational account of the origins of disease and makes no mention of supernatural or religious causes of death or disease. While the scientific community conducted empirical investigation into the causes of disease, it was not common among the general public to make rational connections between the environment and health outcomes. As poverty has always been a risk factor for disease development, theologians, politicians, and even some physicians believed that diseases arose, at least in part, from consequences of laziness, weak constitutions, fear, impiousness, blasphemy, or other moral failings that were often imputed to people living in poverty.

During the early history of epidemiology, infectious diseases caused the largest burden of **morbidity** and **mortality**.[11] Two thousand years after Hippocrates, in 1662, John Graunt published *The Nature and Political Observations Made Upon the Bills of Mortality*, which was the first epidemiologic study of weekly trends in natality and mortality among residents of London. This was one of the first applications of descriptive methods to compare population rates between important demographics such as age and sex and to quantify seasonal variation in disease occurrence. Graunt identified higher mortality rates among men compared to women and higher infant mortality compared to the general population. His work was an important foundational study not just for epidemiology but also the practical application of statistics to describe health issues.

John Snow and Cholera in London

Few epidemiology texts omit a discussion of John Snow's investigation of cholera in London in the mid-1800s. At the time, the scientific community had no knowledge of germ theory, and the causes of the major infectious diseases were therefore unknown. Physicians and health officials believed the miasma theory, which followed that stagnant, foul-smelling air was the mechanism through which cholera and other mortal diseases infected humans. This line of thinking was common and had a long history. For example, in Hippocrates' treatise *On Airs, Waters and Places* (quoted above), the weather and the air were the first major risk factors discussed. Physician John Snow hypothesized that, contrary to popular belief, infected water was the source of cholera outbreaks, though he did not have the technology to isolate the infectious agent, the bacterium *Vibrio cholerae*. Through keen observations and application of the scientific method, Dr. Snow identified that the proportion of deaths in the 1854 London cholera outbreak correlated with the source of people's water. Specifically, neighborhood residents whose municipal water systems were sourced upstream of London had dramatically lower rates of cholera mortality compared to residents whose water system was from sources downstream, which included the unfiltered sewage of London residents. Based on the results of this natural experiment, and a door-to-door investigation of water-drinking behavior, illness, and death due to cholera in the Soho neighborhood of London, Dr. Snow convinced officials to remove the handle on the Broad Street water pump to remove the source of disease transmission. This series of epidemiologic investigations resulted in one of the first and most well documented evidence-based epidemiologic interventions. John Snow has since been called the father of modern epidemiology.

Epidemiologic Transition

Because of improved living conditions, sanitation, and public health interventions such as vaccines, the major causes of morbidity and mortality in most of the world have transitioned from infectious in nature to non-infectious, or chronic disease. The Framingham Heart Study, which began in 1948, was an early and influential longitudinal study in which investigators assembled a cohort of almost 5,200 healthy, non-diseased residents of Framingham, Massachusetts, to evaluate the links between risk factors and chronic diseases. Seventy years later, this study continues and has provided the foundation for much of what we know about the links between lifestyle and morbidity and mortality due to cardiovascular disease.[12] Since the 1950s and 1960s, researchers have established the causal link between smoking and lung cancer and diseases of almost all of the systems of the body. Smoking is, by far, the leading single cause of preventable death in the world.[13] In the United States, smoking and secondhand smoke are responsible for almost 500,000 deaths per year.[6]

▶ Modes of Practice of Epidemiology

Epidemiology is concerned with the distribution and determinants of health and diseases, morbidity, injuries, disability, and mortality in populations. It is of utmost importance that the decisions made by population health practitioners are based on sound evidence. Public and private hospital administrators, health department employees, payers, and other employees working for health industries need to make decisions about the distribution of resources to focus on services that best utilize the skills and training of practitioners, meet the health needs of populations, reduce the burden of disease, and increase the quality of life for members of populations. Epidemiologic methods are integral to determining the best evidence to inform decisions.

Quantification

In order to make evidence-based decisions to improve population health, risk factors and disease outcomes must be quantified empirically. The central aim of epidemiologic methods is to quantify the evidence underpinning public health decisions. Although qualitative research is also important, epidemiologic investigations are never complete without quantifying the distribution or determinants of disease. Health professionals need to measure the number of health "events" in order to determine a risk or rate, which summarizes the extent of the problem. Often health professionals start out by counting the cases of disease that occur among a certain population; this is the numerator, describing the frequency of the event during a certain time interval. The denominator is the number of individuals in the population who were at risk of being a case during the same time interval. The next step might be to further summarize the data by demographic subgroups such as age, gender, race, socioeconomic status, and very importantly, exposure category (whether or not cases were exposed to some particular risk factor).

At the heart of epidemiologic investigations are the research questions and the data necessary to address those questions. Many types of data are used to build evidence that influences health-related decisions. Below are some important examples of epidemiologic data sources.

Sources of Epidemiologic Data

Vital Registration System

Data from the Vital Registration System is routinely collected on births and deaths in the United States. Death, or mortality data in the United States, is reliable because we have the system infrastructure to record practically all deaths in the United States. Death certificates include demographic information and facts about the primary, secondary, and tertiary causes of death— these are deemed immediate causes, underlying causes, and contributing factors, respectively. Parts of the death certificate are completed at the time of death by the attending physician, medical examiner or coroner, and funeral director; then the local registrar checks the certificate for completeness and sends a copy to the state registrar (who checks it again) and sends it to the National Center for Health Statistics (NCHS). NCHS compiles and aggregates mortality data from localities in the United States and uses it for **disease surveillance** through the National Vital Statistics System (NVSS). NVSS makes aggregated mortality rates by disease, demographics, and geographic location publicly accessible so that individuals and organizations can use these data for research, program planning, evaluation, and policymaking purposes.

Mortality data in the United States are systematically collected at local levels and compiled by states. These data are reliable, but there are some limitations.[14] The certification of the cause of death is not always straightforward, as sometimes there are primary, secondary, tertiary (and so on, ad infinitum) causes of death.

Here is an example that describes these limitations. A 60-year-old man died at a local hospital from pulmonary embolism, and the attending physician completed a death certificate. The physician lists pulmonary embolism and total hip replacement surgery as the immediate causes of death. However, the patient also had pneumonia, epistaxis, atrial fibrillation, hypertension, diabetes, and asbestosis. How did the physician determine the immediate cause of death and decide what was a contributing factor? In this case, it might be difficult to determine which cause is listed as the primary cause.[15] Another limitation to mortality data might be stigma associated with certain diseases. For example, if the patient died of chronic alcoholism or AIDS and was a friend of the attending physician, there might be reluctance to note these causes of death because death certificates are publicly accessible. There also may be individual or systematic errors in recording of particular death certificates. Changes in coding complicate analyses of death certificate data, especially since the International Classification of Disease (ICD) system has changed many times over the past 75 years. The ICD system is an international classification scheme for coding morbidity and mortality and is organized by the World Health Organization (WHO). ICD guidelines provide definitions of diseases, including symptoms and metrics, so that practitioners can diagnose disease in a standardized way throughout the world. Establishment of this code allows epidemiologists to measure and compare the burden of disease among countries through international initiatives such as the global burden of disease project.

Over the past 75 years, the ICD has been revised 10 times and, each time, some disease codes have changed. When analyzing mortality data over time, one needs to consider changes in codes and nomenclature so as not to incorrectly attribute a sudden drop in a disease code to a decrease in mortality due to a particular cause of death. Such a decrease may simply reflect a change in how the disease is coded.

Birth certificates and fetal death certificates are nearly complete in their coverage documenting birth events in the U.S. population. Birth certificates include much information about the conditions present during birth, including demographic information about the mother, birth weight, length of gestation, and fetal developmental conditions.

Electronic Medical Records

The Patient Protection and Affordable Care Act (ACA) required that all public and private hospitals transition away from their paper-based medical record systems and demonstrate "meaningful use" of electronic medical records (EMR) by January 1, 2014. EMRs are a major source of data for epidemiologic investigation. Hospital systems use EMR data to characterize the primary conditions affecting their patients or the major services that their practitioners are providing. In addition, this source of data characterizes the population of patients who are served by the hospital system. These data should not be confused with the hospital's catchment area, which is composed of the people who live in areas in which the hospital serves, and is determined by geographic locality, services provided, and historical and cultural factors that impact the characteristics of patients.[16] While EMR data are not population-representative, researchers and stakeholders are increasingly using it for innovative surveillance of patient populations.[17]

Population-Based Surveys

The majority of what we know about health beliefs, behaviors, and prevention of disease among the full U.S. population has been determined not through medical records, but through paper and electronically administered surveys. The federal government, state, and local agencies; regional health systems; and even many nonprofits collect self-reported survey data to describe the health of populations. Because populations typically contain large numbers of individuals, the total sample of individuals who complete health surveys is less than the total number in the full populations. Typically, researchers do not collect data on everyone within a population because of the administrative and logistical burden required to collect that amount of data. Epidemiologists and statisticians use probability sampling to select a *sample* of the population that, based on demographics, is representative of the full population. After surveys are conducted, researchers apply weights to the sample responses to up-weight subpopulations that are under-represented in the sample and down-weight subpopulations that are over-represented, so that responses of these individuals count for more or less, respectively, than one individual. Multistage sampling is sometimes used to ensure that individuals are selected with equal distribution by a geographic unit, such as regions, states, counties, or zip codes, and/or other group characteristics, like voting districts, school districts, or even schools within districts. This process ensures that the sample data collected for large population-based surveys adequately represents the population as a whole.

U.S. Census

Every 10 years the U.S. Census Bureau conducts the census, the most comprehensive source of data about the characteristics of people in the country. The decennial census collects data about demographics, income, labor, and education from individuals and families among U.S. residents by geographic locations. This source is useful for epidemiologic purposes because the population coverage is complete; practically everyone is counted in the survey. Additionally, because the data can be described by geographic locations (state, city, zip code, census tract, census block group) these data often form the denominator for epidemiologic rate calculations. Researchers use these data to identify the population at risk of developing disease.

▶ Epidemiology in Practice

As the scope of epidemiologic investigation is quite extensive, it may be helpful to summarize some important terminology and methods utilized in applied epidemiology. We break this section up into methods related to descriptive epidemiology and analytic epidemiology for ease of categorization.

Descriptive Epidemiology: Quantifying Disease among Populations

Descriptive epidemiologic studies identify the extent to which disease is present in populations. Examples of descriptive studies are those that identify the burden of infectious diseases, chronic diseases, disability, injury, mortality, health behaviors, and other major risk factors by geographic area or among subpopulations of people within urban or rural areas (**BOX 2-1**).

BOX 2-1 Descriptive Method: Hotspotting

Hotspotting is a unique descriptive approach that researchers and health systems are using to identify geographic clusters of the neediest patients—those with comorbid conditions with poorly coordinated care, who often account for a disproportionate amount of medical services and costs.[18] Researchers such as Jeffrey Brenner from the Camden Coalition of Healthcare Providers in New Jersey have found that these patients have challenging economic and social situations and often live in close proximity to one another in poor neighborhoods with few health resources and little support. Once identified, teams of case managers, social workers, nurses, doctors, and other practitioners can coordinate health and social services for those "super-utilizers" in the geographic hotspots. In the Camden Coalition case, this coordinated effort reduced the utilization of healthcare services and cost of these patients' care by almost half.[19] Comprehensive use of electronic medical records and improved capabilities of geographic information systems (GIS) has made the identification of hotspots and coldspots—areas with very limited health and social service resources[20,21]—an increasingly utilized descriptive epidemiologic method for identifying patients and geographic locations on which resources need to be focused.

BOX 2-2 Celiac Disease: The Difficulty of Measuring Burden

Celiac disease is an autoimmune disorder in which the small intestines are damaged by ingestion of foods containing gluten, a naturally occurring protein contained in wheat, barley, and rye. The immune reaction resulting from ingestion of gluten damages the lining of the small intestines and prevents proper absorption of nutrients. Therefore, in addition to the short-term effects of intestinal pain, discomfort, and bloating, celiac disease can result in long-term chronic diseases such as malnourishment, anemia, osteoporosis, diabetes, cancer, infertility, and resulting behavioral health disorders such as depression. The only treatment for celiac disease is for patients to abstain from eating foods containing gluten. After 1 to 6 months of no gluten exposure, the damaged intestinal lining heals and begins adequate absorption of nutrients.

The clinical picture of celiac disease is complex because the symptoms are non-specific, and screening is complex, requiring a serum antibody test and a confirmatory endoscopy.[22] Celiac disease symptoms often manifest differently in different people. Common symptoms include acute stomach pain, diarrhea, weight loss, or even headaches and irritability. The list of symptoms is quite extensive.[23]

While current estimates suggest that 0.5 to 1% of the U.S. general population has celiac disease,[24–26] only 12% of those who have the disease are diagnosed.[27] The burden of the disease may be quite high, but unfortunately, due to the nature of the disease symptoms, limitations of screening tests, and lack of knowledge about celiac disease among providers and the general public, reducing the burden of the disease has proved challenging in the U.S. population.

Epidemiologists measure the burden of disease among populations in a number of ways, including morbidity and mortality rates, economic indicators such as cost, or trends over time (**BOX 2-2**). Epidemiologists calculate many different types of rates, including prevalence, incidence, morbidity, mortality, and attack rates. Over the past 50 years, epidemiologists have developed very useful measures of disease burden that combine the number of years that people are afflicted with a disabling condition with the premature death caused by that condition. These measures are quality-adjusted life years (QALYs) and disability-adjusted life years (DALYs). As mentioned earlier, the ICD system provides the foundation for diagnoses of all diseases.

Rates

Rates are the main way that epidemiologists quantify the burden of disease among populations. Simply counting the number of cases of disease does not say anything about the burden of the disease in the population or the risk of development of disease among individuals. Rates are important because they identify the number of cases of disease but also relate this number to the size of the population being studied. Rates are composed of numerators (the number of cases of disease), denominators (the number of people at risk of developing the disease), and the time period the data describe (per month or per year). It is important to distinguish between *morbidity* and *mortality*—morbidity designates illness, and mortality refers to deaths of individuals during a certain time period.

Mortality Rates

Mortality rates quantify the burden of deaths overall or due to specific diseases among populations. Below is an example of a crude mortality rate calculation.

10 deaths due to all causes per 1,000 people in Pennsylvania in 2014

(a)   (b)

Melonie Heron, Ph.D., Division of Vital Statistics, Deaths: Leading Causes for 2015, National Vital Statistics Reports, Volume 66, Number 5, CDC, 2015.

Let us dissect this rate piece by piece. First, the crude mortality rate is calculated by dividing the number of deaths due to all causes during the year 2014 (e.g., 127,773) by the number of people at risk of dying (in this case, the whole population) during the year 2014 (e.g., 12,787,209). Because 127,773/12,787,209 would be a fraction that is less than 1 (specifically, 0.01), this would mean the population experienced 0.01 deaths per 1 person living in Pennsylvania in 2014. Because there is no such thing as a fraction of a death, we need to multiply this fraction by a number that will allow the rate to make sense intuitively. This number is called the "multiplier," and this is labeled as (a) above. After we multiply the fraction by the multiplier, we can make the statement, *for every 1,000 people in Pennsylvania, there were 10 deaths in the year 2014.*

The label (b) above identifies the rate that denotes place and time, as all rates should be labeled with elements of person (i.e., deaths by all causes), place (i.e., Pennsylvania), and time (i.e., 2014). Further, it is important to think about how the denominator is identified. The Commonwealth of Pennsylvania is said to be *dynamic* (i.e., people are constantly moving to and from Pennsylvania), so it is impossible to get an accurate snapshot of the people who would be eligible to have died during a time period that is larger than 1 day. Therefore, it is best practice for epidemiologists to use the population denominator that represents the population at risk during the midpoint of the year, or July 1, 2014.

Prevalence

Prevalence refers to the number of existing cases of a disease or health issue at some designated time. This is one of the most frequently used measures to describe health-related phenomena in population health. Prevalence data indicate the extent of a health problem within a designated population, and it can be expressed as a number, a percentage, or a number of cases per unit size of population.

Prevalence describes the burden of a health problem in a population during a particular time or estimates the frequency of an exposure. In population health, prevalence is used by decision makers to influence the allocation of health resources, such as funding for programming or other services. It is important to note that the designated time period can be specified or unspecified. When it is unspecified, this is called *point prevalence*, which describes the burden of a health problem during a specific point in time—for example, *11.6 cases of influenza per 100 people in Ellettsville, Indiana, on April 15, 2011.*

A second type of prevalence is the *period prevalence*, which shows the number of cases of a disease that existed during a specific period of time (a week, month, year, or longer). To determine this, one must combine the number of cases at the beginning of the time period with the new cases that occur during the period. Because the period prevalence occurs during a time interval, the denominator may change due to individuals' entering or leaving the population during the period. Because of this, we use the average population during that period as our denominator for calculation of the period prevalence: *15.5 per 100 adults smoked cigarettes every day in the United States in 2016.*

Incidence

The **incidence**, or *incidence rate*, describes the rate of development of *new cases* of disease among people in a group over a certain time period and contains three elements: a numerator, which is the number of newly developed cases during the time period; a denominator, which is the population at risk during the time period; and the time period under study. The population at risk is the denominator for the calculation of incidence rates, and it excludes those individuals who have already had the disease or couldn't develop it. Here's an example of the calculation of an incidence rate, taken from a popular epidemiologic training manual by the CDC[28]:

> Incidence of AIDS in the U.S. in 2003:
>
> In 2003, 44,232 new cases of acquired immunodeficiency syndrome (AIDS) were reported in the United States.[29] The estimated mid-year population of the U.S. in 2003 was approximately 290,809,777. The incidence rate of AIDS in 2003 was:
>
> Numerator = 44,232 new cases of AIDS
> Denominator = 290,809,777 estimated mid-year population
> Multiplier used is 100,000
>
> $$\text{Incidence rate} = \frac{44,232}{290,809,777} \times 100,000$$
>
> = 15.21 new cases of AIDS per 100,000 population in the U.S. in 2003

Epidemic

Epidemiologic terms such as *epidemic* and *outbreak* are often used in the media to describe emerging health issues that affect populations. It is important to define these terms so that the public can distinguish among terminology. An **epidemic** is the occurrence of cases of an illness, health-related behavior, or other health-related event at a higher rate than expected within a population and derived from a common source.[9]

Outbreak is often used synonymously with *epidemic*, but outbreaks are localized to a small geographic area, such as a neighborhood, city, or region. A key characteristic of an epidemic or an outbreak is that the number of new cases of disease must be clearly in excess of expectancy compared to the relative frequency of the disease.

Naturally, diseases are *endemic* within a population—that is, there is a constant presence of the disease within the population. For example, influenza is endemic in many populations and follows distinct seasonal patterns. When the number of cases of influenza exceeds the normal frequency of the disease, an epidemic may be occurring.

A **pandemic** is an epidemic affecting populations of an extensive region, country, or continent. Examples of pandemics are the 1918 or 2009 flu pandemics. In 2009 the world experienced a pandemic of H1N1, or swine flu, because the epidemic was on a worldwide scale. Though it crossed international borders, the 2014–2016 epidemic of Ebola in West Africa was not a pandemic because it was localized to West Africa.

Disease Surveillance

Our discussion of epidemics highlights the importance of disease surveillance. The CDC and other state and local governments collect surveillance data to identify the usual frequency of disease and risk factors. These data are very important to collect because they serve as a baseline for determining whether a disease epidemic is under way among a certain population. *Disease surveillance* is the systematic collection of data pertaining to the occurrence of specific diseases, as well as the analysis and dissemination of surveillance results. Public health agencies, health systems, payers, and other organizations continually monitor the health of populations through a number of methods. Governments at the federal, state, and local level receive reports about cases of specific diseases that are mandatory for healthcare practitioners to report. Most of these are acute infectious diseases in nature, but the lists of notifiable diseases include cancer (in many states), HIV, among others. The federal government mandates that states report diseases to federal agencies. States also have specific lists of notifiable disease that practitioners must report. Lists of notifiable diseases vary by state.

▶ **Analytic Epidemiology: Searching for the Causes of Disease among Populations**

Many of the efforts of epidemiologists focus on searching for the determinants of diseases—this is the branch of analytic epidemiology. Epidemiologists employ a range of study types used to identify and explain mechanisms underlying the development of disease. There are two major categories of analytic study designs: experimental and observational studies.

Experimental Studies

The randomized control trial (RCT) is considered by epidemiologists to be the gold standard for experimental designs to study etiology. RCTs are experimental trials where people in a cohort (subjects) are randomly assigned to one of two groups: an experimental group or a control group. *Randomization* of study subjects refers to a process in which chance determines the likelihood of subjects' assignment to the experimental or control groups in the study. Subjects in the experimental group are given a drug, treatment, or intervention; subjects in the control group are not. Researchers then follow the groups over time to identify which subjects develop the health-related outcome in question. Researchers compare the proportion of subjects who reach the outcome in the experimental group to the proportion of subjects who reach it in the control group in order to evaluate the impact of the drug, treatment, or intervention on the occurrence of the outcome in question. **Experimental studies** allow investigators to maintain the greatest control over the research setting; the investigator manipulates both the study factor (drug, treatment, or intervention) and randomly assigns subjects to the exposed and non-exposed groups (**FIGURE 2-2**).

Observational Studies

It would not be ethical to conduct experimental studies that expose subjects to substances, activities, or other exposures that have been previously linked to onset of disease. For example, it would not be ethical to require an experimental group to smoke cigarettes and a control group to abstain from cigarettes in order to identify which group is more likely to develop

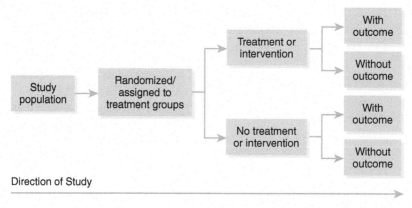

FIGURE 2-2 **Experimental Study.** The researchers control the selection of study subjects and their allocation into study groups for the treatment or intervention of interest. At the end of the study, researchers compare the study groups on the occurrence of the outcome of interest. The study direction proceeds from exposure to outcome.

cardiovascular disease. Because of the characteristics of many of the risk factors and health outcomes that epidemiologists study, the most frequently conducted epidemiologic studies are observational as opposed to experimental in nature. In an **observational study**, researchers do not intervene to impose an exposure on subjects or randomize study subjects. Instead, epidemiologists "observe" the natural exposure categories or disease diagnoses that characterize people and assign them to groups based on these characteristics. These types of studies measure patterns of exposure in populations to draw inferences about cause and effect.

Two types of observational studies commonly used for exploring etiology are *case-control studies* and *cohort studies*.

Case-Control Studies

Case-control studies group people as *cases* (those who have the health outcome) or *controls* (those who do not have the health outcome), and collect data, usually via survey, among these subjects about exposure

to risk factors. Data about exposure are only collected at one point in time. Researchers can then compare the proportion of cases that reported being exposed to the proportion of controls that reported being exposed. This comparison would identify whether the cases are more or less likely than the controls to have been exposed to a potential risk factor (**FIGURE 2-3**).

Cohort Studies

Cohort studies are different from case-control studies because they are prospective; that is, they follow people over a period of time to determine the exposure/disease relationship. As opposed to case-control studies, cohort studies start out with non-diseased individuals only. At baseline (when the study begins) the subjects in the cohort are assessed (surveyed, examined) to identify their exposure status. Researchers then follow the cohort over time to identify if and when they develop a particular health status (e.g., presence of disease, disease severity, or death). Researchers can then compare

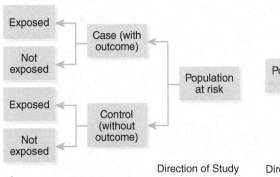

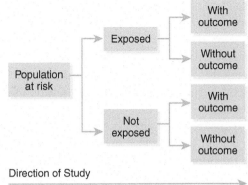

FIGURE 2-3 Case-Control Study. Researchers identify and recruit subjects on the basis of the occurrence of the outcome of interest. Researchers then identify whether or not subjects experienced the exposure of interest and compare the presence of exposure among the cases to the presence of exposure among the controls (usually by calculating an odds ratio). The study direction proceeds from outcome to exposure.

FIGURE 2-4 Cohort Study. Researchers identify and recruit a cohort of study subjects without the outcome of interest. Researchers then classify them by the presence or absence of the exposure of interest, and follow them forward in time to see who experiences the outcome of interest. Researchers then compare the development of disease between the exposed and unexposed. The study direction progresses from exposure to outcome.

the proportion of exposed people who developed the disease to the proportion of unexposed people who developed the disease, in order to identify the strength and direction of the relationship between exposure and disease. Despite being more time consuming and expensive than case-control studies, cohort studies have a major advantage: temporality. Because researchers begin with non-diseased people and assess exposure at baseline, researchers know that exposure happened before the development of the disease. In case-control studies, because the cases have already acquired the disease at baseline, it is not clear whether the exposure that they report happened before or after development of disease. Thus, results showing a relationship between the exposure and outcome in cohort studies more strongly support causation than those derived from case-control studies (**FIGURE 2-4**).

Epidemiology and Population Health

The passage and implementation of the ACA have raised the importance of epidemiology in health system planning, allocation of resources, and service provision. Health systems are no longer responsible just for treating disease at the individual level; now, at least in part, they are responsible for assuring the health of the populations they serve. Hospital systems are not just responsible for treating the health of patients that walk through their doors but also for assessing and working to improve the health of the broader populations that are geographically proximal to their hospitals and clinics. The ACA requires that each non-profit hospital in the United States perform a population health assessment to identify the major health problems in communities. Hospitals are responsible for creating programs to reach out to these populations and work to prevent diseases among the communities in which their patients live. The ACA has created a framework by which hospital systems are not evaluated strictly on the number of patients they treat or tests that they perform but on the quality of the services that they provide and their impact on improving the health of the populations in their catchment area.

This shift from the focus on the individual services provided by health systems to population-focused measures will require health systems to regularly monitor community-level health data and evaluate the system-wide impact on the community. Performing both of these functions will require health systems to monitor social determinants of health in addition to medical outcomes.

Integrating Social Determinants of Health in EMR

Institutions involved with the provision of population health services in the United States are increasingly acknowledging the influence of social determinants in shaping individual and group-level health outcomes. Recently, based on recommendations from the National Academy of Medicine (NAM, formerly the Institute of Medicine, or IOM)[30,31] and the National Quality Forum (NQF),[32] there has been a movement to integrate patient-level EMR with social determinants of health data. There are two major functions of this integration. First, after being linked to data in the electronic health record, socioeconomic and geographic data can help practitioners understand the social and environmental context in which their patients reside. Second, aggregate geography-based measures

can help health system decision makers assess the major health issues experienced by patient sub-groups and those residing in specific geographic areas.

▶ The Future of Epidemiology in Population Health

"The reports of my death are greatly exaggerated." (Mark Twain, responding to his mistakenly posted obituary)

And so it is also true of epidemiology. In a 1981 essay published in the *New England Journal of Medicine*, the renowned epidemiologist Kenneth Rothman highlighted a number of growing concerns about the practice of epidemiology that could lead to its demise.[33] He presented epidemiology's epitaph: "an unpleasant science, providing frequent reminders that ... no action is without some risk"; a science that flourished for a few decades and "is now nearly gone." He cited the increased bureaucratic and regulatory demands on researchers, making it increasingly difficult to conduct epidemiologic studies. New investigators found it difficult to complete enough studies to earn tenure. And yet, Rothman cites as epidemiology's legacy the demise of major 20th-century epidemics attributable to tobacco, dietary fats, and some carcinogens in the workplace and environment.

In a follow-up commentary published in 2007, Rothman clarified that his original essay was "not intended to predict the future of epidemiology," but more to warn that bureaucratic impediments to conducting epidemiologic studies would overwhelm and neuter the discipline.[34] It is important to note that while epidemiology has methodologic and bureaucratic challenges, the need for epidemiology to inform population health action has not been greater. In 2016, 15% of U.S. adults still smoked. The prevalence of adult obesity was approximately 40% in 2015–2016.[35] Workplace health-related problems continue, although the research focus has shifted from carcinogenic chemicals to the sedentary nature of many jobs. According to the a recent meta-analysis exploring sitting time, activity levels, and associated mortality, those who sat for more than eight hours per day, who do not offset this behavior with exercise, had risk of dying similar to the risk posed by obesity or smoking.[36] Our major health issues have not been resolved. And we have not defeated infectious disease. We live in a world with newly emerging (SARS, AIDS, Ebola) and reemerging antibiotic-resistant (e.g., tuberculosis, methicillin-resistant *Staphylococcus aureus*) infectious diseases. According to the CDC, U.S. life expectancy has declined over the past few years,[37] primarily due to the opioid epidemic and obesity. This means that for the first time in history, U.S. children may live shorter, sicker lives than their parents.

And yet, there were those who felt that the rise of genomics, proteomics, and the other technological and scientific advances would render epidemiology irrelevant. After all, if we can identify people most susceptible to disease, haven't we solved most of the exposure/disease problem? However, according to a report issued by the Bureau of Labor Statistics, "Employment of epidemiologists is projected to grow 9 percent from 2016 to 2026, about as fast as the average for all occupations. Epidemiologists are likely to have good job prospects overall."[38] This report reveals that, apparently, the need for epidemiologists is also reflected in the job market.

Perhaps the persistent need for epidemiologists is in part due to the fact that only a small percentage (30%) of premature mortality seen in society is due to genetics.

Social, economic, and behavioral factors account for approximately 70% of what kills us before we reach our life expectancy. Recent work by Dwyer-Lindgren et al.[39] shows "inequalities in life expectancy among counties are large and growing, and much of the variation in life expectancy can be explained by differences in socioeconomic and race/ethnicity factors, behavioral and metabolic risk factors, and health care factors." Epidemiology is the only branch of science equipped to quantify the absolute and relative impact of these risk factors and guide the development of interventions to improve health and reduce mortality.

Both the National Cancer Institute and the National Heart, Lung and Blood Institute conducted multi-year discussions and strategic planning on the future of their epidemiologic priorities.[39] Although these activities were conducted separately for each institute, a number of overlapping themes emerged. There was a recognition that, moving forward, epidemiologic studies should be conducted by multidisciplinary/interdisciplinary teams to account for the fact that population health is due to a combination of biological, environmental, and social factors.

Also, in this era of "big data," there is a need to learn how to leverage all of this new information along with the growth and development of ever more sophisticated technology. There is also the need to leverage the existing cohorts and new cohorts being created (e.g., the Precision Medicine Initiative) so that the best, most efficient, and most effective use can be made of them. A statement from the National Cancer Institute strategic planning initiative stands out: "Develop and design rational cost-effective epidemiologic studies and resources to optimize funding, accelerate translation, and maximize health impact."[40] In one sentence, they express the need for more efficient resources and charge epidemiology with not only reporting results but also translating the results into understandable and usable information that can more directly impact the health of populations.

It is apparent that the need for epidemiology continues to grow, not shrink. As we move forward in this 21st century, the need grows to not only identify risk factors but also to use that knowledge to target appropriate care to the right individuals at the correct time (what is now being referred to as "precision medicine").[41]

Study and Discussion Questions

1. Why is epidemiology important to the provision of population health services?

2. What are the key differences between descriptive and analytic epidemiology?

3. What makes epidemiology distinct compared to the provision of medicine?

4. How are experimental studies different from observational studies?

Suggested Readings and Websites

Readings

Berkman LF, Kawachi I, Glymour MM. *Social Epidemiology* (2nd ed.). New York: Oxford University Press; 2014.

Friis RH, Sellers TA. *Epidemiology for Public Health Practice* (5th ed.). Sudbury, MA: Jones and Bartlett Learning; 2014.

Gordis L. *Epidemiology* (5th ed.). Philadelphia, PA: Elsevier Saunders; 2014.

Keyes KM, Galea S. *Epidemiology Matters*. New York, NY: Oxford University Press; 2014.

Koch T. *Cartographies of Disease: Maps, Mapping and Disease*. Redlands, CA: ESRI Press; 2005.

Marmot M. The health gap: The challenge of an unequal world. New York, NY: Bloomsbury Press; 2015.

Merrill RM. *Introduction to Epidemiology* (7th ed.). Burlington, MA: Jones & Bartlett Learning; 2013.

Rothman K, Greenland S, Lash TL. *Modern Epidemiology* (3rd ed.). Philadelphia, PA: Lippincott Williams & Wilkins; 2008.

Szklo M, Nieto, FJ. *Epidemiology: Beyond the Basics* (4th ed.). Burlington, MA: Jones and Bartlett Learning; 2019.

Websites

Journals

International Journal of Epidemiology: https://academic.oup.com/ije

American Journal of Epidemiology: https://academic.oup.com/aje/

American Journal of Public Health: https://ajph
.aphapublications.org/
Cancer Epidemiology: https://www.journals.elsevier
.com/cancer-epidemiology

Training Courses and Programs
Centers for Disease Control and Prevention —
Epidemiology Training and Resources: https:
//www.cdc.gov/eis/request-services
/epiresources.html
Centers for Disease Control and Prevention Center
for Surveillance, Epidemiology, and Laboratory
Services (CSELS) — Division of Scientific
Education and Professional Development:
https://www.cdc.gov/csels/divisions/dsepd
/index.html
Centers for Disease Control and Prevention — Public
Health 101 Series, Introduction to Epidemiology:
https://www.cdc.gov/publichealth101
/epidemiology.html

Supercourse — Epidemiology, the Internet, and
Global Health: http://www.pitt.edu/~super1
/index.htm

Blog
The Epidemiology Monitor: https://www.epimonitor
.net/

Data Sources
Centers for Disease Control and Prevention
Wide-ranging Online Data for Epidemiologic
Research (WONDER): https://wonder.cdc.gov/
The HealthMap Project (online informal sources
for disease outbreak monitoring and real-time
surveillance of emerging public health threats):
https://www.healthmap.org/en/
World Health Organization — Epidemiology:
https://www.who.int/topics/epidemiology/en/

References

1. Centers for Disease Control and Prevention. Ten great public health achievements–United States, 1900-1999. *MMWR Morb Mortal Wkly Rep.* 1999;48(12):241.
2. National Center for Health Statistics. Health, United States, 2016: with Chartbook on Long-term Trends in Health. Hyattsville, MD. 2017.
3. Last JM. Determinant. *A Dictionary of Public Health*. Oxford University Press. 2007:90.
4. American Cancer Society. *Cancer Facts & Figures 2016*. Available at https://www.cancer .org/content/dam/cancer-org/research/cancer -facts-and-statistics/annual-cancer-facts-and -figures/2016/cancer-facts-and-figures-2016.pdf (accessed February 22, 2019).
5. U.S. Department of Health and Human Services. *Healthy People 2020*. Available at https://www .healthypeople.gov/ (accessed February 22, 2019).
6. U.S. Department of Health and Human Services. *The Health Consequences of Smoking—50 Years of Progress*. 2014. Available at https://www.cdc.gov /tobacco/data_statistics/sgr/50th-anniversary /index.htm (accessed February 22, 2019).
7. World Health Organization. *Constitution of the World Health Organization*. Geneva, Switzerland: Author; 2005. Available at http://apps.who.int /gb/bd/PDF/bd47/EN/constitution-en.pdf?ua=1 (accessed May 10, 2019).
8. Keyes KM, Galea S. *Epidemiology Matters*. New York, NY: Oxford University Press; 2014.
9. Gordis L. *Epidemiology* (5th ed.). Philadelphia, PA: Elsevier Saunders; 2014.
10. Hippocrates. On Airs, Waters, and Places. In: Adams F (ed./transl.). *The Genuine Works of Hippocrates*. London: Sydenham Society; 1849.
11. Martin PM, Martin-Granel E. 2,500-year evolution of the term epidemic. *Emerging Infectious Diseases*. 2006;12(6):976.
12. Mahmood SS, Levy D, Vasan RS, Wang TJ. The Framingham Heart Study and the epidemiology of cardiovascular disease: a historical perspective. *Lancet.* 2014;383(9921):999–1008.
13. World Health Organization. WHO report on the global tobacco epidemic, 2017: monitoring tobacco use and prevention policies. 2017. Available at https://www.who.int/tobacco /global_report/2017/en/ (accessed February 22, 2019).
14. Glasser JH. The quality and utility of death certificate data. *Am J Public Health.* 1981;71(3):231–233.
15. Sehdev AES, Hutchins GM. Problems with proper completion and accuracy of the cause-of-death statement. *Arch Intern Med.* 2001;161(2):277–284.

16. Gilmour SJ. Identification of hospital catchment areas using clustering: an example from the NHS. *Health Serv Res*. 2010;45(2):497–513.

17. Paul MM, Greene CM, Newton-Dame R, Thorpe LE, Perlman SE, McVeigh KH, Gourevitch MN. The state of population health surveillance using electronic health records: a narrative review. *Population Health Mgmt*. 2015;18(3):209–216.

18. Gawande A. The hot spotters. *The New Yorker*. 2011;86(45):40–51.

19. Kaufman S, Ali N, DeFiglio V, Craig K, Brenner J. Early efforts to target and enroll high-risk diabetic patients into urban community-based programs. *Health Promotion Pract*. 2014;15(2_suppl):62S–70S.

20. Westfall JM. Cold-spotting: linking primary care and public health to create communities of solution. *J Am Board Fam Med*. 2013;26(3):239–240.

21. Liaw W, Krist AH, Tong ST, Sabo R, Hochheimer C, Rankin J, Grolling D, et al. Living in "cold spot" communities is associated with poor health and health quality. *J Am Board Fam Med*. 2018;31(3): 342–350.

22. Robert ME, Crowe SE, Burgart L, Yantiss RK, Lebwohl B, Greenson JK, et al. Statement on best practices in the use of pathology as a diagnostic tool for celiac disease: A guide for clinicians and pathologists. *Am J Surg Pathol*. 2018 Sep;42(9):e44–e58.

23. Beyond Celiac. Celiac Disease Symptom List. 2018. Available at https://www.beyondceliac.org/celiac-disease/symptoms/ (accessed February 25, 2019).

24. Fasano A, Berti I, Gerarduzzi T, Not T, Colletti RB, Drago S, et al. Prevalence of celiac disease in at-risk and not-at-risk groups in the United States: a large multicenter study. *Arch Internal Med*. 2003;163(3): 286–292.

25. Dubé C, Rostom A, Sy R, Cranney A, Saloojee N, Garritty C, et al. The prevalence of celiac disease in average-risk and at-risk Western European populations: a systematic review. *Gastroenterology*. 2005;128(4):S57–S67.

26. NIH Consensus Development Conference on Celiac Disease. NIH Consensus and State of the Science Statements. 2004;21:1–23.

27. Rubio-Tapia A, Kyle RA, Kaplan EL, Johnson DR, Page W, Erdtmann F, et al. Increased prevalence and mortality in undiagnosed celiac disease. *Gastroenterology*. 2009;137:88–93.

28. Centers for Disease Control and Prevention. *Principles of Epidemiology in Public Health Practice, Third Edition: An Introduction to Applied Epidemiology and Biostatistics, Lesson 3 Measures of Risk*. Available at https://www.cdc.gov/ophss/csels/dsepd/ss1978/lesson3/section2.html (accessed February 25, 2019).

29. Hopkins RS, Jajosky RA, Hall PA, Adams DA, Connor FJ, Sharp P, et al. Summary of notifiable diseases — United States, 2003. *MMWR Morb Mortal Wkly Rep*. 2005 Apr 22;52(54):1–85.

30. National Academy of Medicine (formerly the Institute of Medicine). *Capturing social and behavioral domains and measures in electronic health records: Phase 1*. 2014. Washington, DC: The National Academies Press.

31. National Academy of Medicine (formerly the Institute of Medicine). *Capturing social and behavioral domains and measures in electronic health records: Phase 2*. 2014. Washington, DC: The National Academies Press.

32. National Quality Forum. Multi-stakeholder input on a national priority: improving population health by working with communities—action guide 1.0. Washington, DC: National Quality Forum; 2014.

33. Rothman KJ. The rise and fall of epidemiology, 1950–2000 A.D. *N Engl J Med*. 1981;304:600–602. Available at http://doi.org/10.1056/NEJM198103053041010 (accessed February 25, 2019).

34. Rothman KJ. Commentary: epidemiology still ascendant. *Int J Epidemiol*. 2007;36.4(2007):710–711. Available at https://doi.org/10.1093/ije/dym151 (accessed February 25, 2019).

35. Hales CM, Carroll MD, Fryar CD, Ogden CL. Prevalence of obesity among adults and youth: United States, 2015–2016. NCHS data brief, no. 288. Hyattsville, MD:

National Center for Health Statistics, 2017. Available at: Available at https://www.cdc .gov/nchs/products/databriefs/db288.htm (accessed March 18, 2019).

36. Ekelund U, Steene-Johannessen J, Brown WJ, Fagerland MW, Owen N, Powell KE, et al. Lancet Sedentary Behaviour Working Group. Does physical activity attenuate, or even eliminate, the detrimental association of sitting time with mortality? A harmonised meta-analysis of data from more than 1 million men and women. *Lancet.* 2016;388(10051):1302–1310.

37. Centers for Disease Control. CDC Director's Media Statement on U.S. Life Expectancy. 2018. Available at https://www .cdc.gov/media/releases/2018/s1129-life -expectancy.html (accessed February 2, 2019).

38. U.S. Bureau of Labor Statistics. Life, physical, and social science occupations. Available at: Available at https://bls.gov/physical-and-social

-science/print/home.htm (accessed March 18, 2019).

39. Dwyer-Lindgren L, Bertozzi-Villa A, Stubbs RW, Morozoff C, Mackenbach JP, vanLenthe FJ, et al. Inequalities in life expectancy among counties, 1980 to 2014: temporal trends and key drivers. *JAMA Intern Med.* 2017;177(7):1003–1011.

40. National Cancer Institute Epidemiology and Genomics Research Program. Trends in 21st Century Epidemiology: From Scientific Discoveries to Population Health Impact [workshop summary]. Available at https:// epi.grants.cancer.gov/events/century-trends/ (accessed May 10, 2019).

41. Khoury MJ. Planning for the future of epidemiology in the era of big data and precision medicine. *Am J Epidemiol.* 2015;182(12):977– 979. Available at https://doi.org/10.1093/aje /kwv228 (accessed May 10, 2019).

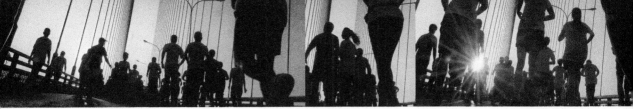

CHAPTER 3

On the Path to Health Equity

Rosemary Frasso
Martha Romney
Jillian Baker
Jennifer Ravelli
Livia Frasso Jaramillo

EXECUTIVE SUMMARY

"Good health begins in the places where we live, learn, work and play."

While access to quality medical care is necessary and should be a population health goal, it is not enough to keep us well. Population health efforts to improve patient outcomes start with a recognition that clinical care is only part of the key to ensuring health. In fact, clinical care is estimated to account for only 20% of the modifiable contributors to overall health. The remaining 80% is attributed to social and economic factors, including poverty (40%), health behavior (30%), and the physical environment (10%).[1–4]

As we care for patients, we must consider everything that influences their health: economic stability, education, social and community realities, neighborhood characteristics, and the built environment.[3,5] Providers and health systems must consider looking beyond the clinical presentation and see the patient holistically and in context and recognize, acknowledge, and address the social determinants of health (SDOH) with the goal of achieving health equity. Additionally, we must consider the social and political context—that is, the other forces that affect healthcare access, quality of care, and trust in providers and the system at large. These include linguistic and cultural barriers and overt, subtle and unconscious bias and discrimination.

This chapter will address the non-biomedical influences on health that impact health equity and summarize some current efforts to address these influences in concert with the provision of healthcare services. The chapter is broken down into four sections: we first explore the meaning of health equity. Second, we move on to issues like racism and discrimination that interfere with our goal of achieving health equity. Next, we share information about cultural competency, a key step toward achieving health equity, and finally, we share some ways in which health systems are trying to achieve health equity by addressing the SDOH.

LEARNING OBJECTIVES

1. Describe non-biomedical influences on health.
2. Discuss current efforts to address the SDOH in the healthcare setting.
3. Explain some key drivers of health disparities.
4. Recognize the impact that racism, trust, stigma, and bias may have on health.
5. Consider how current efforts to address the SDOH may be applied to the work you do or hope to do when you complete your training.

KEY TERMS

Allostatic load
Community health workers
Cultural competency
Health disparities
Health equity

Healthy People 2030
Medical-legal partnerships
Patient navigators
Social determinants of health
 (SDOH)

Stigma
Structural racism
Weathering

▶ Introduction

The U.S. healthcare system is at the heart of a multibillion-dollar industry that has captured the attention of government and the public as they struggle to contain the costs associated with healthcare services. It is important to remember, however, that health is largely impacted by non-medical factors outside of this complex system. That is, health is impacted by where we live, work, learn, and play and the realities of life that influence health behaviors and interactions among patients, providers, and the healthcare system (**FIGURE 3-1**). [1–4]

Health status is dependent on the degree to which we practice *healthy behaviors*, the *environmental determinants* to which we're exposed, and our *educational and economic status and opportunities*. All of these factors and determinants play a role in positively supporting our health (**FIGURE 3-2**). [6,7]

Healthy behaviors include getting adequate sleep, healthy nutrition, routine physical activity, avoidance of adverse substances, preventive screening, timely immunizations, and annual physical examinations.

Environmental determinants include the availability of safe and habitable housing, healthy food, clean water and air, and access to parks and public transportation.

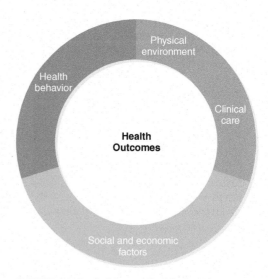

FIGURE 3-1 What Influences Health Outcomes?

Economic Stability	• Poverty • Employment • Food security • Housing stability
Education	• High school graduation • Enrollment in higher education • Language and literacy • Early childhood education and development
Social and Community Context	• Social cohesion • Civic participation • Discrimination • Incarceration
Health and Health Care	• Access to health care • Access to primary care • Health literacy
Neighborhood and Built Environment	• Access to healthy food • Quality of housing • Crime and violence • Environmental conditions

FIGURE 3-2 A Closer Look at the Drivers of Health.
Healthy People 2020 DPHP Campaign.

Educational and economic status and opportunities are comprised of healthy neighborhoods and positive workplaces; access to affordable education from early childhood through 12th grade, as well as opportunities for college or technical training; healthy interactions with public servants, including the police; and personal relationships free from violence.

Every 10 years, the U.S. Department of Health and Human Services (HHS) publishes the *National Health Promotion and Disease Prevention Objectives*. A recent HHS document, **Healthy People 2030**, confirms that achieving health and well-being requires eliminating **health disparities**, attaining health literacy, and achieving **health equity**.[8] This requires a holistic look at the individual in context; that is, we must

consider and address the realities and conditions in which we live. Even when access to health care is "equal," context explains, in part, "why some Americans are healthier than others and why Americans more generally are not as healthy as they could be."[1] *Healthy People 2030* identifies the importance of addressing the **social determinants of health (SDOH)**, through programs that "Create social and physical environments that promote good health for all."[8] HHS is not the only entity that highlights the nonclinical contextual realities that influence health. This priority is shared by other U.S. health initiatives such as the National Partnership for Action to End Health Disparities[9] and the National Prevention and Health Promotion Strategy.[10] Additionally, in 2008, the World Health Organization's (WHO) Commission on Social Determinants of Health published a report entitled Closing the gap in a generation: *Closing the Gap in a Generation: Health Equity Through Action on the Social Determinants of Health*.[2,11]

To ensure that all Americans have that opportunity to be as healthy as possible, we need advances in health care, education, child care, social justice, business, media, planning, transportation, housing, agriculture, and social environmental justice. The SDOH cannot be addressed in isolation but must be addressed at the patient's side and in the community.

This chapter is broken down into four sections: the first explores health equity; the second, race; the third, **cultural competency**; and finally, we share some ways in which health systems are trying to achieve health equity by addressing the SDOH.

As we move forward with our discussion, it is important to understand some key terms:

1. *Health Disparities*: The Centers for Disease Control and Prevention (CDC) defines *health disparities* as "the differences in health outcomes and their causes among groups of people."[1] These differences are closely linked to social, educational, physical, economic, and community exposures, as well as environmental disadvantage, and current and historical discriminatory policies and actions.[1,9,12–14]

2. *Social Determinants of Health (SDOH)*: The social determinants of health are the conditions in which people are born, grow, live, work, and age. These circumstances are shaped by the distribution of money, power, and resources at the global, national, and local levels.[15]

According to the National Academy of Medicine (NAM, formerly the Institute of Medicine or IOM), there are five things we should know about SDOH[15]:

- As a determinant of health, medical care is insufficient for ensuring better health outcomes.
- SDOH are influenced by policies and programs and associated with better health outcomes.
- New payment models are prompting interest in the SDOH.
- Frameworks for integrating SDOH are emerging.
- Experiments are occurring at the local and federal level.

3. *Health Equity*: HHS defines *health equity* as "the attainment of the highest level of health for all people."[10,16] Equality and equity are not synonymous. If we settle for an equal system, then everyone is treated the same and provided the same access to services, information, and health care. However, "same access" is not necessarily what is needed. For a patient who only speaks Mandarin, sharing *The Patient's Guide to a Healthy Diet* in English will not provide the information in a way that enables that patient to understand and follow the recommendations. Unlike health equality, health equity not only requires that all persons have equal access but also necessitates actions to ensure that

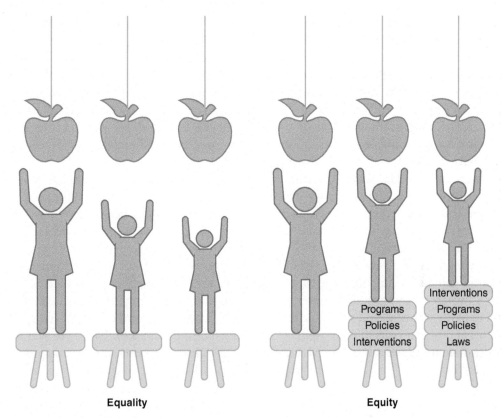

FIGURE 3-3 Equality and Equity.

added obstacles are addressed for vulnerable groups. This often requires policy interventions that level the playing field and remove obstacles created by factors including poverty and discrimination (**FIGURE 3-3**).[12,13]

▶ Health Equity

To mitigate health disparities and achieve health equity, medical practice must extend its reach to the community, and SDOH must be front of mind. However, as the NAM points out, there are many variables to consider. How do we best set priorities when it comes to addressing the

SDOH? What are the costs associated with addressing SDOH, and equally important, what are the costs truly associated with failing to address them? Which SDOH have the greatest effect on total population health and well-being, healthcare expenditures, and health equity?[14,15]

The problem is complex and has far-reaching consequences, as evidenced by differences of 10–15 years in life expectancy between more affluent and lower-income communities. In large cities like Philadelphia, New York, and Chicago, life expectancy drops from 78 to 63 years based upon economic status, even in neighboring zip codes.[17-19] Healthcare costs and healthcare debt far too often exacerbate income disparities and might lead to poorer health outcomes.[20,21] Being uninsured or underinsured has led many Americans into bankruptcy, exacerbating the link between poverty and health.[22,23] Even with coverage under the Patient Protection and Affordable Care Act (ACA), Americans living at or near the poverty line have less access to care and have higher out-of-pocket expenses for services than their wealthier counterparts. In the United States, far too many people still must choose between paying for prescriptions or medical care and food, housing, or utilities.[24,25]

Without consideration of SDOH, the ground gained in the clinical setting can be lost when a patient returns home, leading to costly, stressful, and avoidable treatments and return visits to the hospital.[26–29] According to the Centers for Medicare and Medicaid Services (CMS), one in five Medicare patients return to the hospital within 30 days of discharge. CMS estimates that readmissions costs for Medicare patients is around $26 billion per year, and more than half of that cost can be attributed to potentially preventable rehospitalizations.[30,31] These visits tax hospital systems, impact public health budgets, and compromise the patient's quality of life on multiple levels.

Despite increased attention to the SDOH, clinical care providers are far too often left "between a rock and a hard place." They know addressing non-clinical issues is important to their patients, but they often are not prepared—nor do they have the time—to do so in an effective way. While the SDOH have long been embedded in nursing and social work education, medical schools have only recently begun to weave these issues into their tightly packed curricula, leaving the medical workforce lacking skills in this area.[32–36]

Results of a 2018 survey conducted by healthcare consulting group Leavitt Partners confirms that while physicians appreciate the importance of non-biomedical determinants of health, most are unsure how to properly address the SDOH, many believe it is beyond the scope of their professional responsibilities and, of course, time is an issue.[26]

Additionally, providers often fail to appreciate the link between the SDOH, health factors, and health outcomes and are not at the table when policies and programs are developed to improve these outcomes.[26] The focus is often on access to care and quality of care. While these are important, they only account for 20% of what matters in terms of impact on health outcomes (FIGURE 3-4). Failure to identify social challenges can lead to inappropriate work-ups, misdiagnosis, discounting of symptoms, inappropriate treatment plans, readmissions, and ultimately poor health outcomes despite access to a provider.[27,31,37,38] For example, treating a patient for chronic pain but failing to identify exposure to violence or recommending that a patient add walking to his or her daily activities without appreciating community-level barriers that may keep him or her housebound can affect short- and long-term health.

Programs that consider SDOH central to their approach offer the potential to reduce readmission rates and improve patient outcomes. For example, Community-Based Care Management Models are improving outcomes for a small segment of the population (known as "super utilizers") that account for a large volume of unnecessary emergency room visits.[39–41] These models look beyond the clinical needs of the patients and provide support that addresses their SDOH. Home

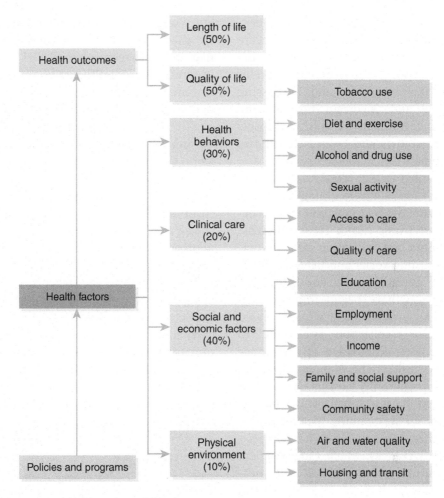

FIGURE 3-4 County Health Rankings & Roadmaps.

Reproduced from County Health Rankings & Roadmaps, http://www.countyhealthrankings.org/our-approach (accessed March 28, 2019).

visits enable the team to explore complex needs and connect patients to important non-clinical resources including utility services, transportation, lead abatement resources, and programs like Meals on Wheels or the Women, Infants and Children (WIC) nutrition program.[39,41–43] The Camden Coalition of Healthcare Providers (Camden Coalition), the first to document the impact of high-intensity care management for super utilizers, is a leader in this space.[39,42–44] The Camden Coalition's work aligns with the goals of accountable care

organizations and has transitioned from a small-scale program to an exemplar of an effective approach to addressing the SDOH. Their model has been duplicated across the nation, and evaluations have shown efficacy.[45,46]

Across disciplines and roles, healthcare leaders are increasingly focused on SDOH and employing a range of approaches to address them. HHS has described the SDOH as a key driver of population health and healthcare costs.[3] The Centers for Medicare and Medicaid

Innovation (CMMI), charged with testing the efficacy of innovative healthcare payment and delivery models, is currently investigating whether systematically screening for and addressing Medicare and Medicaid beneficiaries' social determinants of health impacts healthcare costs and reduces healthcare utilization.[47]

To enhance providers' knowledge of patient's social status to ultimately inform clinical care the NAM recommends structuring electronic health records (EHRs) to support the collection of information regarding social and behavioral factors.[48-50] Private payers and providers, like Optum, have begun implementing innovative social determinants–based information collection strategies to advance their knowledge of their population's health. The National Association of Community Health Centers has developed an assessment tool called the Protocol for Responding to and Assessing Patients' Assets, Risks, and Experiences (PRAPARE), which gauges patient social health status.[51] PRAPARE's measures focus on actionable conditions and templates exist for several EHR systems, including eClinicalWorks, Epic, GE Centricity, and NextGen.[51,52]

While health policymakers and thought leaders are increasingly interested in addressing the SDOH as a means to improve quality of care and reduce healthcare costs, their ability to do so hinges on providers. Providers are well positioned to advance health equity because of their access to the patient population, contextual knowledge of the patient's medical status, and their role as the "team leader" in the healthcare industry. A new and clearer appreciation of the role of the SDOH has led to a reimagining of healthcare delivery and a call to enhance the provider's reach. Patient-centered care is critical to the population health response to SDOH and any progress toward health equity.

In patient-centered care, the patient defines his or her health needs and desired health outcomes. Patient goals are the driving force behind all healthcare decisions. Patients become partners with their providers, and providers treat patients not only from a clinical perspective but also from an "emotional, mental, spiritual, social, and financial perspective."[53-55] This approach should not be reserved solely for the super utilizers discussed above, as there is ground to gain when this lens is applied broadly. Poverty, social isolation, lack of transportation, stress, poor childcare, under-employment, lack of autonomy, power imbalances, and low health literacy can hinder health outcomes for many patients.

▶ Racism, Trust, Stigma, and Bias

Despite major advances in medicine and public health, disparities persist by race, ethnicity, income, and educational attainment—and in some cases they are increasing.[56] These disparities are driven, both directly and indirectly, by gender bias, stereotyping, unconscious bias, and **structural racism**. If health is to be an earnest goal in the population health era, we must remember that disadvantage is complicated and still hard to talk about.

Despite a renewed interest in how the SDOH can be addressed to improve health outcomes, there is still far too little being done to address racism as a driver of health inequities.[13,57] Racial minorities have higher rates of morbidity and mortality than their majority counterparts, and while SDOH account for some of this, they do not explain all that we see.[13,28,58-60] For example, recent studies have documented that individuals who report experiencing racism have greater rates of several chronic and acute medical conditions, and race is associated with a host of poor health outcomes independent of SDOH, including housing, insurance status, and literacy.[61-67]

The discussion has moved from considering racism on the individual level to exploring it on a structural level. Structural racism refers to "the totality of ways in which societies foster racial discrimination through mutually reinforcing systems of housing, education, employment, earning, benefits, credit, media, health care and criminal justice. These patterns and practices in turn reinforce discriminatory beliefs, values and distribution of resources"[68] that all potentially impact health. Structural racism has resulted in reduced access to care, lower-quality care, denial of services (including recommended diagnostic tests and treatments), fewer referrals to clinical research programs, and delivery of unneeded and harmful interventions.[68,69]

Blacks or African Americans (referred to as blacks in this chapter) are the third-largest racial/ethnic population in the United States, after whites and Hispanics,[70] and while the life expectancy gap is narrowing, there are still very worrisome challenges to health equity. For example, disparities in the leading causes of death for blacks compared with whites are pronounced by early and middle adulthood, especially deaths from violence, homicide, and chronic diseases including heart disease and diabetes.[65,71] In addition, blacks in the United States have the highest death rate and shorter survival rate for all cancers combined compared to their white counterparts.[66,67] The route of these disparities is not completely clear. However, structural and interpersonal racism, bias, and discrimination in and out of the healthcare settings can directly, and indirectly, affect health.[68] These experiences are most certainly stressful and together create what many researchers refer to as **allostatic load**, or "the cumulative wear and tear on the body's systems owing to repeated adaptation to stressors."[72] Arline Geronimus and her coauthors developed the "**weathering**" hypothesis, which posits that black Americans' health deteriorates more rapidly than other groups because they bear a heavier allostatic load. "These effects may be felt particularly by black women because of 'double jeopardy' (gender *and* racial discrimination)."[72] Infant mortality, cervical cancer, asthma, diabetes, and cardiovascular disease all disproportionately affect black Americans.[72-74] While it has been many years since the NAM released a report titled *Unequal Treatment: Confronting Racial and Ethnic Disparities in Health Care,*[75] which documented systematic and pervasive bias in the treatment of minorities in the healthcare system, researchers are continuing to document this finding.[73,74,76-79]

If patients perceive a healthcare system as discriminatory, this can lead to decreased levels of healthcare utilization.[80] Trust in providers and the healthcare system remains a complicated issue, embedded in a history of social, medical, and research abuses, from slavery to the Tuskegee Syphilis Experiment, which continues to inform minorities' interactions with the medical system and fuel distrust and suspicion.[69,81-84] Unconscious bias by healthcare professionals undermines quality of care and reinforces minority patients' negative perceptions of providers.[61] Despite advances in research and training, according to a recent survey, the majority of medical students and residents reported believing the fallacious stereotypes that black patients experience less pain than white patients do.[85] Likely, as a result, several studies have found that in comparison to white patients, black patients are less likely to receive pain medication at all and are often prescribed lower doses when they do receive it.[85-90]

These disparities in pain treatment also occur among children. A study of almost one million children diagnosed with appendicitis showed that in comparison to white children, black children were less likely to receive any pain medication (the standard treatment for severe pain).[85,90] Due to cumulative discriminatory experiences with healthcare systems, as well as the larger society, minority patients may also be especially sensitive to interpersonal cues from their healthcare providers that convey a message of caring, trustworthiness, and partnership, or not.[76,91-93] Despite modest improvements following the ACA, research has repeatedly demonstrated health disparities in access and quality of care overall for minority patients.[94-98]

Cultural sensitivity and trust can facilitate patient satisfaction, which has a positive influence on quality of health care received and health outcomes of patients.[99] In addition, race-concordant medical visits have been found to be more satisfying, more participatory, include more positive patient affect, and to be longer.[100-102] Minority patients in race-discordant patient-provider relationships report less involvement in medical decisions, less partnership with physicians, and less

satisfaction with healthcare.[103-105] Despite efforts to diversify the healthcare workforce, minorities are underrepresented in many medical and nursing training programs across the United States.[103-105]

Bias is not limited to issues of race; researchers have documented bias associated with gender, sexual identity, physical and intellectual disabilities, weight, ethnicity, and culture, resulting in everything from reduced referrals for screening among people who identify as transgender and variation in medication recommendations for women, to limited access to mammography for people with mobility impairments.[106-110]

An examination of stigma yields an important understanding of population health inequalities.[111,112] **Stigma** is defined as "the co-occurrence of labeling, stereotyping, separation, status loss, and discrimination in a context in which power is exercised."[113-115] Stigma overlaps with racism and discrimination, but it differs from these constructs in important ways. While race and ethnicity are stigmatized statuses, the notion of stigma as a concept encompasses multiple statuses and characteristics, such as sexual orientation, gender roles, disability, age, and obesity. Stigma addresses a broader scope of issues than racism.[113-115] However, discrimination at the individual level and at the structural level (structural racism) is a byproduct of stigma.[113-116] Efforts to address these challenges begin with attempts to address cultural competency in medical, nursing, and allied professional education.

Cultural Competence

Cultural competence has been defined as "a set of congruent behaviors, attitudes, and policies that come together in a system, agency or among professionals and enable that system, agency or those professions to work effectively in cross-cultural situations."[117-119] The Campinha-Bacote model, one of the many that explores cultural competency, describes the constructs as cultural awareness, cultural knowledge, cultural skill, cultural encounters, and cultural desire.[119] There is evidence that improved cultural competency among the healthcare work force is an effective step towards health equity.[119] Recognizing the need to reduce health disparities begins with a recognition of social injustice and discrimination.

The public and private sectors have initiated guidelines, policies, and programs to facilitate the implementation of "culturally and linguistically appropriate services and care."[57] Healthcare professionals who understand and acknowledge the varied cultural traditions, practices, beliefs, and values associated with health, illness, and care-seeking create the opportunity to have a more productive relationship with their patients. This leads to better health outcomes, decreased disparities, and, ultimately, health equity.[119] While becoming an expert on every culture and subculture is not feasible, becoming committed to employing a culturally competent lens can build trust, improve communication, and ultimately, enhance patient care.[119]

Cultural humility, a component of cultural competency, involves ongoing self-reflection about one's attitudes, values, beliefs, communications, and behaviors.[120,121] Culturally competent care also requires providers to be cognizant of power imbalances, attentively listen to patients, and respect their perspectives, beliefs, and decisions without judgment, even when they differ from their own.[120,121] Additionally, providers must recognize the challenges that patients and families encounter when interacting with health systems. These include navigating the facilities,

understanding signage, completing administrative and insurance forms, and communicating with different professionals.

Recognizing that a systematic approach to achieving cultural competency is also necessary, the federal and state governments have enacted statutes and issued regulations and guidelines that address cultural competency, and semi-regulatory organizations (e.g., The Joint Commission's National Quality Forum) have developed quality measures related to cultural and linguistic standards.[122,123] HHS has identified elimination of health disparities as a goal and specifically addresses language access and cultural accommodations in its guidelines. HHS's Office of Minority Health has issued National Standards for Culturally and Linguistically Appropriate Services (National CLAS Standards),[124] and the Agency for Healthcare Research and Quality (AHRQ) has developed toolkits and other resources to support integration of health literacy and cultural competency in healthcare organizations[125] (**FIGURE 3-5**). The CLAS Standards identify strategies for organizations implementing system policies, procedures, and initiatives to support and improve access to health care and advance health equity for the diverse populations they serve.[124]

The provision of culturally competent care also depends on an appreciation of the literacy demands in the healthcare space. Specifically, health literacy, defined as "the degree to which individuals have the capacity to obtain, process, and understand basic health information and services needed to make appropriate health decisions,"[100,125] has been associated with health outcomes. An estimated 36% of adults in the United States have low health literacy, and while there is a

National Standards for Culturally and Linguistically Appropriate Services (CLAS) in Health and Health Care

The National CLAS Standards are intended to advance health equality, improve quality, and help eliminate health care disparities by establishing a blueprint for health and health care organizations to:

Principal Standard:
1. Provide effective, equitable, understandable, and respectful quality care and services that are responsive to diverse cultural health beliefs and practices, preferred languages, health literacy, and other communication needs.

Governance, Leadership, and Workforce:
2. Advance and sustain organizational governance and leadership that promotes CLAS and health equity through policy, practices, and allocated resources.
3. Recruit, promote, and support a culturally and linguistically diverse governance, leadership, and workforce that are responsive to the population in the service area.
4. Educate and train governance, leadership, and workforce in culturally and linguistically appropriate policies and practices on an ongoing basis.

Communication and Language Assistance:
5. Offer language assistance to individuals who have limited English proficiency and/or other communication needs, at no cost to them to facilitate timely access to all health care and services.
6. Inform all individuals of the availability of language assistance services clearly and in their preferred language, verbally and in writing.
7. Ensure the competence of individuals providing language assistance, recognizing that the use of untrained individuals and/or minor as interpreters should be avoided.
8. Provide easy to understand print and multimedia materials and signage in the languages commonly used by the populations in the service area.

Engagement, Continuous Improvement, and Accountability:
9. Establish culturally and linguistically appropriate goals, policies, and management accountability, and infuse them throughout the organization's planning and operations.
10. Conduct ongoing assessments of the organization's CLAS-related activities and integrate CLAS-related measures into measurement and continuous quality improvement activities.
11. Collect and maintain accurate and reliable demographic data to monitor and evaluate the impact of CLAS on health equity and outcomes and to inform service delivery.
12. Conduct regular assessments of community health assets and needs and use the results to plan and implement services that respond to the cultural and linguistic diversity of populations in the service area.
13. Partner with the community to design, implement, and evaluate policies, practices, and services to ensure cultural and linguistic appropriateness.
14. Create conflict and grievance resolution processes that are culturally and linguistically appropriate to identify, prevent, and resolve conflicts or complaints.
15. Communicate the organization's progress in implementing and sustaining CLAS to all stakeholders, constituents, and the general public.

FIGURE 3-5 National Standards for Culturally and Linguistically Appropriate Services (CLAS) in Health and Health Care.

The National CLAS Standards, United States Department of Health and Human Services.

disproportionate prevalence in low-income families, a 2016 study found disparities in health literacy across socioeconomic and demographic groups.[126] Low health literacy has been shown to be an independent predictor of poor health outcomes, misuse of prescriptions, failure to comply with screening protocols, and underuse of preventative healthcare services, as well as poor obstetric, diabetic, cancer, cardiac, and other outcomes.[99,100,127–129]

AHRQ recommends that health systems and providers take a "universal precautions" approach and make no assumptions about the health literacy levels of their patients rather than screening for low health literacy.[130] AHRQ calls for the use of plain language in all forms of communication.[129,130] Governmental and nongovernmental cultural competency and health literacy training programs have been developed and integrated into educational, training and licensure programs across the country.[119,131]

Language barriers must also be addressed if one is committed to providing culturally competent care. There are statutory (e.g., Patient Protection and Affordable Care Act) and semi-regulatory (e.g., The Joint Commission) provisions and standards regarding the accessibility of medically certified interpreters or interpreter services rather than relying on family members and staff to translate for patients whose English language skills are limited.[132,133] Ensuring that certified medical interpretation services are accessible is an essential component of culturally competent care.

In 2012, the Institute of Medicine (now the National Academy of Medicine) released the Ten Attributes of Health Literate Health Care Organizations to identify components and strategies for health systems to integrate health literacy policies, procedures, and resources to improve communication, patient-centered care, and outcomes.[100] The ten attributes are:

1. Has leadership that makes health literacy integral to its mission, structure, and operations
2. Integrates health literacy into planning, evaluation measure, patient safety, and quality improvement
3. Prepares the workforce to be health literate and monitors progress
4. Includes populations served in the design, implementation, and evaluation of health information and services
5. Meets the needs of populations with a range of health literacy skills while avoiding stigmatization
6. Uses the health literacy strategies in interpersonal communications and confirms understanding, at all points of contact
7. Provides easy access to health information and services and navigation assistance content
8. Designs and distributes print, audiovisual, and social media content that is easy to understand and act on
9. Addresses health literacy in high-risk situations, including care transitions and communication about medicine
10. Communicates clearly what health plans cover what individuals will have to pay for services

Efforts to eliminate health disparities and establish health equity begin with a clear understanding of the SDOH, the impact of structural racism and stigma, and the value of culturally competent care. Because patients interact with a healthcare system on multiple levels and in a variety of ways, this most certainly requires creative thinking and a team-based approach.[134-136] While there is a growing body of evidence linking teamwork in hospitals to improved patient outcomes and patient safety, more studies need to be done.[137-139]

It Will Take the Entire Team and Some New Players

Hospitals around the nation are implementing innovative strategies to reduce disparities, including multidisciplinary team approaches and engaging individuals in new roles like **patient navigators** (PNs) and **community health workers** (CHWs). Working side by side with clinicians (MDs, DOs, PAs, NPs), nurses, and social workers, PNs and CHWs are addressing the SDOH. People working in these roles are generally lay members of communities who work as paid employees or as volunteers, and when possible, they share ethnicity, culture, language, and life experiences with the patient population or communities they serve.

CHWs are also known as community health advisors, lay health advocates, *promotoras* ("health promoters" in Spanish), outreach educators, peer health educators, or community health representatives. CHWs offer interpretation and translation services, provide culturally tailored health education, and help community members connect with needed resources inside and outside the health system.[140,141] CHWs and PNs help patients negotiate appointments, transportation, address prevention, and conduct health education programs and a host of non-traditionally billable activities that simply help people get well, stay well, and do well. Many health systems have begun to screen patients to get a sense of their non-clinical needs and then PNs, CHWs, or other staff or hospital volunteers then connect patients to non-clinical community-based resources, including student tutoring programs, diaper donations, and services that help patients address debt, secure housing, avoid eviction, or keep the utilities on.[142,143]

While PNs generally focus on what happens inside the health systems, CHWs often bridge health systems and communities by helping address the SDOH while also being part of the team approach to culturally competent care. PNs and CHWs serve important roles on the healthcare team; by addressing the SDOH, they allow others to operate at the top of their license.

However, it is important to note, that does not free other players from focusing on the SDOH, and this issue is not simply one for the primary care providers. Specialists, taught to hyper-focus on their area of expertise, may need additional training in order to assure they provide care that is sensitive to the SDOH. For example, complex medication regimens to deal with heart failure may be particularly hard to manage for a patient with low literacy and little social support.

Certainly, an understanding of SDOH allows primary care doctors and specialty providers to provide care in context and to be effective advocates for health system investments in non-clinical resources (often not billable) to improve health outcomes. These include staff training, culturally and linguistically appropriate and accessible patient educational resources and bridge programs that may engage players that are not traditionally seen as members of the healthcare team, like lawyers.

Medical-legal partnerships (MLPs) are formal collaborations between attorneys and healthcare systems to address those SDOH for which there are civil law remedies.[144,145] MLPs were established to facilitate providers' timely referrals of low-income patients to attorneys to address issues that impact patients' health and are beyond the scope of providers' and social workers' professional responsibilities. In this model, attorneys are based in health facilities, ideally easily accessible to the providers and patients. Attorneys conduct needs assessments and develop screening tools based upon the needs of the designated patient population. The medical screening tools incorporate the SDOH impacting their patients' health, safety, and quality of life, including loss of insurance, food insecurity, housing issues, utility cut-offs, domestic violence, and family issues. There are no costs to patients or to health systems.

In addition to providing patients with direct legal services, the MLP staff train healthcare providers and hospital staff regarding the laws that relate to their patients' needs. They also help patients and providers complete governmental and organizational documents related to patients' accessing care, benefits, utilities and other resources, and, when appropriate, they open legal cases. [144,145]

There are currently more than 300 active MLPs in hospitals and health centers in 46 states. The types of legal issues handled by MLP attorneys vary based upon the clinics' mission, the needs of the patient populations, the number of MLP attorneys, their areas of expertise, and provisions of their funding. Common legal issues include public benefits, domestic violence, immigration status, housing, food insecurity, utility terminations, family matters, special education and consumer rights. MLPs will also work with local law firms as needed. [144,145]

The benefits of MLPs to patients are many and documented in the literature. Another key benefit of MLPs are the relationships that develop between healthcare providers and attorneys who educate and train each other to assess for social determinants, intervene to address current problems, work to prevent recurrences, and identify issues before they become problems. [144,145]

▶ Conclusion

As we conclude this chapter, it is important to underscore the value of data. Most hospitals collect demographic information (race, ethnicity, age, social support, primary language) and some are screening for SDOH when the patient arrives at the clinic, provider's office, or emergency room. These data, along with outcome measures, can assist providers and health systems committed to health equity and community-based prevention by affording organizations the ability to monitor trends and patterns that might point to opportunity to improve services and promoting institutional accountability for addressing SDOH.

These data, augmented by qualitative inquiry, can paint a more complete picture of how well efforts to reduce disparities are working and can be used to identify new and emerging opportunities to intervene and improve health outcomes. Importantly, hospitals and health systems can better engage the communities they serve if they authentically embed and engage stakeholders. Health systems can work to understand diverse cultures by seeking advice from their neighbors—that is, individuals, community organizations, and social groups who know and understand the needs of the community better than any other entity. These constituencies can help hospitals develop educational materials, improve access to services for patients, enhance trust, and facilitate connections. Health professionals, including physicians, social workers, CHWs, PNs, nurses, NPs, and PAs, collaborating with lawyers, community organizers, and public health professionals, must work together to address the SDOH, remove bias and discrimination in health care, create and support culturally competent environments, and improve communication with the goal of achieving health equity.

Study and Discussion Questions

1. What are the main influencing factors on health?
2. Define the SDOH and discuss how they impact access and equity.
3. How can racism, trust, stigma, and bias potentially impact health?
4. How can cultural competency improve health equity?
5. How do health systems engage non-clinicians in efforts to improve health equity?

Suggested Readings and Websites

Readings

Braveman P, Egerter S, Williams DR. The social determinants of health: coming of age. *Annu Rev Public Health*. 2011;32:381–398.

National Academy of Medicine (formerly the Institute of Medicine); (US) Committee on Understanding and Eliminating Racial and Ethnic Disparities in Health Care. Unequal treatment: confronting racial and ethnic disparities in health care. Smedley BD, Stith AY, Nelson AR, editors. Washington (DC): National Academies Press (US); 2003.

Kumaş-Tan Z, Beagan B, Loppie C, MacLeod A, Frank B. Measures of cultural competence: examining hidden assumptions. *Acad Med*. 2007 Jun;82(6):548–557.

Murphy JS, Lawton EM, Sandel M. Legal care as part of health care: the benefits of medical-legal partnership. *Pediatr Clin North Am*. 2015 Oct;62(5):1263–1271.

The National Prevention and Health Promotion Strategy. The National Prevention Strategy: America's Plan for Better Health and Wellness [archived]. Available at https://web.archive.org/web/20190411071840/https://www.surgeongeneral.gov/priorities/prevention/strategy/index.html.

The ROI of Addressing Social Determinants of Health. Available at: https://www.ajmc.com/contributor/ara-ohanian/2018/01/the-roi-of-addressing-social-determinants-of-health

Websites

Healthy People: An Opportunity to Address the Societal Determinants of Health in the United States. Available at http://www.healthypeople.gov/2010/hp2020/advisory/SocietalDeterminantsHealth.htm

Legal Services Corporation. 2017, *The Justice Gap: Measuring the Unmet Civil Needs of Low-Income Americans*. Available at: https://www.lsc.gov/sites/default/files/images/TheJusticeGap-FullReport.pdf

National Partnership for Action: HHS Action Plan to Reduce Racial and Ethnic Health Disparities Available at:. https://minorityhealth.hhs.gov/npa/

United States Department of Health and Human Services Office of Minority Health. Available at: https://www.minorityhealth.hhs.gov

World Health Organization, Commission on Social Determinants of Health. Closing the Gap in a Generation: Health equity through action on the social determinants of health. Available at: http://www.who.int/socialdeterminants/en

References

1. Centers for Disease Control and Prevention. CDC Health Disparities & Inequalities Report (CHDIR) 2013. Available at https://www.cdc.gov/minorityhealth/chdireport.html (accessed September 1, 2018).

2. World Health Organization. Social determinants of health. Available at: http://www.who.int/social_determinants/en/ (accessed September 1, 2018).

3. Healthy People 2020. Social determinants of health. Available at https://www.healthypeople

.gov/2020/topics-objectives/topic/social -determinants-of-health (accessed July 2, 2018).

4. Heiman HJ, Artiga S. Beyond health care: the role of social determinants in promoting health and health equity. 2015. *The Kaiser Commission on Medicaid and the Uninsured,* The Henry J. Kaiser Family Foundation, Washington, DC.

5. World Health Organization, Commission on Social Determinants of Health. Closing the gap in a generation: health equity through action on the social determinants of health. Available at: http://www.who.int/socialdeterminants/en (accessed January 31, 2019).

6. Healthy People. Development of Healthy People 2030: Healthy People 2030 framework. Available at https://www.healthypeople.gov/2020/About -Healthy-People/Development-Healthy -People-2030/Framework (accessed March 19, 2019).

7. World Health Organization. Health Impact Assessment: the determinants of health. Available at https://www.who.int/hia/evidence/doh/en/ (accessed March 19, 2019).

8. Healthy People. Planning for Healthy People 2030. Available at https://www .healthypeople.gov/2020/About-Healthy -People/Development-Healthy-People-2030 (accessed March 19, 2019).

9. National Partnership for Action to End Health Disparities. HHS Action Plan to Reduce Racial and Ethnic Health Disparities (2011); National Stakeholder Strategy for Achieving Health Equity (2011). Available at: https://www.minorityhealth. hhs.gov/npa (accessed November 29, 2018).

10. U.S. Department of Health and Human Services. Surgeon General. The National Prevention Strategy: America's Plan for Better Health and Wellness. 2011 [archived]. Available at https://www .surgeongeneral.gov/priorities/prevention /strategy/index.html(accessed May 16, 2019).

11. World Health Organization. Commission on Social Determinants of Health, Final Report. Closing the gap in a generation: health equity through action on the social determinants of health. 2008. Available at https://www .who.int/social_determinants/thecommission /finalreport/en/ (accessed March 19, 2019).

12. Healthy People 2020. Disparities. Available at https://www.healthypeople.gov/2020/about /foundation-health-measures/Disparities (accessed September 29, 2018).

13. Centers for Disease Control and Prevention. Strategies for reducing health disparities 2016. Available at https://www.cdc.gov /minorityhealth/strategies2016/index.html (accessed September 1, 2018).

14. Braveman P. What are health disparities and health equity? We need to be clear. Nursing in 3D: workforce diversity, health disparities, and social determinants of health. *Public Health Reports.* 2014;suppl 2(129):5–8.

15. Magnan S. Social Determinants of Health 101 for Health Care: Five Plus Five. *NAM Perspectives.* Discussion Paper, 2017. National Academy of Medicine, Washington, DC.

16. Department of Health and Human Services. National Stakeholder Strategy for Achieving Health Equity. Available at https: //minorityhealth.hhs.gov/npa/files/Plans/NSS /CompleteNSS.pdf (accessed March 19, 2019).

17. Robert Wood Johnson Foundation. Could where you live influence how long you live? Available at https://www.rwjf.org/en/library/interactives /where youliveaffectshowlongyoulive.html (accessed March 19, 2019).

18. Greenberg MR. Healthography. *American Journal of Public Health,* 2014;*104*(11):2022.

19. Robert Wood Johnson Foundation Commission to Build a Healthier America. Metro Map: New Orleans, Louisiana. 2013. Available at www.rwjf.org/en/library/infographics/new -orleans-map.html (accessed March 19, 2019).

20. Chokshi DA. Income, poverty, and health inequality. *JAMA.* 2018;319(13):1312–1313.

21. Lynch JW, Kaplan GA, Shema SJ. Cumulative impact of sustained economic hardship on physical, cognitive, psychological, and social functioning. *N Engl J Med.* 1997;337(26):1889–1895.

22. Himmelstein DU, Thorne D, Warren E, et al. Medical bankruptcy in the United States, 2007: results of a national study. *Am J Med.* 2009;122: 741–746.

23. Sullivan TA, Warren E, Westbrook JL. *The Fragile Middle Class: Americans in Debt.* New Haven, CT: Yale University Press; 2000.

24. Truesdale BC, Jencks C. The health effects of income inequality: averages and disparities. The Annual Review of Public Health. 2016. Available at https://www.annualreviews.org/doi/full/10 .1146/annurev-publhealth-032315-021606 (accessed March 20, 2019).

25. Federal Reserve Bank, Corporation for Enterprise Development. What it's worth: strengthening the financial future of families, communities and the nation. 2015. Available at http://www.strongfinancialfuture.org/wp-content/uploads/2015/12/What-its-Worth_Full.pdf (accessed March 20, 2019).

26. Winfield L, DeSalvo K, Muhlestein D. Social Determinants Matter, But Who Is Responsible? Leavitt Partners. 2018 May. Available at https://sirenetwork.ucsf.edu/tools-resources/resources/social-determinants-matter-who-responsible (accessed March 20, 2019).

27. Lax Y, Martinez M, Brown NM. Social determinants of health and hospital readmission. *Pediatrics*. 2017;140(5): e20171427. Available at https://pediatrics.aappublications.org/content/pediatrics/early/2017/10/16/peds.2017-1427.full.pdf (accessed May 16, 2019).

28. Dickman SL, Himmelstein DU, Woolhandler S. Inequality and the health-care system in the USA. *Lancet*. 2017;389(10077):1431–1441.

29. Ohanian A. The ROI of addressing social determinants of health. AJMC Managed Markets Network. January 11, 2018. Available at https://www.ajmc.com/contributor/ara-ohanian/2018/01/theroi-of-addressing-social-determinants-of-health (accessed March 20, 2019).

30. Brennan N. Findings from recent CMS research on Medicare. Centers for Medicare and Medicaid Services; 2012. Available at https://kaiserhealthnews.files.wordpress.com/2014/10/brennan.pdf (accessed March 20, 2019).

31. Jencks SF, Williams MV, Coleman EA. Rehospitalizations among patients in the Medicare fee-for-service program. *N Engl J Med*. 2009;360(14):1418–1428.

32. Mahony D, Jones EJ. Social determinants of health in nursing education, research, and health policy. *Nurs Sci Q*. 2013;26(3):280–284.

33. Moniz C. Social work and the social determinants of health perspective: a good fit. *Health Soc Work*. 2010;35(4):310–313.

34. Browne T, Keefe RH, Ruth BJ, Cox H, Maramaldi P, Rishel C, et al. Advancing social work education for health impact. *Am J Public Health*. 2017;107(S3): S229–S235.

35. Stanhope V, Videka L, Thorning H, McKay M. Moving toward integrated health: an opportunity for social work. *Soc Work Health Care*. 2015;54(5):383–407.

36. Rine CM. Social determinants of health: grand challenges in social work's future. *Health Soc Work*. 2016;41(3):143–145.

37. Murray TA. Outside the hospital walls: the social determinants and population health. *J Nurs Educ*. 2017;56(6): 319–320.

38. Kangovi S, Grande D. Hospital readmissions–not just a measure of quality. *JAMA*. 2011;306(16): 1796–1797.

39. Truchil A, Dravid N, Singer S, Martinez Z, Kuruna T, Waulters S. Lessons from the Camden Coalition of Healthcare Providers' first Medicaid shared savings performance evaluation. *Popul Health Manag*. 2018;21(4):278–284.

40. Grabowski F. Camden Coalition of Healthcare Providers: A Community Model. *AADE in Pract*. 2013;1(1):18–24.

41. Mautner D, Pang H, Brenner J, Shea J, Gross K, Frasso R, Cannuscio C. Generating hypotheses about care needs of high utilizers: lessons from patient interviews. *Popul Health Manag*. 2013;16(1):S26–S33.

42. Vaida B. For super-utilizers, integrated care offers a new path. *Health Aff*. 2017;36(3):394–397.

43. Camden Coalition of Healthcare Providers. About the Camden Coalition. Camden, NJ: Author. Available at https://www.camdenhealth.org/about-camden-coalition/

44. Bodenheimer T. Strategies to reduce costs and improve care for high-utilizing Medicaid patients: reflections on pioneering programs. San Francisco, CA: Center for Health Care Strategies, Inc.; 2013. Available at http://www.chcs.org/media/HighUtilizerReport_102413_Final3.pdf (accessed March 20, 2019).

45. Hu J, Wang F, Sun J, Sorrentino R, Ebadollahi S. A healthcare utilization analysis framework for hot spotting and contextual anomaly detection. *AMIA Annu Symp Proc*. 2012;2012:360–369.

46. Grover CA, Crawford E, Close RJH. The efficacy of case management on emergency department frequent users: an eight-year observational study. *J Emerg Med*. 2016;51(5):595–604.

47. Centers for Medicare and Medicaid Services. Accountable Health Communities Model. Available at https://innovation.cms.gov/initiatives/ahcm/ (accessed May 16, 2019).

48. National Academy of Medicine (formerly the Institute of Medicine). Recommended social and behavioral domains and measures for

electronic health. Washington, DC: National Academies Press; 2014. Available at http://nationalacademies.org/HMD/Activities/PublicHealth/SocialDeterminantsEHR.aspx.

49. National Academy of Medicine (formerly the Institute of Medicine), Committee on the Recommended Social Behavioral Domains and Measures for Electronic Health Records. *Capturing Social and Behavioral Domains and Measures in Electronic Health Records, PHASE 2.* Washington, DC: National Academies Press; 2014.

50. Gold R, Bunce A, Cowburn S, Dambrun K, Dearing M, Middendorf M, et al. Adoption of social determinants of health EHR tools by community health centers. *Ann Fam Med.* 2018;16(5):399–407.

51. National Association of Community Health Centers, Inc., Association of Asian Pacific Community Health Organizations, Oregon Primary Care Association. PRAPARE. Bethesda, MD: National Association of Community Health Centers; 2016. Available at http://www.nachc.org/research-and-data/prapare (accessed March 20, 2019).

52. LaForge K, Gold R, Cottrell E, et al. How 6 organizations developed tools and processes for social determinants of health screening in primary care: an overview. *J Ambul Care Manag.* 2017;41(1):2–14.

53. Langston C, Undem T, Dorr D. (2014). Transforming primary care: what Medicare beneficiaries want and need from Patient-Centered Medical Homes to improve health and lower costs. Washington, DC: The John A. Hartford Foundation.

54. Chu LM, Tu YL, Sayles JN, Sood N. The impact of patient-centered medical homes on safety net clinics. *Am J Manag Care.* 2016;22(8):532–538.

55. Friedberg MW, Rosenthal MB, Werner RM, Volpp KG, Schneider EC. Effects of a medical home and shared savings intervention on quality and utilization of care. *JAMA Intern Med.* 2015;175(8):1362–1368. Available at http://archinte.jamanetwork.com/article.aspx?articleid=2296117 (accessed March 25, 2019).

56. Jackson CS, Garcia JN. Addressing health and healthcare disparities: the role of a diverse workforce and the social determinants of health. *Public Health Rep.* 2014;129(Suppl 2):57–61.

57. van Ryn M, Burgess DJ, Dovidio JF, Phelan SM, Saha S, Malat J, et al. The impact of racism on clinician cognition, behavior, and clinical decision making. *DuBois Rev.* 2011;8(1):199–218.

58. National Academies of Sciences, Engineering, and Medicine. Communities in Action: Pathways to Health Equity. Washington, DC: The National Academies Press; 2017. Available at https://doi.org/10.17226/24624.

59. Agency for Healthcare Research and Quality. 2015 National Healthcare Quality and Disparities Report and 5th Anniversary Update on the National Quality Strategy. Rockville, MD: Author; 2016. AHRQ Pub. No. 16-0015. Available at https://www.ahrq.gov/research/findings/nhqrdr/nhqdr15/index.html (accessed March 25, 2019).

60. Smedley BD, Stith AY, Nelson AR (eds.). National Academy of Medicine (formerly the Institute of Medicine) (US) Committee on Understanding and Eliminating Racial and Ethnic Disparities in Health Care. *Unequal Treatment: Confronting Racial and Ethnic Disparities in Health Care.* Washington (DC): National Academies Press (US); 2003.

61. Williams DR, Wyatt R. Racial bias in health care and health: challenges and opportunities. *JAMA.* 2015 Aug 11;314(6):555–556.

62. Feagin J, Zinobia B. Systemic racism and US health care. *Soc Sci Med.* 2014;103:7.

63. Lhachimi SK, Bala MM, Vanagas G. Evidence based public health. *Biomed Res Int.* 2016;2016:1.

64. Paradies Y, Ben J, Denson N, Truong M, Gupta A, Pieterse A, et al. Racism as a determinant of health: a systematic review and metaanalysis. *PLoS One.* 2015;10(9):e0138511.

65. Mensah GA, Mokdad AH, Ford ES, Greenlund KJ, Croft JB. State of disparities in cardiovascular health in the United States. *Circulation* 2005;111:1233–1241.

66. Jemal A, Ward EM, Johnson CJ, Cronin KA, Ma J, Ryerson B, et al. Annual report to the nation on the status of cancer, 1975–2014, featuring survival. *J Natl Cancer Inst.* 2017;109(9). doi: 10.1093/jnci/djx030.

67. Cunningham TJ, Croft JB, Liu Y, Lu H, Eke PI, Giles WH. Vital signs: racial disparities in age-specific mortality among blacks or African Americans — United States, 1999–2015. *MMWR Morb Mortal Wkly Rep.* 2017;66:444–456.

68. Baily ZD, Krieger N, Agenor M, Graves J, Linos N, Bassett MT. Structural racism and health inequities in the USA: evidence and interventions. *Lancet*. 2017;389(10077):1453–1463.

69. Robinson W, Finegold K. The Affordable Care Act and African Americans. U.S. Department of Health and Human Services. 2012. Available at https://aspe.hhs.gov/report/affordable-car-act-and-african-americans (accessed March 25, 2019).

70. Colby SL, Ortman JM. Projections of the size and composition of the U.S. population: 2014 to 2060. Washington, DC: US Department of Commerce, Economics and Statistics and Administration, Bureau of the Census; 2014.

71. National Center for Health Statistics. Health, United States 2015: with special feature on racial and ethnic disparities. Hyattsville, MD: U.S. Department of Health and Human Services, CDC, National Center for Health Statistics, 2015.

72. Geronimus AT, Hicken M, Keene D, Bound J. Weathering and age patterns of allostatic load scores among blacks and whites in the United States. *Am J Public Health*. 2006;96(5):826–833.

73. Artiga S, Foutz J, Cornachione, Garfield R. Key facts on health and health care by race and ethnicity. Menlo Park, CA: Kaiser Family Foundation; 2016. Available at http://files.kff.org/attachment/Chartpack-Key-Facts-on-Health-and-Health-Care-by-Race-and-Ethnicity (accessed March 25, 2019).

74. Choi K, Martinson M. The relationship between low birthweight and childhood health: disparities by race, ethnicity, and national origin. *Ann Epidemiol*. 2018;28(10):704–709.

75. National Academy of Medicine (formerly the Institute of Medicine). Unequal treatment: confronting racial and ethnic disparities in health care. Washington, DC: The National Academies Press; 2003.

76. Shavers VL, Fagan P, Jones D, Klein WM, Boyington J, Moten C, Rorie E. The state of research on racial/ethnic discrimination in the receipt of health care. *Am J Public Health*. 2012;102:953–966.

77. Flores G. Racial and ethnic disparities in the health and health care of children. *Pediatrics*. 2010;125:e979–1020.

78. Blair IV, Havranek EP, Price DW, Hanratty R, Fairclough DL, Farley T, et al. Assessment of biases against Latinos and African Americans among primary care providers and community members. *Am J Public Health*. 2013;103:92–98.

79. Puumala SE, Burgess KM, Kharbanda AB, Zook HG, Castille DM, Pickner WJ, Payne NR. The role of bias by emergency department providers in care for American Indian children. *Med Care*. 2016;54:562–569.

80. Doescher MP, Saver BG, Franks P, Fiscella K. Racial and ethnic disparities in perceptions of physician style and trust. *Arch Fam Med*. 2000;9(10):1156–1163.

81. Hoffman KM, Trawalter S, Axt JR, Oliver MN. Racial bias in pain assessment and treatment recommendations, and false beliefs about biological differences between blacks and whites. *Proc Natl Acad Sci USA*. 2016;113(16):4296–4301.

82. Agency for Healthcare Research and Quality. National Healthcare Disparities Report, 2006 [archived]. Available at https://archive.ahrq.gov/qual/nhdr06/nhdr06.htm (accessed November 26, 2018).

83. Corbie-Smith G, Thomas SB, St George DMM. Distrust, race, and research. *Arch Intern Med*. 2002;162(21):2458–2463.

84. Reverby SM. Ethical failures and history lessons: The U.S. Public Health Service research studies in Tuskegee and Guatemala. *Public Health Rev*. 2012;34(1):13. doi:10.1007/BF03391665. Available at https://publichealthreviews.biomedcentral.com/track/pdf/10.1007/BF03391665 (accessed May 17, 2019).

85. Hoffman K, Trawalter S, Axt J, Oliver M. Racial bias in pain assessment and treatment recommendations, and false beliefs about biological differences between blacks and whites. *Proc Natl Acad Sci USA*. 2016;16:4296–4301.

86. Stone VE. Optimizing the care of minority patients with HIV/AIDS. *Clin Infect Dis*. 2004 Feb 1;38(3):400–404.

87. Anderson KO, Green CR, Payne R. Racial and ethnic disparities in pain: causes and consequences of unequal care. *J Pain*. 2009;10(12):1187–1204.

88. Bonham VL. Race, ethnicity, and pain treatment: striving to understand the causes and solutions to the disparities in pain treatment. *J Law Med Ethics*. 2001;29(1):52–68.

89. Morrison CA. Pain and ethnicity in the United States: a systematic review. *J Palliat Med*. 2006;9(6):1454–1473.

90. Cleeland CS, Gonin R, Baez L, Loehrer P, Pandya KJ. Pain and treatment of pain in minority patients with cancer. *Ann Intern Med.* 1997;127(9):813–816. Available at https://annals.org/aim/fullarticle/710937/pain-treatment-pain-minority-patients-cancer-eastern-cooperative-oncology-group (accessed March 25, 2019).

91. Todd KH, Deaton C, D'Adamo AP, Goe L. Ethnicity and analgesic practice. *Ann Emerg Med.* 2000;35(1):11–16.

92. Krieger N, Sidney S. Racial discrimination and blood pressure: the CARDIA Study of young black and white adults. *Am J Public Health.* 1996;86(10):1370–1378.

93. LaVeist TA, Nickerson KJ, Bowie JV. Attitudes about racism, medical mistrust, and satisfaction with care among African American and white cardiac patients. *Med Care Res Rev.* 2000;57 Suppl 1:146–161.

94. Thomas SB, Quinn SC. The Tuskegee Syphilis Study, 1932 to 1972: implications for HIV education and AIDS risk education programs in the black community. *Am J Public Health.* 1991;81(11):1498–1505.

95. Todd KH, Deaton C, D'Adamo AP, Goe L. Ethnicity and analgesic practice. *Ann Emerg Med.* 2000;35(1):11–16.

96. Doty MM, Gunja MZ, Collins SR, Beutel S. Coverage gains among lower-income Blacks and Latinos highlight ACA's successes and areas for improvement, *To the Point,* The Commonwealth Fund, Aug. 15, 2017. Available at https://www.commonwealthfund.org/blog/2017/coverage-gains-among-lower-income-blacks-and-latinos-highlight-acas-successes-and-areas?redirect_source=/~/media/6cc83971f17c48189e1d9e51f00e0446.ashx (accessed May 17, 2019).

97. Doty MM, Gunja MZ, Collins SR, Beutel S. Latinos and Blacks have made major gains under the Affordable Care Act, but inequalities remain. *To the Point,* The Commonwealth Fund, Aug. 18, 2016. Available at https://www.commonwealthfund.org/blog/2016/latinos-and-blacks-have-made-major-gains-under-affordable-care-act-inequalities-remain?redirect_source=/~/media/acde1f17ebd245bc9389675555a6fa1f.ashx (accessed May 17, 2019).

98. Agency for Healthcare Research and Quality. Access and disparities in access to health care. In 2015 National Healthcare Quality and Disparities Report and 5th Anniversary Update on the National Quality Strategy. Rockville, MD: Author. Available at https://www.ahrq.gov/research/findings/nhqrdr/nhqdr15/access.html (accessed March 25, 2019).

99. Gant L, Green W, Stewart P, Wheeler D, Wright E. HIV/AIDS and African Americans: assumptions, myths, and realities. Social workers speak out on the HIV/AIDS crisis: voices from and to African-American communities. Pp 1-12. Praeger Publishers, Inc., Westport, CT; 1999.

100. National Academy of Medicine (formerly the Institute of Medicine) (US) Roundtable on Health Disparities. Challenges and successes in reducing health disparities: workshop summary. Washington (DC): National Academies Press (US); 2008.

101. Cooper LA, Roter DL, Carson KA, Beach MC, Sabin JA, Greenwald AG, Inui TS. The associations of clinicians' implicit attitudes about race with medical visit communication and patient ratings of interpersonal care. *Am J Public Health.* 2012;102(5):979–987.

102. Martin KD, Cooper LA. Maximizing the benefits of "we" in race-discordant patient-physician relationships: novel insights raise intriguing questions. *J Gen Intern Med.* 2013;28(9):1119–1121.

103. Bouye KE, McCleary KJ, Williams KB. Increasing diversity in the health professions: reflections on student pipeline programs. *J Healthc Sci Humanit.* 2016;6(1):67–79.

104. Office of the Assistant Secretary for Health (OASH). HHS action plan to reduce racial & ethnic health disparities: a nation free of disparities in health and health care. Washington, DC: Office of the Assistant Secretary for Health; 2011.

105. Williams SD, Hansen K, Smithey M, Burnley J, Koplitz M, Koyajma K, Bakos A. Using social determinants of health to link health workforce diversity, care quality and access, and health disparities to achieve health equity in nursing. *Public Health Rep.* 2014;129(Suppl 2):32–36.

106. New Mexico Department of Public Health 2018. Addressing the Health Needs of Sex and

Gender Minorities in New Mexico [June; 2018]; Available at https://nmhealth.org/publication/view/report/4514.

107. Okoro CA, Hollis ND, Cyrus AC, Griffin-Blake S. Prevalence of disabilities and health care access by disability status and type among adults — United States, 2016. *MMWR Morb Mortal Wkly Rep.* 2018;67:882–887.

108. Centers for Disease Control and Prevention. Disability and access to health care. Available at https://www.cdc.gov/features/disabilities-health-care-access/index.html (accessed March 25, 2019).

109. Angus J, Seto L, Barry N, Cechetto N, Chandani S, Devaney J, et al. Access to cancer screening for women with mobility disabilities. *J Cancer Educ.* 2012;27(1):75–82.

110. Hafeez H, Zeshan M, Tahir MA, Jahan N, Naveed S. Health care disparities among lesbian, gay, bisexual, and transgender youth: a literature review. *Cureus.* 2017;9(4):e1184.

111. van Ryn M, Burke J. The effect of patient race and socio-economic status on physicians' perceptions of patients. *Soc Sci Med.* 2000;50(6):813–828.

112. Kamen C, Vorasarun C, Canning T, Kienitz E, Weiss C, Flores S, et al. The impact of stigma and social support on development of post-traumatic growth among persons living with HIV. *J Clin Psychol Med Settings.* 2016;23(2):126–134.

113. Hatzenbuehler ML, Phelan JC, Link BG. Stigma as a fundamental cause of population health inequalities. *Am J Public Health.* 2013;103(5):813–821.

114. Link BG, Phelan JC. Conceptualizing stigma. *Annu Rev Sociol.* 2001;27(1):363–385.

115. Phelan JC, Link BG, Dovidio JF. Stigma and prejudice: one animal or two? *Soc Sci Med.* 2008;67(3):358–367.

116. Centers for Disease Control and Prevention. National Prevention Information Network. Cultural competence. Available at https://npin.cdc.gov/pages/cultural-competence (accessed March 25, 2019).

117. Cross T, Bazron B, Dennis K, Isaacs M. *Towards a Culturally Competent System of Care*, Volume I. Washington, DC: Georgetown University Child Development Center; 1989.

118. Knibb-Lamouche J. *Leveraging Culture to Address Health Inequalities.* Washington, DC:

National Academies Press; 2012. Available at https://www.ncbi.nlm.nih.gov/books/NBK201298/ (accessed February 10, 2019).

119. Campinha-Bacote J. The proces of cultural competence in the delivery of healthcare services: a model of care. *J Transcult Nurs.* 2002;13(3):181–184.

120. Tervalon M, Murray-Garcia J. Cultural humility versus cultural competence: a critical distinction in defining physician training outcomes in multicultural education. *J Health Care Poor Underserved.* 1998;9(2):117–125, 118.

121. Kumas-Tan Z, Beagan B, Loppie C, MacLeod A, Frank B. Measures of cultural competence: examining hidden assumptions. *Acad Med.* 2007;82(6):548–557.

122. The Joint Commission with Assistance from the Health Determinants & Disparities Practice at SRA International. A Crosswalk of the National Standards for Culturally and Linguistically Appropriate Services (CLAS) in Health and Health Care to the Joint Commission Hospital Accreditation Standards. July 2014. Available at https://www.jointcommission.org/assets/1/6/Crosswalk-_CLAS_-20140718.pdf (accessed May 16, 2019).

123. U.S. Department of Health and Human Services Office of Minority Health. Think cultural health: the National Standards for Culturally and Linguistically Appropriate Services (CLAS) in Health and Health Care. Available at https://www.thinkculturalhealth.hhs.gov (accessed March 25, 2019).

124. Brega AG, Barnard J, Mabachi NM, Weiss BD, DeWalt DA, Brach C, Cifuentes M, Albright K, West DK. AHRQ Health Literacy Precautions Toolkit. 2nd Edition. Agency for Healthcare Research and Quality Pub. No. 15-0023-EF. Rockville, MD: AHRQ; 2015.

125. Neilsen-Bohlman L, Panzer AM, Kindig DA, National Academy of Medicine (formerly the Institute of Medicine) (U.S.) Committee on Health Literacy. *Health Literacy: A Prescription to End Confusion.* Washington, DC: National Academies Press; 2004.

126. Rikard RV, Thompson MI, McKinney L, Beauchamp A. Examining health literacy disparities in the United States: a third look at the National Assessment of Adult Literacy. *BMC Public Health.* 2016;16:975.

127. Adsul P, Wray R, Gautuam, Jupka K, Weaver N, Wilson K. Becoming a health literate organization: formative research results from healthcare organizations providing care for underserved communities. *Health Serv Manag.* 2017;30(4):188–196.

128. Hudak PL, Wright JG. The characteristics of patient satisfaction measures. *Spine.* 2000;25(24):3167–3177.

129. Brach C, Keller D, Hernandez LM, Baur C, Parker R, Dreyer B, et al. Ten attributes of health literate health care organizations. IOM Roundtable on Health Literacy, discussion paper. 2012. Available at http://nam.edu /wp-content/uploads/2015/06/BPH_Ten _HLit_Attributes.pdf (accessed March 27, 2019).

130. Agency for Healthcare Research and Quality. AHRQ Healthcare Literacy Universal Precautions Toolkit, 2nd ed. Available at https:// www.ahrq.gov/professionals/qualitypatient -safety/quality-resources/tools/literacy-toolkit /index.html (accessed March 27, 2019).

131. Dao DK, Goss AL, Hoekzema AS, Kelly LA, Logan AA, Mehta SD, et al. Integrating theory, content, and method to foster critical consciousness in medical students: a comprehensive model for cultural competence training. *Acad Med.* 2017;92:335–344.

132. U.S. Congress. Patient Protection and Affordable Care Act. 42 U.S.C. § 18001 (2010). Available at https://www.congress.gov/111/plaws/publ148 /PLAW-111publ148.pdf (accessed March 27, 2019).

133. The Joint Commission. Standards interpretation. Available at https://www .jointcommission.org/standards_information /jcfaq.aspx (accessed March 27, 2019).

134. Babiker A, El Husseini M, Al Nemri A, Al Frayh A, Al Juryyan N, Faki MO, et al. Health care professional development: working as a team to improve patient care. *Sudan J Paediatr.* 2014;14(2):9–16.

135. Schottenfeld L, Petersen D, Peikes D, Ricciardi R, Burak H, McNellis R, et al. Creating patient-centered team-based primary care. AHRQ pub. no. 16-0002-EF. Rockville, MD: Agency for Healthcare Research and Quality; March 2016.

136. World Health Organization. HEARTS Technical package for cardiovascular disease management in primary health care: team-based care. Geneva: World Health Organization; 2018 (WHO/NMH / NVI/18.4). Licence: CC BY-NC-SA 3.0 IGO. Available at https://www.who.int /cardiovascular_diseases/hearts/Hearts _package.pdf (accessed May 17, 2019).

137. Sun R, Marshall DC, Sykes MC, Maruthappu M, Shalhoub J. The impact of improving teamwork on patient outcomes in surgery: a systematic review. *Int J Surg.* 2018;53:171–177.

138. Proia KK, Thota AB, Njie GJ, Finnie RKC, Hopkins DP, Mukhtar Q, et al. Team-based care and improved blood pressure control: a Community Guide systematic review. *Am J Prev Med.* 2014;47(1):86–99.

139. Miller CJ, Kim B, Silverman A, Bauer MS. A systematic review of team-building interventions in non-acute healthcare settings. *BMC Health Services Research* 2018;18:146. Available at https://doi.org/10.1186/s12913 -018-2961-9 (accessed March 27, 2019).

140. U.S. Department of Health and Human Services. Community Health Worker National Workforce Study. 2007. Available at https://bhw.hrsa.gov/sites/default/files/bhw /nchwa/projections/communityhealth workforcebibliography.pdf (accessed March 27, 2019).

141. Damio G, Ferraro M, London K, Pérez-Escamilla R, Wiggins N. Addressing Social Determinants of Health through Community Health Workers: A Call to Action, Hispanic Health Council Policy Brief, Hartford CT; 2017. Available at https://www. cthealth.org /wp-content/uploads/2018/01/HHC-CHW -SDOH-Policy-Briefi-1.30.18.pdf (accessed March 27, 2019).

142. U.S. Department of Health and Human Services, Centers for Medicare & Medicaid Services. (2017, September 05). Accountable Health Communities Model. Available at https://innovation.cms.gov/initiatives /ahcm.

143. Billioux A, Verlander K, Anthony S, Alley D. Standardized Screening for Health-Related Social Needs in Clinical Settings: The Accountable Health Communities Screening Tool. National Academy of Medicine. 2017. Available at https://nam.edu/wp-content /uploads/2017/05/Standardized-Screening

-for-Health-Related-Social-Needs-in -Clinical-Settings.pdf (accessed March 27, 2019).

144. Tobin-Tyler E, Teitelbaum JB. Medical-legal partnership: a powerful tool for public health and health justice. *Public Health Rep.* 2019 Mar/Apr;134(2):201-205. doi: 10.1177/0033354918824328.

145. Murphy JS, Lawton EM, Sandel M. Legal care as part of health care: the benefits of medical-legal partnership. *Pediatr Clin North Am.* 2015;62(5):1263–1271.

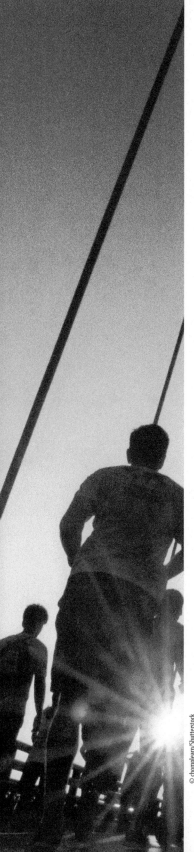

© chomplearn/Shutterstock

PART II

The Population Health Ecosystem

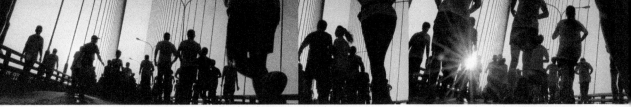

CHAPTER 4

Structure, Systems, and Stakeholders

Justin Beaupre
Myles Dworkin
Alexis Skoufalos
Willie H. Oglesby

EXECUTIVE SUMMARY

Population health is heavily influenced by the unique structure, systems, and stakeholders of the U.S. healthcare system and the way in which they interact. Health is not just a function of new technologies and therapies to treat and prevent disease, but also of how the system reaches sub-populations, whether each sub-group receives the same benefits, different outcomes that emerge for these groups when given the same treatment, and the degree to which the system itself is functioning efficiently and effectively. In this chapter, we will review the main components of the U.S. healthcare system, with particular emphasis on the history, key stakeholders, and how they interrelate.

When we refer to the structure of the U.S. healthcare system, it is in the context of the elements that are in place to support the delivery of clinical care. Among these elements are clinical service providers, the delivery networks and personnel that support the provision of care, the various settings in which care is delivered, and the technologies that facilitate care delivery. The numbers and types of clinical care providers and support personnel are increasing to support new therapeutic developments and advances in technology that improve patient access to quality care. Government at all levels (federal, state, and local) plays a significant role in establishing procedures for payment, regulation, and policy.

The term *systems* refers to the relationships between these structural elements of the healthcare delivery framework. Providers, for example, may interact with patients, vendors, regulatory agencies, and various technologies across multiple care settings and be supported by various types of healthcare professionals. Whether in the community, hospitals, clinics, or patients' homes, there is a complex network of relationships that directly and indirectly influence how care is provided. Employers and businesses, which bear a large portion of the cost burden of health care, have a major role and a significant stake in population health. Four of the primary factors that define and influence the delivery of health care include payment, insurance, financing, and regulation.

Arguably the most important stakeholders are those whom the system exists to serve: the population of the United States. It is critical to understand how the size, region, demographics, culture, and philosophies of a particular population offer insight into its unique needs and expectations, as well as the nature of its interaction with the healthcare system. These population characteristics, in the context of the healthcare structure and system, serve to illustrate the current population health dynamics and provide opportunities to improve population health.

LEARNING OBJECTIVES

1. Describe the structure, systems, and stakeholders of the U.S. healthcare system.
2. Describe relationships between the structural components of the U.S. healthcare system.
3. Identify stakeholders in the U.S. healthcare system and how they influence the nature of the system.
4. Describe how the nature of the U.S. healthcare system influences population health.

KEY TERMS

Accountable care organizations (ACOs)
Delivery
Financing
Federally Qualified Health Center (FQHC)
Health insurance exchange

Health and Human Services (HHS)
Insurance
Medicaid
Medicare
Patient Protection and Affordable Care Act (ACA)

Payment
Stakeholders
Structure
Systems
Telemedicine

▶ Introduction

The U.S. healthcare system is a complex **delivery** system that has undergone significant changes in recent years. Throughout its history, there have been many attempts at reform that include aspects such as how patients access care, quality of care, insurance, and the government's role. While many of these attempts at reform failed, several significant events have redefined the American healthcare system over the past two centuries. The history of the U.S. healthcare system can be divided into three time periods: the Preindustrial Era, the Industrial Era, and the Corporate Era.[1]

The Preindustrial Era (Mid-18th to Late 19th Century)

Although the first American hospital opened in 1751, widespread development of formalized hospital **systems** did not occur until the 1880s.[2] There has been a long history of government engagement with the healthcare system. The first attempt at federal government involvement occurred following the Civil War, when the first system of national medical care was created in the South with the construction of 40 hospitals staffed by 120 physicians.[3] The poor and severely ill received care from government-run almshouses, or poorhouses, which were public welfare agencies that functioned primarily as shelters with infirmaries for the sick.[4] In the 1800s, medicine was practiced similarly to other trades of the time—that is, with little in the way of overarching professional standards.[5] Training was typically performed through apprenticeships rather than formal university education. The shift toward a standardized system of clinical training occurred over the next century, as more medical schools opened and the number of formally educated physicians grew to outnumber those trained in the apprenticeship system.[6]

As a result of the disorganization and a lack of institutional centers, most Americans in the 1800s relied on professionals other than physicians to provide care.[7] Health care was an unregulated free-market economy with a fee-for-service **payment** system. As such, consumer sovereignty dictated demand. Communities frequently turned to traditional home remedies and so-called healers, as opposed to medical doctors, in large part due to lack of access and high costs.[1] Demand for healthcare services remained low until the formalization of education led to an increase in trained physicians, which in turn legitimized the medical field; cost structures then began to change from a fee-for-service model to insurance-based payments. The quality of training began to improve with the formation of the American Medical Association (AMA) in 1847 and the implementation of licensing laws and education reforms in the 1870s. The education system went through additional changes in 1876 with the formation of the

Association of American Medical Colleges, which helped monitor medical education programs. These collective efforts to enhance education and require licensing further legitimized the field of medicine.[8]

One of the earliest healthcare reforms during this time period was the 1854 Bill for the Benefit of the Indigent Insane. It was vetoed by the 14th president, Franklin Pierce, who argued that the government should not be involved in or commit itself to social welfare.[3] As the nation approached the 1900s, health-care access and affordability would greatly change in America with advances in the medical field. Starting in the 1890s, this would largely be orchestrated by hospitals.[1] Although there were only a few dozen hospitals in 1875, the number would grow to over 4,000 by the early 1900s.[9]

The Industrial Era (Late 19th to Late 20th Century)

From 1880 to 1930, the medical profession in the United States experienced a cultural and economic growth that dramatically changed the way that physicians practiced. Earlier, physicians competed not only against each other but also against other alternative healers in an unregulated medical marketplace. However, as the field progressed in the late 1800s and into the 1900s, the reorganization of commercial medical schools began to produce numerous graduates with greater knowledge and skills than in previous decades. By the end of the 1800s, hospitals were shifting from care centers for the poor to centers of scientific inquiry. As the culture of medicine changed to focus more on laboratory science and medical discovery, there was a call for stricter state regulations involving physicians and hospitals. The healthcare economy grew with the construction of more hospitals and an increased number of physicians, and gradually led to a change in the way in which people accessed and thought about health care. By the 1930s, health care was one of the largest industries in the United States, with Americans spending nearly $3.5 billion on medical services, despite the Great Depression.[10]

The first attempt to create a national health insurance model similar to what was available in many European countries began in the early 1900s. Theodore Roosevelt introduced the first draft of a plan for universal health care during his presidency (1901 to 1909); however, attempts to pass a bill were unsuccessful because of a fear of the rise of socialism resulting from too much government control. From 1916 to 1918, 16 state legislatures attempted to create legislation that would require employers to provide health insurance; these attempts also failed.[11] Funding for healthcare programs was authorized by Congress in 1933 as part of President Franklin D. Roosevelt's landmark Social Security legislation, but it stopped short of universal health care.[3]

Changes to Social Security and public funding for health care led to the emergence of private insurance companies. In 1929, Justin F. Kimball, vice president of Baylor Health, began one of the first hospital insurance plans for teachers in Texas. The model of allowing a patient to pay a small fee per month to cover the cost of a 21-day hospital stay created the blueprint for companies like Blue Cross.[12] This model expanded over the course of the next several years from single-hospital insurance plans to larger group-sponsored hospital plans. This development created the first opportunity for consumer choice in health care and became widely supported by the American Hospital Association. By 1946, Blue Cross had been extended to 43 states, serving nearly 20 million people.[11] As this model grew in popularity, commercial (for-profit) insurance began to grow, resulting in over 700 different companies selling insurance by the 1950s.

Employer-sponsored health insurance became more popular around the time of World War II, largely in response to wage freezes during the war. Many employers offered health insurance to compensate their employees for lost wages. Moving into the 1950s, the federal government and U.S. Supreme Court ruled that employee benefits were part of a union-management negotiation, and therefore, health insurance became part of collective bargaining agreements between unions and employers. In 1954, employer-paid health insurance became non-taxable under the new Internal Revenue Code. This had a significant economic value because it was equivalent to getting an increase in salary without having to pay taxes on it.[11] As more Americans gained health insurance coverage through their employers, the debate around the need for a national health insurance model resurfaced, especially as a means to provide access to health care for the elderly and the poor. The American Medical Association lobbied against national health insurance out of concern for the impact on private practice physicians, private hospitals, and healthcare delivery. As a result of this resistance, in 1965, the federal government made legislative amendments to the Social Security Act that created **Medicare** and **Medicaid**. Through intense debate and grass roots-level organizing, a system emerged that consisted of a three-part program that included hospital and nursing home coverage for the elderly and insurance for the impoverished.[9] Medicare, funded by a Social Security tax, was widely accepted by the public. Medicaid, on the other hand, was stigmatized as public welfare and faced some opposition from providers. Medicare had strict universal standards for care and payment. Medicaid was controlled by the states and therefore varied widely in terms of cost, access, and coverage.[11] In 1970, Richard Nixon attempted to introduce a plan to create a national health insurance program, but the effort failed. Health insurance would continue to be debated over the next several decades, which resulted in many significant changes in access to care, quality, costs and payment for care, and innovation.

The Corporate Era (Late 20th Century to the 21st Century)

The advances of the 20th century added a number of new aspects to the U.S. healthcare system. These new participants and players required novel approaches in organization and management that would help to monitor the quality and cost of care. The first of these new strategies was proposed by the Nixon Administration through the Health Maintenance Organization Act of 1973.[13] The object of this initiative was to encourage employers to offer prepaid medical plans that would be less expensive than traditional fee-for-service practices.[1] Soon, other care network management approaches were developed, such as Preferred Provider Organizations (PPOs) and Exclusive Provider Organizations (EPOs). In 1973, Medicare was expanded to cover nonelderly disabled people who had been receiving Social Security for the previous 24 months and provided coverage

to individuals with end-stage renal disease who needed dialysis or a kidney transplant.[11]

The Advent of Managed Care

By the late 1980s, the United States had nearly 44 million uninsured Americans and was experiencing an epidemic of HIV/ AIDS. The cost of health care rose significantly above the rate of inflation, which led to the first national rise in health insurance premiums among employer-sponsored health plans. In 1983, legislation was passed to control Medicaid spending as the cost of services rose. The federal government would follow similar guidelines used under Medicare by paying a set fee based on 467 diagnosis-related groups (DRGs).[14] Another attempt to control healthcare costs during this time was the creation of the Health Maintenance Organization (HMO), an organized **structure** of groups of providers and networks from which patients would receive their care. This model of managed care led to many health systems becoming more integrated in order to offer a variety of health services from different providers within one geographic location. Integrated healthcare systems allowed patients to use any physician within the hospital system's network without having to worry whether their care would be covered by their insurance. This model gave rise to a variety of integrated health networks including Kaiser Permanente and Geisinger Health System.

Despite the growing number of integrated health systems and health alliances, healthcare spending was still rising rapidly. President Clinton developed legislation in 1993 focused on major health reform, lowering costs, and providing access to care for all Americans. The Clinton administration's health plan had a "bedrock assumption that all Americans must be guaranteed health coverage that, in President Clinton's words, can never be taken away."[15] President Clinton believed that coverage for all would produce better health and well-being for all of society and could do so more efficiently than any past or present system.

President Clinton's reform plan was focused on five principles; savings, choice, quality, simplicity, and responsibility.[15] The Health Security Act maintained the rule that Americans, not the government or their employer, should have a right to choose where they receive their health care. Individuals would also be able to choose their "price point" for coverage, their own providers, and their own insurance package. Because there were existing state and federal health programs, the reform plan focused on developing national rules that would create consistency across state lines with respect to **financing**, establishing comprehensive benefits packages, insurance reform rules, guidelines for which employers could operate their own systems, and rules regarding controls on healthcare costs.[15]

Additionally, states were given leeway to choose alternative delivery models, define alliances and structures for health plans, and create long-term benefit care arrangements. The Health Security Act had a strong emphasis on preventative care in the comprehensive package of benefits and would create two new benefits designed to fill gaps in Medicare prescription drug coverage and long-term care in order to provide for home and community-based care instead of nursing home care for those with severe disabilities. No American could be denied coverage for preexisting conditions; there would be

no waiting periods to get insurance; and Americans working for larger companies would receive their health insurance from health alliances that would require employers to pay 80% of the average premium costs. Smaller companies and public employees and dependents would contribute 80% of the weighted average premium in a regional alliance for each employee. Individuals and families would pay the difference between the 80% of the average premium and the cost of the plan they chose.[15] The health alliances and reform would replace competition between health plans based on risk with competition based on quality; it would equitably spread risk by moving to a community rating system, maximize consumer choice, consolidate purchasing power, simplify choices for consumers, increase consumer cost-consciousness, reduce administrative costs, enhance insurance portability for consumers, and eliminate coverage restrictions.[15] Funding for this program would have come from employers and families, as well as from government sources. Savings earned from Medicaid and Medicare, new government revenues, and an increased tax on tobacco were to provide the appropriate funding for the healthcare reform plan. However, the plan did not pass because many felt there was too much government involvement and it would eventually lead to a single-payer system. Others felt that their health would not be improved under the Clinton plan and that the cost savings would be neither attainable nor sustainable. Nearly 63% of Americans disapproved of managed care plans or HMOs, and many felt that the corporate health alliances that would be created would be similar to those of HMOs. By the end of 1994, President Clinton had lost nearly all support for the health reform plan.

By the year 2000, health care spending was rapidly increasing. The Centers for Medicare and Medicaid Services (CMS) was formed, and Medicare implemented DRG or "bundled" payments for services to control costs and spending. By the mid 2000s, CMS was beginning to restructure the payment model to focus on value-based care. Value-based programs reward healthcare providers with incentive payments for the quality of care they give to Medicare beneficiaries. These programs are part of a larger quality strategy to reform how health care is delivered and paid for. Value-based programs also support the Triple Aim: better care for individuals, better health for populations, and lower costs.[16]

Recognizing the need to insure more Americans, reduce excessive spending, and curb the rising costs of medical expenditures, the federal government began drafting legislation for a more comprehensive healthcare reform bill. Under President Obama, the **Patient Protection and Affordable Care Act** of 2010 (ACA) was passed, resulting in 21 million Americans receiving health insurance for the first time.

The ACA was the first piece of comprehensive healthcare reform legislation since the implementation of Medicare and Medicaid, passed with the goal of ensuring healthcare access to all Americans. It expanded on the model of bundled payments, provided funding for electronic medical records, and sought to create greater efficiency, quality, and transparency in the healthcare system. The ACA focused on changing eight major aspects of healthcare delivery[17]:

1. *Access*, addressed by expanding Medicaid and creating a national health exchange

2. *Cost control*, by creating **accountable care organizations (ACOs)**, bundled payments, and a "Cadillac Tax" on employer-sponsored health benefits in situations where the monetary value of the benefits exceeds legally specified thresholds

3. *Quality improvement*, focused on reducing in-hospital infections and readmissions

4. *Prevention*, which included coverage for preventative services (essential health benefits) without copayments

5. *Workforce development* to train new physicians and health professionals

6. *Revenue* earned on devices, cosmetic surgery, and tanning salons

7. *Changes to administrative billing and costs*, that is, saving overhead costs through simplification of administrative tasks

8. *Creation of the Center for Medicare and Medicaid Innovation (CMMI)* to design, implement, and test new payment models.[17]

The 21st century has seen significant developments in how and where people receive their care. Healthcare systems are becoming larger and more integrated, offering a wider range of services and for a lower cost. Allowing patients to stay in one network for care has improved access, coordination, and quality by standardizing delivery requirements within the network. Technology has also greatly changed how Americans access care. Many healthcare networks are using **telemedicine** to extend access to specialty care in remote (rural) communities and to provide 24-hour on-demand health care for patients via a smartphone or PC.

▶ The Evolution of Health Insurance

The United States is the only industrialized nation without universal health insurance.[18] Throughout the early 20th century, advocates of social welfare programs, working in concert with the American Association of Labor Legislation, pushed for the adoption of national health insurance policies. Health insurance plans in the United States are either private (commercially funded) or public (government supported); both have different coverage options. Approximately 56% of the population is covered under private insurance while 36% of Americans have public insurance.[19] Despite the expansion of health insurance coverage of both types under the ACA, 9% of the population in the United States (approximately 28.9 million people) still lack coverage.[20] These individuals are forced to pay for services out of pocket and suffer from worse health outcomes.[21] The next section highlights the key concepts of each payer system.

Commercial and Employer-Sponsored Insurance

Private health insurance is the most common type in the United States. Most people obtain coverage through their place of employment under a group plan, but individuals can also purchase coverage on their own. Employer-provided insurance is significantly less expensive because the risk is spread over a group as opposed

to a (potentially high-risk) individual. Also, health insurance benefits purchased through employers are not taxed, in contrast to the after-tax income that is required to purchase individual plans.[22]

There are a number of private options available for both employers and individuals. Group insurance involves a number of individuals coming together to purchase insurance from an insurance company. These groups are typically formed by businesses, unions, or other professional organizations.[1] They function by spreading the risk among all of the individuals in the group in order to lower costs. In a self-insurance plan, large groups (such as employers) act as their own insurance company. Instead of outsourcing coverage responsibility to a *third-party payer*, these organizations budget a certain amount of yearly income for health expenditures for their employees and use commercial insurers as *third-party administrators* to process and manage the claims. Self-insurance is very common among larger companies; 94% of businesses with over 5,000 employees participated in self-insurance in 2016.[23] The benefit for employers rests in the tax benefits they gain and their ability to avoid the regulation required of other health insurance plans that can lead to higher costs. For example, the ACA mandates that require insurance plans to include essential health benefits[24] (e.g., hospitalization, newborn and maternity care, lab services, preventive care, etc.) do not apply to self-insurance plans.[25] Another common form of employer-based insurance is the high-deductible health plan (HDHP).[26] As healthcare costs have risen in recent years, these plans have become more popular due to the lower premiums associated with them. However, until the deductible is reached, patients must pay out of pocket for services (except for preventive services, which are covered in full) before plan benefits are paid.

Medicare

Medicare is a federal program that provides health insurance to individuals over the age of 65, those with certain disabilities, and patients with end-stage renal disease. There are currently 58.5 million people covered under this program.[27] Coverage under Medicare is organized into four parts.[28] Part A is the hospital insurance portion that covers hospitalization, short-term nursing facilities, hospice care, and inpatient rehabilitation facilities. Medicare Part A is provided to all individuals over the age of 65 as long as they have paid at least 10 years of Medicare taxes (all others are subject to a monthly premium for benefits). Part B covers outpatient expenses, such as physician appointments, medical equipment, laboratory tests, and preventive care. This coverage is optional and paid for partly by tax revenues and premium contributions. Medicare typically covers 80% of costs, and individuals must pay for the remainder out of pocket unless they purchase coverage under a supplemental plan ("Medigap"). Medicare Part C, also known as Medicare Advantage, provides beneficiaries with additional choices in coverage through managed care organizations (MCOs). Individuals enrolled in Medicare Advantage receive Medicare Part A and Part B through these MCOs and, depending on the plan, may also receive additional benefits (e.g., vision, dental, hearing, and prescription drugs) not covered under traditional Medicare. Medicare Advantage, however, may require higher premiums and impose restrictions on access and utilization of services based on the specifications of the plan. Finally, Medicare Part D provides prescription drug coverage and assists with payment for outpatient medications.

Medicare has developed several alternative reimbursement strategies. One such strategy bases payments on a resource-based relative value scale (RBRVS). This scale establishes various relative value units (RVUs) for different aspects of medical care. RVUs are created for providers that factor in time, skill, and intensity of work required to complete a given service. RVUs are also established for the cost of practice, malpractice insurance, and overhead-related elements of facilities budgets. The different RVUs are taken into consideration when determining a Medicare Physician Fee Schedule, a price list for a physician's services.[1] While this creates a more equitable payment structure for providers, it contains many of the same problems as fee-for-service plans (providers are still incentivized to provide unnecessary services).

Recently, Medicare has begun using value-based reimbursements.[16] This method provides incentives for providers to reduce cost and improve quality of care.

Medicaid

Medicaid is a state-run program funded through matching contributions from the state and federal governments.[29] It provides health insurance to low-income Americans based on eligibility requirements set by each state. There are currently 65.9 million people insured through Medicaid throughout the United States.[30] Federal guidelines mandate that all families with children receiving support under the Temporary Assistance for Needy Families

(TANF) program, people receiving Supplemental Security Income (SSI), and children or pregnant women whose family income is at or below 133% of the Federal Poverty Level (FPL) are eligible for Medicaid.[1] Individual states can then set their own regulations for inclusion of other groups for consideration. One of the major components of the ACA included a mandate requiring state expansion of Medicaid. However, this was struck down by the Supreme Court in June, 2012,[31] leaving states to choose whether to expand Medicaid to include all citizens under the age of 65 with income up to 138% of the FPL. As of mid 2019, 36 states and the District of Columbia have chosen to expand coverage, which has helped many low-income individuals access needed care.[32]

Veterans Affairs and TRICARE

The Military Health System is a program directed by the U.S. Department of Defense (DoD) and provides medical services to all active duty and retired members of the armed forces and their families. This healthcare institution is completely operated by the DoD and provides care around the world to 9.4 million people.[33] The specific insurance provided by the Military Health System is TRICARE, which allows beneficiaries to access care at either DoD-sponsored medical facilities or private providers. Military members who leave the armed forces may continue to be eligible for TRICARE but are typically offered benefits through the Veterans Administration (VA). The VA manages a complicated system of hospitals, outpatient offices, and health centers that provide care to veterans and certain dependents. Although it was originally established to provide care to veterans with

service-related conditions, the VA now cares for over 9 million "previous service" men and women.[34]

Children's Health Insurance Program and American Indian and Alaska Native

Uninsured children whose family income exceeds the Medicaid threshold are eligible for the Children's Health Insurance Program (CHIP). Each state receives a federal block grant to create programs to cover all children under the age of 19. CHIP has been shown to successfully increase coverage and access to coverage for low-income children.[35]

Another vulnerable population segment that receives public insurance coverage is American Indian and Alaska Native (AIAN) tribes. They are provided services through the federal Indian Health Service (IHS) administration. This division of the Department of Health and Human Services provides services to this population through systems of hospitals, outpatient clinics, and health centers. These are essential for AIAN tribes, who often live in remote settings and may lack access to other healthcare options.

High-Deductible Health Plans (HDHP)

High-deductible health plans (HDHPs, also known as consumer-driven health plans or CDHPs) have become more common in recent years. As mentioned earlier, the distinguishing features of these plans is that they have a higher deductible (and typically lower premiums) than a traditional insurance plan. A high-deductible plan (HDHP) is frequently combined with a health savings account (HSA) or health reimbursement account (HRA). Funds set aside in these accounts by plan members can be accessed to pay for certain medical expenses with money free from federal taxes. According to the Healthcare .gov website, an HDHP is defined by the IRS as "as any plan with a deductible of at least $1,350 for an individual or $2,700 for a family."[36] Total yearly out-of-pocket expenses related to in-network services (including deductibles, copayments, and coinsurance) are limited to $6,650 for an individual or $13,300 for a family, but any out-of-network services are not included in this maximum amount.[36] As of 2018, 70% of large employers offered at least one HDHP to employees, either in addition to or as a replacement for traditional plans.[37] Many companies are only offering high-deductible options, leaving workers no choice in the matter.[38]

▶ Healthcare Delivery Systems

The delivery of healthcare services involves a complex, multidimensional system that requires engagement and interaction among providers, payers, and patients. Legislative and regulatory changes, particularly in the past 20 years, have had a significant impact on the way in which healthcare services are accessed and delivered in America. At the beginning of the 20th century, nearly all healthcare services were received in the hospital and were only accessible to those who were able to pay a fee for these services. The creation of health insurance, Medicare and Medicaid, the expansion of employer-sponsored insurance, and the **health insurance**

exchanges created under the ACA have allowed millions of Americans access to preventative and life-saving care. Americans are receiving health care in hospitals, **Federally Qualified Health Centers (FQHCs)**, ambulatory care centers (including retail clinics, urgent-care facilities and same-day surgical centers), and through virtual visits using telemedicine applications. Healthcare systems have become large, integrated networks providing comprehensive care in innovative ways, while maintaining quality and affordability.

Healthcare Providers

Healthcare services are provided by a wide variety of clinicians, including physicians, nurses, physician assistants, pharmacists, advanced practice professionals, and community health workers. In 2017, this workforce accounted for 9.1% of total employment[39] and 17.9% of the nation's Gross Domestic Product (GDP).[40] These numbers are predicted to rise as a result of the country's aging population, advances in research and technology, disease trends, and changes in delivery models.[1] Additionally, passage of the ACA increased the number of U.S. citizens with health insurance, necessitating a proportionate rise in the supply of healthcare providers. These increased numbers, however, have yet to be realized.[41]

Physicians

There are over one million actively licensed physicians in the United States.[42] Primary care physicians (PCPs), or generalists, are physicians trained in family medicine, internal medicine, and pediatrics, although others may practice general medicine as well.[43] Primary care focuses on preventative services and the treatment of common illnesses and diseases. PCPs are typically a patient's first point of contact with the healthcare system and often serve as gatekeepers or managers, referring patients to specialized services if needed. A recent epidemiologic study found a significant decrease in PCPs from 2005 to 2015.[44] In this study of the distribution of PCPs and its impact on population-level mortality, it was found that for every 10 additional PCPs per 100,000 population, there was a 51.2-day increase in life expectancy.[44] Since 2005, the density of PCPs, however, has decreased from 46.6 to 41.4 per 100,000 population. By contrast, adding 10 specialists per 100,000 population increases life expectancy by only 19 days.[44] The findings from this study are concerning because it highlighted the important role that PCPs play on managing the health of the population and reducing mortality. As the number of medical students entering the field of primary care decreases, the risk for higher mortality rates related to health conditions that are managed by a PCP may occur. PCPs are often in limited supply or entirely unavailable in rural counties, and the number per 100,000 population has continued to decrease since 2005.

Since the adoption of the Affordable Care Act (ACA), more incentives have been made available to encourage medical students to choose primary care. There continues to be mounting evidence associating access to PCPs with improved population health outcomes. The ACA created a strong emphasis on covering primary care services such as preventative services and wellness visits for Medicare beneficiaries. Under the ACA, PCPs who provide 60% of services in qualifying evaluation and managed could receive a 10% bonus in Medicare

payments for five years.[45] The ACA also led to the creation of patient-centered medical homes (PCMHs), ACOs, and increased federal funding for community health centers and federally qualified health centers (FQHCs), which improve access to preventative health services and allow people to establish a relationship with a PCP.[45] This model has helped to reduce healthcare costs by shifting from a fee-for-service model to a value-based care practice that provides incentives for physicians to provide high-value care for their patients.

Nursing

Nurses constitute the largest group of healthcare providers in the United States.[46] They are responsible for direct (i.e., hands-on) patient care and typically manage most day-to-day healthcare needs of their patients. In response to a longstanding problem of physician shortages, the Advanced Nursing Education Expansion Program was established as part of the ACA to help train nurses to perform these much-needed services. Nurses work in hospitals, outpatient offices, hospice care, and long-term care facilities and conduct home visits.[1] The ACA's changes and the increase in access to primary care services have led many nurses to pursue advanced degrees to become nurse practitioners (NPs). As the number of PCPs declines, NPs are likely to fill these gaps by providing primary care services. Healthcare systems are investing in hiring more NPs to address this shortage for patients who will need primary care. Primary care NPs are more likely to practice in urban settings and provide a wider range of clinical services than PCPs working in similar geographic areas.[47] Additionally, the NPs are more likely to treat Medicaid patients and treat the healthcare needs of vulnerable populations. Unfortunately, due to stringent regulations for NPs, many of them see fewer patients than PCPs in the same settings and are unable to admit and perform rounds on patients without a physician's signature.[47] This requirement has implications in underserved areas because, as the shortage of PCPs continues, it creates challenges for NPs to treat and refer patients to advanced care settings. States that have experienced significant expansion in Medicaid under the ACA are struggling to connect patients with PCPs; NPs have been able to fill some of those vacancies. However, without a significant change in state and federal regulations for NP practice standards, many patients who already face barriers to accessing primary care may have no access to primary care at all.

Recent data have shown that the United States is projected to experience a shortage in nurses as a result of an aging workforce and a decrease in the number of nursing school graduates.[48] The National Council of State Boards of Nursing reported that nearly 55% of the RN workforce is over the age of 50 and projects that nearly 1 million nurses will be eligible for retirement in the next decade.[48] This may have negative impacts on population health because of nurses' important role in managing chronic conditions. Research from CMS has shown that when there is a lower patient-to-nurse ratio, the cost of healthcare services is lower and there is a decrease in post-surgical infections and hospital readmissions.[48] In the coming years, it will be important for healthcare systems to recruit and retain nurses to reduce healthcare costs and avoid negative health outcomes for patients.

Advanced Practitioners

Advanced practitioners (APs) are clinicians who function in many similar primary care roles as physicians. The demand for these services is increasing in the United States due to an expanding population and physician shortages. As such, the need for APs such as NPs, clinical nurse managers, and physician assistants (PAs) is also on the rise.[6] The term "allied health professionals" refers to professionals who have obtained degrees in health or applied sciences in order to use evidence-based methods to provide direct patient care while considering broader public health outcomes.[49] This large group of providers is typically broken into either technicians/assistants or therapists/technologists, based on level of education.[1] Some examples of technicians/assistants include physical therapy assistants and certified occupational therapy assistants. Meanwhile, examples of therapists/technologists include physical therapists and occupational therapists.

Pharmacists

Pharmacists are healthcare providers responsible for dispensing medication and providing patient education regarding its proper use. Pharmacists can practice in a number of settings, including community pharmacies, private hospitals, and large corporations. Their role is continuously evolving due to changes in demand and the growing complexity of medical management. For example, the passage of the Omnibus Budget Reconciliation Act of 1990 mandated that pharmacists provide education to all patients regarding drug information and potential misuse. This has enabled pharmacists to take on a larger role in patient management.

Community Health Workers

The World Health Organization (WHO) introduced the theory that Community Health Workers (CHWs) in rural and underserved communities could be used as advocates for distributing health information, educating the population about healthy behaviors, and leading community-based participation. Arguably, CHWs have greater influence primarily in remote or rural areas because they are often the only available source for healthcare services.[50] CHWs who met with low-income, underserved individuals and families were able to give a voice to people who once felt powerless and unable to influence change.[51] The WHO recently updated guidelines for countries to adopt the use of CHWs. Community health workers are seen as an essential link between connecting health systems and communities in order to increase coverage of essential health services such as preventative care, health promotion, and curative services.[51] Employing CHWs will help to improve equity, which will result in a decrease in deaths, illnesses, and lowering disease burdens. There is evidence to support the notion that using CHWs in communities that collaborate with local health systems has improved maternal health care, child health, mental health, and sexual and reproductive health and has resulted in a reduction of communicable and noncommunicable diseases through education and training.[52] The WHO has developed policy recommendations for health systems and communities to use when implementing CHWs. These

recommendations focus on levels of education and training and build on a person's preexisting knowledge and experiences, while also incorporating institutional and operational requirements. The training is based upon expected preventative, promotive, diagnostic, and treatment and care services that are important to specific communities, populations, and regions. Last, the role of CHWs should be transformative and able to adapt and evolve over time as the epidemiologic profile of populations and the needs of each health delivery system change.[52]

Types of Delivery Systems
Integrated Health Networks

As the healthcare landscape began to change in the late 1990s, more hospitals, physician groups, and healthcare service providers began to merge to create integrated care delivery systems (IDS). As MCOs became increasingly popular, inpatient and outpatient service organizations started merging, offering greater access to a multitude of healthcare services to patients in one geographic location (and often in one insurance network). The adoption of the ACA led to the requirement for healthcare organizations to be accountable for people's health outcomes.[11] This led to an increase in healthcare organizations' merging into larger integrated delivery systems. Today the two most common types of healthcare systems are Integrated Delivery Systems (IDS) and ACOs.[11] An IDS is a group of several organizations under ownership or a contractual agreement that provides multiple healthcare services to large communities. Geisinger and Kaiser Permanente are two examples of IDS that offer one-stop shopping environments that are centered at one or more hospitals. These large health networks include both inpatient and outpatient services, surgical centers, hospice care, and a variety of specialty care clinics. An IDS may also include imaging centers, rehabilitation hospitals, and mental health centers. In 2016, 81% of acute care hospitals in the United States were affiliated with an IDS.[53] When IDS are created, they result in lower patient discharge costs, a reduction in average length of stay, higher caseloads for inpatient and outpatient services, and increased revenue because of the availability of a greater number of services. Similar to an ACO, IDS are able to reduce the costs associated with health care by having a streamlined standard of care, clinical integration, and the elimination of duplicating services for patients.

Other unique structures of an IDS may include an insurance plan for members who utilize the system. Healthcare systems such as Geisinger and Kaiser Permanente, which were mentioned earlier, are examples of an open (Geisinger) versus closed (Kaiser Permanente) IDS. Both Geisinger and Kaiser Permanente have their own health insurance plans, referred to as Geisinger Health Plan (GHP) and Kaiser Health Plan, respectively. As an open IDS, Geisinger accepts patients who have health insurance plans other than GHP. This organizational structure allows patients to move in and out of Geisinger for care. Many patients who utilize Geisinger for care have primary care physicians who are not Geisinger physicians. However, those physicians may refer their patients to Geisinger providers, assuming the patient's insurance is part of their network. Similarly, Geisinger physicians may refer patients outside of the Geisinger network to other physicians for specialty care that may not be available within GHP. This is an example of an *open integrated delivery system.*

Conversely, Kaiser Permanente, the largest non-profit IDS in the nation, operates very differently. Kaiser Permanente operates in nine states and the District of Columbia, with over 8.7 million members, 150,000 employees, and an annual revenue of $38 billion.[54] This IDS consists of three main components; (1) Kaiser Foundation Health Plans, (2) Kaiser Foundation Hospitals, and (3) Permanente Medical Groups. Each component has a unique role in how patients access and utilize services. The health plan is a nonprofit, public-benefit corporation that contracts with individuals and groups for prepaid, comprehensive healthcare services. The health plan contracts exclusively with Permanente Medical Groups and Kaiser Foundation Hospitals for medical and hospitals services for members. Kaiser Foundation Hospitals are a nonprofit, public-benefit corporation that owns and operates community hospitals in several states. They own outpatient facilities and provide or arrange hospital services in other states. Last, Permanente Medical Groups are partnerships or professional corporations of physicians represented by the Permanente Foundation. These groups of providers contract exclusively with the Kaiser Foundation Health Plans to arrange or provide medical services to its members.[54] This system is considered a *closed IDS* because consumers purchase a Kaiser Health Plan that allows them to only use healthcare services at Kaiser Foundation Hospitals and from providers who are part of the Permanente Medical Groups. Providers who are a part of this IDS can only refer patients within the system across the nine states and District of Columbia. Consumers who have this health plan are also unable to seek treatment that will be covered by their insurance from other healthcare systems. Both open and closed IDS are still much more effective at providing high-quality, low-cost care to patients because of their ability to consolidate multiple services under a larger umbrella system. Patients who use IDS often report better health outcomes and higher patient satisfaction and are likely to use the same IDS for all of their healthcare services.

Managed Care Organizations

Managed care organizations (MCOs) are integrated healthcare delivery systems that focus on reducing cost and improving quality while controlling utilization by patients. They have three main approaches toward payment. The first is the *preferred provider* approach, in which fees for services are negotiated directly with specific clinicians in order to keep costs down in exchange for patient referrals. The second is *capitation*, in which providers are given a set fee for each patient in the organization regardless of that patient's utilization of their services. Finally, the third strategy involves MCOs' directly employing providers and paying them a regular salary with bonuses.[55]

Accountable Care Organizations

Accountable Care Organizations (ACOs) are integrated groups of providers that include hospitals, physicians, and post-discharge care delivery organizations that work together to deliver coordinated care that is focused on quality, efficiency, and value.[11] The Affordable Care Act originally established this model of care as a new category for Medicare because it utilizes coordinated care that helps to ensure that patients get the right care at the right time with the goal of avoiding unnecessary duplication of services and preventing errors.[56] The adoption of ACOs has changed the model for payment by reducing or eliminating the fee-for-service model to a payment structure that incentivizes good health and high quality rather than treating illness and managing a high volume of patients. To ensure this model is effective, there are over 33 quality measures that ACOs must meet in four domains: patient/caregiver experience, care coordination/patient safety, preventative health, and care of at-risk populations.[56]

ACOs were originally designed for the Medicare system; however, they are on the rise in the private and public sectors. The payer side is encouraging healthcare systems to adopt this model through incentives for providing coordinated care for patients that is focused on quality. This model decreases costs in care provision by partnering and sharing risk with providers by using one clinical model of care in an organization. The goals of an ACO include empowering patients to take charge of their health and engaging in shared decision making with providers that results in eliminating waste and excessive spending. The ACO model also allows patients to have greater access to preventative care by incorporating quality measures for reducing illness and chronic conditions.[57] When the ACA was implemented, it embraced the concept of ACOs because it provided financial incentives for clinical integration that shifted from siloed healthcare delivery systems to coordinated care using value-based models for patients, providers, and payers.[57]

A distinguishing feature of an ACO is its people-centered foundation that aims to engage patients in their own health by providing education and resources to help them navigate the healthcare system, improve their healthcare experiences, and measure and monitor their health status. Also recognized as *health homes*, ACOs seek to optimize primary care services and coordinate each patient's overall care across the full range of healthcare settings with a focus on creating high-value delivery provider networks (e.g., appropriate specialists, outpatient centers, hospitals).

By using population health data to inform their clinical decision making, ACOs can help improve health outcomes for their patients. The data can also be used to leverage advanced financial and clinical technology integration.[57] Since 2012, over 560 ACOs have participated in the Medicare Shared Savings Program (MSSP), with provider participation exceeding 1,678%. Currently, 51% of ACOs are physician-led, compared with 33% that have been led by hospitals alone.[11]

Veterans Administration

Founded in 1930, the Veterans Administration (VA) system is the largest integrated healthcare system in the United States. It provides healthcare services for active military members and those who have been honorably discharged from the U.S. armed forces.[58] The VA system is funded through federal taxes and is widely recognized as a national health service specifically for veterans. In the 1970s, the VA had a reputation for providing care that was inefficient, costly, and had a high rate of medical errors. However, in recent years, the VA has reported better outcomes, higher performance ratings, and better quality rankings than the rest of the U.S. healthcare system.[58] The median age of veteran men is 65 years old, and the median age for female veterans is 51.[59] The current racial/ethnic breakdown of VA patients for male veterans is 78% white; for female veterans, it is 65% white; the remaining patients are nonwhite/non-Hispanic. Veterans are more likely to live at or above 400% of the federal poverty level than their non-veteran counterparts and are likely to have both public and private health insurance, resulting in very few male and female veterans being uninsured (2.8% vs. 3.8%). Recent quality improvement changes and new measures have found that VA patients received significantly better overall care, chronic care, and preventive care among a sample of 596 VA patients and 992 non-VA patients.[58] The VA is constructed of 21 Veterans Integrated Service Networks that are each responsible for healthcare planning and resource allocation across particular geographical regions in the United States. Providers for the VA are employed by the federal government and provide a variety of inpatient and outpatient health services. Access to these services is free for active duty military personnel and retired military personnel, and their families receive TRICARE insurance, which is financed by the Department of Defense. TRICARE also allows its members to receive private medical care. Currently, the VA provides healthcare services to over 9.6 million individuals across 1,100 sites, including nearly 153 hospitals, 807 ambulatory and community-based clinics, 135 nursing homes, 209 counseling centers, 47 residential care facilities, and 73 home healthcare programs.[11]

Federally Qualified Health Centers

Federally qualified health centers (FQHCs) were formed in 1965 by President Lyndon Baines Johnson as a healthcare delivery component of his Great Society initiative and its War on Poverty.[60] FQHCs are centered in areas with a large distribution of underserved populations (people who are on Medicaid, are uninsured, or are underinsured). FQHCs are often referred to as safety net clinics because they provide care to patients regardless of their insurance status or ability to pay for services. According to regulations, 51% of the FQHC governing board that regulates the clinics must represent the population that the center serves.[60] The Health Resources and Services Administration (HRSA) regulates and administers the government FQHC program and requires that each center's strategic vision is driven by consumer input. FQHCs and FQHC "look-alikes" currently provide comprehensive healthcare services to 20 million Americans in 38 states. Nearly 85% of the patients using these centers are on Medicaid or are uninsured.[61] Many of the patients who utilize FQHCs struggle with low health literacy levels, housing insecurity, and food insecurity, which can complicate their health outcomes; these patients often have complex health problems. Patients using FQHCs are also more likely to face depression, to be obese, to live in impoverished zip codes, and to be diagnosed with multiple comorbidities.[61]

Telehealth

Telehealth or telemedicine refers to the use of medical information that is exchanged from one site to another through electronic communications to improve a patient's health.[62] The use of "smart" technology—electronic health records (EHRs) and health apps—has led to a growth in telehealth over the past several years. Telehealth is another potential tool to assist with achieving the goals of the Quadruple Aim: improving the patient experience of care, improving the health of populations, reducing the per capita cost of health care, and improving the provider experience of care.[62] The use of telehealth technologies and tools is becoming an integrated component of care delivery in large healthcare systems like Kaiser Permanente, Geisinger, and Intermountain Healthcare. Telehealth use is projected to grow to 60% of all healthcare systems and 40% to 50% of all hospitals in the coming years.[62] The benefits of telehealth for patients include real-time access to care, after-hours clinical care, and reducing the need to travel for non-emergency care for those living far from a hospital. Many patients are using telehealth to refill prescriptions and schedule appointments. Nearly all health insurance providers reimburse telehealth services; however, Medicare continues to be more restrictive, only allowing reimbursement for telehealth services for rural patients. In the next decade, telehealth will likely be used as a continuous source for innovation in consumer health technology, provide advancements in the data collected and accessed in the EHR, influence clinical decision making for more integrated health, and address the growing shortages of healthcare professionals.[62] Some patients are using telehealth for real-time video consultations in the areas of cardiology, dermatology, psychiatry and behavioral health, gastroenterology, infectious disease, rheumatology, oncology, and peer-to-peer mentoring.[62] Other benefits of telehealth include the ability for wireless monitoring of vital signs, the development of mobile health apps that store important health information for patients and providers, and social media platforms that can connect patients with providers and services. Telehealth may lead to improvements in patient engagement with their providers by changing the nature of the relationship that exists between them. As more providers and patients use telehealth technology, it is believed that patients will assume a more active role in their health management through regular discussions with their providers via smart devices.[62]

▶ Stakeholders

The **stakeholders** in health care all have a unique role to play in managing population health in diverse settings. Each stakeholder in the healthcare industry brings a unique set of skills and knowledge that helps to improve health outcomes, reduce costs, identify gaps in care and delivery, and facilitate better coordination of care for patients and consumers. Under a population health paradigm, stakeholders use value-driven population health interventions to address the social determinants that affect health outcomes in their targeted population. The goal is to influence the distribution of care and services by working collaboratively to create more equitable policies, initiatives, interventions, and services to address health disparities and ultimately lead to improved health. The following is a brief list of the primary stakeholders in healthcare delivery and their role in managing population health.[63]

Patients/Consumers

Patients and consumers are perhaps the most important stakeholders in the healthcare system. It is important to understand why and how patients choose their healthcare system, services, and providers and how they define satisfaction. There are many factors that inform the decisions consumers make about their health that are essential for healthcare systems to understand. These factors include costs, insurance, accessibility, quality, and value. Consumers have become more aware of the cost of healthcare services and are choosing insurance plans that allow them to stay in their network and have lower premiums and lower out-of-pocket expenses but still allow for flexibility and choice in the providers they see.

Because of the significant rise in healthcare costs, consumers are also more aware of what their insurance will cover and are asking more questions about the treatments, services, and necessity of care they will receive from their providers. Consumers are increasingly holding their providers and healthcare systems accountable for the services for which they are being charged and asking questions about how particular treatments will improve their health in the long term. Those consumers with commercial plans that have larger networks of providers are also more willing to travel farther and to make more informed decisions if they feel their local healthcare system is not transparent, has unwarranted variation in care, or is more expensive than other providers or hospitals within a reasonable distance. As consumer choice expands and patients become more knowledgeable about costs, transparency, and quality, health systems are looking for innovative new ways to engage with patients to improve quality and access and reduce the cost of care.

Providers

Physicians, physician assistants, nurses, and other allied health professionals are responsible for the delivery of medical care and coordination of care for patients in a variety of medical settings. Healthcare providers should strive to deliver quality care that is affordable and accessible. With the adoption of the ACA and new CMS regulations for reimbursement, many providers have shifted their objectives to focus on improving the quality of care, reducing the costs, and eliminating waste within the system (e.g., unnecessary testing and services). Using population health tools, many providers have turned to CMS for guidelines or have adopted more efficient ways of using the electronic medical record to track and manage their patient populations. Providers are using evidence-based medicine to implement new intervention strategies that reduce readmissions, incentivize appropriate use of care and services, and reduce preventable illness and disease. Finally, providers are responsible for analyzing outcomes and costs to promote the use of high-value services and reduce waste by using differential cost-sharing methods to incentivize and encourage behavioral changes in their patients.[63]

Payers

Health insurance companies have a significant impact on how patients are able to access care and receive necessary services. Insurance companies are often regulated by state and federal guidelines that set standards for payment, liability, coverage, and limitation. Since the passage of the ACA, insurance companies have shifted their payment models from fee-for-service reimbursement to bundled payments (in the case of Medicare and Medicaid) to value-driven insurance design that rewards quality over quantity of services. Insurance companies often are the primary driver of the cost of services because hospitals tend to set their pricing scale based on what they know or expect will be reimbursed. Value-based insurance design analyzes cost and outcome data to determine the relative value of a particular type of care. It functions to incentivize and encourage patients to use high-value services that are linked to the most beneficial outcomes relative to cost.[63] Insurance companies are adopting this practice because, from the population health perspective, it leads to an increase in desired behavior changes in patients as well as providers so that there is less wasteful spending, which in turn lowers the overall cost of care. Value-based insurance design provides options for patients to improve their health status, emotional well-being, and functional status by incorporating the best evidence-based treatment and services that extend beyond direct medical care. Insurance companies work with health systems and providers to reduce unwarranted clinical variation and establish care coordination that leads to improved outcomes, reduced costs, and fewer hospitalizations and readmissions for patients.

Pharmaceutical Industry

Pharmaceutical companies play a significant role in the healthcare system because many patients rely on their products for managing their illnesses. Pharmaceutical companies are regulated by the federal government; however, these regulations have not focused on the cost of medications. The prices for prescription drugs have been rising at what many consider to be an alarming rate, and there are no caps in place to prevent them from reaching stratospheric prices. In recent years, many healthcare providers and the federal government have questioned how pharmaceutical companies market, promote, and sell their products to physicians. Since the late 1980s, pharmaceutical companies started hiring young, attractive representatives with no formal training in pharmaceuticals to build social relationships and provide incentives for physicians to prescribe their products, rather than developing expertise in the biomedical literature on the benefits and risks that products may have for patients.[64] As a result, many patients were prescribed medications that were unnecessary or had very limited benefit to the patient's long-term health.

By the mid 1990s, the FDA and the U.S. Patent and Trademark Office created regulations that protected patents for pharmaceuticals and had no price restrictions, which led to a profound investment in pharmaceutical development in the United States.[65] Because there are no price restrictions on medications and it is illegal to purchase pharmaceuticals outside the country, many patients are unable to afford their medication in the United States, although in some cases, the same prescription can cost up to 50% less in other countries. Most patents allow three to five years for pharmaceutical companies to market a brand-name drug before a generic version can be created; however, generic drugs are not always more affordable. Pharmaceutical companies tend

to raise generic drug prices to whatever price the market will sustain regardless of the actual cost to produce the medication.[65] Additionally, many drug companies have found blind spots in the FDA approval and patent process to slightly alter the formulation of generic drugs and remarket them as a new product, which allows for higher pricing. This method has resulted in many patients with chronic illness who have taken a specific generic drug for many years to suddenly find their generic medication is no longer available, forcing them to choose between paying for an expensive "new" drug that is not significantly different from the previous generic and rationing or foregoing their medication—with significant health consequences.

Since the passage of the ACA and the shift to value-based reimbursement, however, pharmaceutical companies have begun to reexamine the costs for both the patient and the healthcare system that is purchasing their products. Pharmacy benefit managers (PBMs) are third-party administrators that work for commercial health plans, self-insured employers, Medicare Part D, and others to develop and maintain formularies, contract with pharmacies, negotiate with pharmaceutical manufacturers, and process prescription drug claims.[66] This model allows for cost savings, efficiency, and enhanced care for patients because the model is based on buying products and drugs that have high value and result in better outcomes.[63]

▶ Conclusion

Health care in the United States is a complex ecosystem of interdependent structures, systems, and stakeholders. Unfortunately, despite the significant cost, the U.S. healthcare system as it is currently organized does not always produce the best outcomes for patients. The professionalization of the field of medicine, the growth of new allied health fields, and the emergence of various forms of health insurance have created dramatic shifts in how the United States organizes, finances, and delivers health services—with some of the most significant changes occurring in the past 50 years. These changes, along with medical innovation, have certainly improved length and quality of life, but they have also created a very complex system of stakeholder groups that continue to react and adapt to each other, in addition to adjusting to population shifts; changes in government regulation; introduction of new technologies; and new ways of organizing, financing, and delivering health services.

Many significant challenges remain intractable, including unwarranted clinical variation and unnecessary expenditures (waste), high prescription drug costs, and disparities in care for vulnerable patient populations. Since the passage of the Affordable Care Act, however, stakeholders have begun to tackle some of these problems using a population health approach.

The new paradigm of population health will also have a transformational impact on the U.S. healthcare system. The continuing shift from "volume" to "value" will not only realign financial incentives for providers to improve outcomes rather than perform more services, but it will also encourage them to improve population health through more effective care coordination, judicious integration of new technologies, and better use of data to inform decision making.

Study and Discussion Questions

1. How have historical changes in the organization, financing, and delivery of health services in the United States impacted how it functions today?

2. How has the growth of the health insurance industry and the "corporatization" of health care changed the practice of medicine?

3. Describe the ways in which health services are financed, and list the pros and cons of each using a population health approach.

4. Characterize differences between the Clinton administration's proposals for healthcare reform and the Affordable Care Act (ACA) enacted under President Obama. What were the principles guiding each, and what were the mechanisms for paying for each of these approaches? Relate these themes to changes in healthcare payment mechanisms over time.

Suggested Readings and Websites

Readings

Emanuel E. *Reinventing American Health Care: How the Affordable Care Act Will Improve Our Terribly Complex, Blatantly Unjust, Outrageously Expensive, Grossly Inefficient, Error Prone System*. New York: PublicAffairs; 2014.

Pearl R. *Mistreated: Why We Think We're Getting Good Health Care – and Why We're Usually Wrong*. New York: PublicAffairs; 2017.

Dzau VJ, McClellan M, Burke S, Coye MJ, Daschle TA, Diaz A, et al. Vital Directions for Health and Health Care: Priorities from a National Academy of Medicine Initiative. *NAM Perspectives*. Discussion Paper, National Academy of Medicine, Washington, DC; 2017. doi: 10.31478/201703e

Websites

Agency for Healthcare Research and Quality: www .ahrq.gov

Commonwealth Fund – www.commonwealthfund .org

Health Affairs Blog: www.healthaffairs.org/blog

Kaiser Health News: www.khn.org

Development of the National Health Promotion and Disease Prevention Objectives for 2030 – Healthy People 2030: https://www.healthy people.gov/2020/About-Healthy-People /Development-Healthy-People-2030

References

1. Shi L, Singh DA. *Delivering Health Care in America: A Systems Approach.* 6th ed. Sudbury, MA: Jones and Bartlett Learning; 2015.
2. Cutter JB. Early hospital history in the United States. *Calif State J Med.* 1922;20(8):272–274.
3. Manchikanti L, Helm SI, Benjamin RM, Hirsch JA. Evolution of US health care reform. *Pain Physician.* 2017;20(3):107–110.
4. Wagner D. *The Poor House: America's Forgotten Institution.* Lanham, MD: Rowman & Littlefield; 2005.
5. Kaufman M. Review of "Review of American Physicians in the Nineteenth Century: From Sects to Science." *J Am History.* 1973;60(1):142–144.
6. Rothstein WG. *American Physicians in the Nineteenth Century: From Sect to Science.* Baltimore, MD: Johns Hopkins University Press; 1972.
7. Rosen G. *The Structure of American Medical Practice 1875–1941.* Philadelphia, PA: University of Pennsylvania Press; 1983.
8. Stevens R. *American Medicine and the Public Interest.* New Haven, CT: Yale University Press; 1971.
9. Wright JW. *The New York Times Almanac.* New York, NY: Penguin Putnam; 1977.
10. Tomes N. Merchants of health: medicine and consumer culture in the United States, 1900–1940. *J Am History.* 2001;88(2):519–547.
11. Shi L, Singh DA. *Essentials of the US Health Care System.* Sudbury, MA: Jones & Bartlett; 2019.
12. Minor D. Kimball, Justin Ford. In: *Handbook of Texas Online.* Austin, TX: Texas State Historical Association; 2010. Available at http://www .tshaonline. org/handbook/online/articles/fki09 (accessed April 16, 2019).
13. Wilson FA, Neuhauser D. *Health Services in the United States.* 2nd ed. Cambridge, MA: Ballinger; 1985.
14. Mistichelli J. Diagnosis related groups (DRGs) and the prospective payment system: forecasting social implications. *Scope Note Series: 4.* Washington, DC: Bioethics Research Library, Georgetown University; 1984. Available at https://pdfs.semanticscholar.org/6 de1/1a9e 69a83aaa68c4dd9325404b1f6e3414de.pdf (accessed June 12, 2019).
15. Zelman WA. The rationale behind the Clinton health care reform plan. *Health Affs.* 1994;13(1):9–29.
16. Centers for Medicare & Medicaid Services. CMS Value-Based Programs. Available at https://www .cms.gov/Medicare/Quality-Initiatives-Patient -Assessment-Instruments/Value-Based -Programs/Value-Based-Programs.html (accessed April 17, 2019).
17. Emanuel E. *Reinventing American Health Care: How the Affordable Care Act Will Improve Our Terribly Complex, Blatantly Unjust, Outrageously Expensive, Grossly Inefficient, Error Prone System.* New York: PublicAffairs; 2014.
18. Vladeck B. Universal health insurance in the United States: reflections on the past, the present, and the future. *Am J Public Health.* 2003;93(1):16–19.
19. The Kaiser Family Foundation. Health insurance coverage of the total population. 2017. Available at https://www.kff.org/other

/state-indicator/total-population/ (accessed April 17, 2019).

20. Cohen RA, Martinez ME. Health insurance coverage: early release of estimates from the National Health Interview Survey, 2008. Washington, DC: American Psychological Association; 2009. Available at https://doi.org/10.1037/e565212009-001 (accessed May 20, 2019).

21. Woolhandler S, Himmelstein DU. The relationship of health insurance and mortality: is lack of insurance deadly? *Ann Intern Med.* 2017;167(6):424.

22. O'Brien E. Employers' benefits from workers' health insurance. *Milbank Q.* 2003;81(1):5–43. Available at https://doi.org/10.1111/1468-0009.00037/ (accessed May 20, 2019).

23. Kaiser Family Foundation. 2016 Employer Health Benefits Survey. 2016. Available at https://www.kff.org/report-section/ehbs-2016-section-ten-plan-funding/ (accessed May 20, 2019).

24. Families USA. 10 essential health benefits insurance plans must cover under the Affordable Care Act. Available at https://familiesusa.org/blog/10-essential-health-benefits-insurance-plans-must-cover (accessed May 20, 2019).

25. Noble A, Chirba M. Individual and group coverage under the ACA: more patches to the federal-state crazy quilt [blog]. *Health Affs.* 2013. Available at https://www.healthaffairs.org/do/10.1377/hblog20130117.027189/full/ (accessed May 20, 2019).

26. Office of Personnel Management. Fast facts: high deductible insurance plans. Available at https://www.opm.gov/healthcare-insurance/fastfacts/high-deductible-health-plans.pdf (accessed May 20,2019).

27. Centers for Medicare & Medicaid Services. Program statistics. 2017 Medicare Enrollment. Available at https://www.cms.gov/Research-Statistics-Data-and-Systems/Statistics-Trends-and-Reports/CMSProgramStatistics/2017/2017_Enrollment.html (accessed May 20, 2019).

28. Rajaram R, Bilimoria KY. Medicare. *JAMA* 2015;314(4):420–420. Available at https://doi.org/10.1001/jama.2015.8049 (accessed April 17, 2019).

29. Komisa HL. Medicaid. *JAMA*. 2006;295(24):2891–2895. Available at https://doi.org/10.1001/jama.295.24.2893 (accessed April 17, 2019).

30. Centers for Medicare and Medicaid Services. December 2018 Medicaid & CHIP Enrollment. Available at https://www.macpac.gov/wp-content/uploads/2018/12/December-2018-MACStats-Data-Book.pdf (accessed May 20, 2019).

31. Rosenbaum S, Westmoreland TM. The Supreme Court's decision on the Medicaid expansion: how will the Federal government and states proceed? *Health Affs*. 2012. Available at https://www.healthaffairs.org/doi/full/10.1377/hlthaff.2012.0766 (accessed May 20, 2019).

32. Kaiser Family Foundation. Status of State Action on Medicaid Expansion Decision. 2019. Available at https://www.kff.org/health-reform/state-indicator/state-activity-around-expanding-medicaid-under-the-affordable-care-act/?currentTimeframe=0&sortModel=%7B%22colId%22:%22Location%22,%22sort%22:%22asc%22%7D (accessed May 20, 2019).

33. Military Health System. Beneficiary Population Statistics. 2019. Available at https://health.mil/I-Am-A/Media/Media-Center/Patient-Population-Statistics (accessed May 20, 2019).

34. Veterans Health Administration [website]. 2019. Available at https://www.va.gov/health/ (accessed May 20, 2019).

35. Paradise J. The impact of the Children's Health Insurance Program (CHIP): what does the research tell us? Kaiser Family Foundation; 2014. Available at https://www.kff.org/medicaid/issue-brief/the-impact-of-the-childrens-health-insurance-program-chip-what-does-the-research-tell-us/ (accessed May 20, 2019).

36. Healthcare.gov. Glossary: High-Deductible Health Plan, Health Savings Account. Available at https://www.healthcare.gov/search/?q=glossary

37. The State of Employee Benefits: Insights and Opportunities Based on Behavioral Data. 2018. Charleston, SC. BenefitFocus.com. http://go.benefitfocus.com/insights/report/the-state-of-employee-benefits-2018/pr?utm_source=web&utm_medium=pr&utm_campaign=report_2018_soeb.

38. Renter E. Should you roll the dice on a high-deductible health plan? US News: Health 2014.

Available at https://health.usnews.com/health-news/health-insurance/articles/2014/11/10/should-you-roll-the-dice-on-a-high-deductible-health-plan (accessed May 20, 2019).

39. Centers for Medicare and Medicaid Services. (2018). National Health Expenditure Data. Available at https://www.cms.gov/Research-Statistics-Data-and-Systems/Statistics-Trends-and-Reports/NationalHealthExpendData/index.html (accessed May 20, 2019).

40. United States Department of Labor. State Occupational Employment and Wage Estimates. 2017. Available at https://www.bls.gov/oes/tables.htm (accessed May 20, 2019).

41. Wishner J, Burton R. How have providers responded to the increased demand for health care under the Affordable Care Act? US Health Reform - Monitoring and Impact. Washington, DC: Urban Institute; November 1, 2017. Available at https://www.rwjf.org/en/library/research/2017/11/how-have-providers-responded-to-the-increased-demand-for-health-care-under-the-aca.html (accessed May 20, 2019).

42. Kaiser Family Foundation. State health facts: professionally active physicians. March 2019. Available at https://www.kff.org/other/state-indicator/total-active-physicians/?currentTimefr ame=0&sortModel=%7B%22colId%22:%22Locat ion%22,%22sort%22:%22asc%22%7D (accessed May 20, 2019).

43. Rich EC, Wilson M, Midtling J, Showstack J. Preparing generalist physicians: the organizational and policy context. *J Gen Intern Med.* 1994;9(4 Suppl 1):S115–S122.

44. Basu S, Berkowitz SA, Phillips RL, Bitton A, Landon BE, Phillips RS. Association of primary care physician supply with population mortality in the United States, 2005-2015. *JAMA Intern Med.* 2019. Available at https://jamanetwork.com/journals/jamainternalmedicine/article-abstract/2724393 (accessed May 20, 2019).

45. Klink K. (2015). Incentives for physicians to pursue primary care in the ACA era. *AMA J Ethics.* 2015;17(7):637–646.

46. National Academy of Medicine (formerly the Institute of Medicine) (US) Roundtable on Evidence-Based Medicine. Leadership Commitments to Improve Value in Healthcare: Finding Common Ground: Workshop Summary. Part II, 6. Washington (DC): National Academies Press (US); 2009.

47. Buerhaus PI, DesRoches CM, Dittus R, Donela K. Practice characteristics of primary care nurse practitioners and physicians. *Nursing Outlook.* 2015;63(2):144–153.

48. Snavely TM. A brief economic analysis of the looming nursing shortage in the United States. *Nursing Econ.* 2016;34(2):98–100.

49. Speyer R, Denman D, Wilkes-Gillan S, Chen Y-W, Bogaardt H, Kim JH, et al. Effects of telehealth by allied health professionals and nurses in rural and remote areas: a systematic review and meta-analysis. *J Rehab Med.* 2018;50:225–235.

50. Schachter K, Ingram M, Jacobs L, DeZapien JG, Hafter H, Carvajal S. Developing an action learning community advocacy/leadership training program for community health workers and their agencies to reduce health disparities in Arizona border communities. *J Health Disparities Res Pract.* 2014;7(2):34–49.

51. Rifkin SB. A framework linking community empowerment and health equity: it is a matter of CHOICE. *J Health Popul Nutr.* 2003;21(3):168–180.

52. WHO guideline on health policy and system support to optimize community health worker programmes. Available at https://www.who.int/hrh/community/guideline-health-support-optimize-hw-programmes/en/ (accessed May 22, 2019).

53. Shi L, Singh DA. *Essentials of the US Health Care System.* Sudbury, MA: Jones & Bartlett Publishers; 2019: 221.

54. McKinsey & Co. What health systems can learn from Kaiser Permanente: An interview with Hal Wolf. *McKinsey Q.* July 2009. Available at https://www.mckinsey.com/industries/healthcare-systems-and-services/our-insights/what-health-systems-can-learn-from-kaiser-permanente-an-interview-with-hal-wolf?reload (accessed May 22, 2019).

55. Berenson RA. (1991). A physician's view of managed care. *Health Affs.* 1991;10(4):106–119.

56. Ulrich B. Accountable care organizations: what they are and why you should care. *Nephrol Nurs J.* 2012;39(6):427–428.

57. DeVore S, Champion RW. Driving population health through accountable care organizations. *Health Affs.* 2011;30(1):41–50.

58. Oliver A. (2007). The Veterans Health Administration: an American success story? *Milbank Q.* 2007;85(1):5–35.

59. United States Department of Veterans Affairs. Profile of veterans 2017. Available at https://www.va.gov/vetdata/docs/SpecialReports/Profile_of_Veterans_2017.pdf (accessed May 22, 2019).

60. Wright B. Who governs federally qualified health centers? *J Health Politics Policy Law.* 2013;38(1):27–55.

61. Goldman LE, Chu PW, Tran H, Romano MJ, Stafford RS. Federally qualified health centers and private practice performance on ambulatory care measures. *Am J Prev Med.* 2012;43(2):142–149.

62. Tuckson RV, Edmunds M, Hodgkins ML. Telehealth. *N Engl J Med.* 2017;377(16):1585–1592.

63. Allen H, Burton WN, Fabius R. Value-driven population health: an emerging focus for improving stakeholder role performance. *Popul Health Manag.* 2017;20(6):465–474.

64. Health care reform: duties and responsibilities of the stakeholders. Institute of Clinical Bioethics Blog, Saint Joseph's University. September 2011. Available at https://sites.sju.edu/icb/health-care-reform-duties-and-responsibilities-of-the-stakeholders/ (accessed May 22, 2019).

65. Rosenthal E. *An American Sickness: How Healthcare Became Big Business and How You Can Take It Back.* New York: Penguin Random House; 2018.

66. Advisory Council on Employee Welfare and Pension Benefits Plans. Report to U.S. Secretary of Labor: PBM compensation and fee disclosure. November 2014. Available at https://www.dol.gov/sites/default/files/ebsa/about-us/erisa-advisory-council/2014-pbm-compensation-and-fee-disclosure.pdf (accessed May 22, 2019).

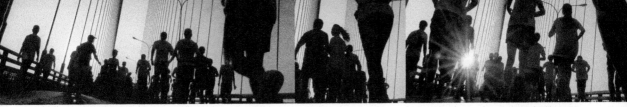

CHAPTER 5

Reimbursement Models to Support Value-Based Care

Michael Kobernick

EXECUTIVE SUMMARY

Health care continues to experience upward price pressure in the cost of medications, treatments, and technology. For example, in 2019, Deloitte predicts a 5.5% increase of pharmaceutical spending and a 20% increase in orphan (rare and very high-cost) drug sales by 2024.[1] PwC predicts an overall trend of a 6% healthcare cost increase in 2019 driven by new health technologies, government regulation, and aging of the population. "Unaddressed social factors such as economic instability and education can impact utilization patterns and care decisions, while poor wellness and prevention habits are drivers of poor health."[2]

In an attempt to curb these trends, alternatives to the predominant fee-for-service reimbursement models are being developed and piloted. Known as *value-based care*, payment under these models not only reimburses for services, it also incorporates outcomes and patient experience into the calculation of payment. Considered along a continuum, these models begin with fee-for-service and end with value-based, full-risk accountable care organizations. A population health approach is essential to the success of the value-based model.

LEARNING OBJECTIVES

1. Discuss the variety of healthcare reimbursement models.
2. Explain the elements on the fee-for-service value-based payment continuum.
3. Define value in economics, health, and health care.
4. Explain the Triple Aim.
5. Discuss the role of population health in supporting value-based payment.

KEY TERMS

Accountable care organization
Administrative services only
Bundled payment
Capitation
Commercial insurance
Demand
Downside risk

Fee-for-service
Medicaid
Medicare
Opportunity cost
Patient-centered medical
     home
Shared savings

Social determinants of health
Supply
Triple Aim
Upside risk
Value
Value equation

▶ Introduction

In order to discuss value-based care, it is necessary to understand the foundational concepts from health economics and insurance. This chapter presents these concepts and defines value and value-based care in the context of the various types of reimbursement models currently in operation. It closes with a review of some of the evidence on value-based reimbursement models and their application to population health.

▶ Definition of Value

Value has been defined by a variety of disciplines. Economics views the value of a good or service as "what an individual would be willing to pay for it in monetary terms or give up in terms of other resources or time to receive it."[3] The concept of *giving up something to purchase another thing* is referred to as the **opportunity cost**. The opportunity cost of sitting in a doctor's office waiting room may be the wage given up for lost time at work. For many, especially those paid by the hour, that cost will be too great, and they will decide to forgo the visit with the doctor. Opportunity cost is an important part of healthcare value to an individual, and it often drives their decisions.

The World Health Organization defines health as "the state of complete physical, mental and social well-being and not merely the absence of disease."[4] This is an important definition in the context of value-based care because it distinguishes between the absence of disease and the overall well-being of the individual. If we are only concerned about the absence of disease, health care treats the sick until the disease is cured or abated. The measure of health is not the individual's return to a state of well-being but rather the return to a "normal" laboratory value or vital sign. It is reasonable to conclude that the definition of value in health care must include the well-being of the individual, and the performance of healthcare delivery must be measured in terms of the value created to the patient.

Noted Harvard economist Michael Porter has discussed value in health care extensively: "… value is defined as the patient health outcomes achieved per dollar spent … value encompasses many of the other goals already embraced in health care, such as quality, safety, patient centeredness, and cost containment, and integrates them."[5] It is the integration of all the elements of health care on behalf of the patient that defines value. As Porter states, "it is the value for the *patient* that is the central goal, not value for other actors per se."[5] These variables may be used to define the **value equation**, where value is equal to outcomes divided by cost or value = outcome/cost. It is this relationship between the outputs (the totality of well-being rather than the absence of illness) and inputs (the resources expended) that defines value, as opposed to defining value as the volume of services provided (which only includes the perspective of the deliverer of healthcare services).

Traditionally, the value of health care has been expressed in terms of profitability and has been measured by the volume of services delivered and reimbursed. Introducing the concept of reimbursement based on the calculation of the value to the patient is a method designed to ensure the highest quality at the best price (value). It defines the oft-discussed "transition from volume to value" and integrates the **Triple Aim** as defined by Berwick and the Institute for Healthcare Improvement (IHI): "the United States will not achieve high-value health care unless improvement initiatives pursue a broader system of linked goals; we call those goals the 'Triple Aim': improving the individual experience of care; improving the health of populations; and reducing the per capita costs of care for populations" (**FIGURE 5-1**).[6,7]

Value-based care reimbursement models are, therefore, dependent upon the integration of the outcomes and cost as embodied in the Triple Aim rather than a strict adherence to a fee reimbursement for every service provided.[8]

Economic Concepts

The field of health economics adds some concepts that aid in understanding value-based reimbursement models. Traditional economics focuses on the interaction

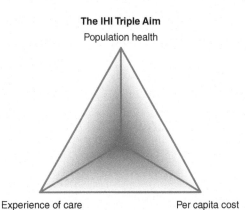

The IHI Triple Aim

Population health

Experience of care   Per capita cost

FIGURE 5-1 The IHI Triple Aim.

The IHI Triple Aim framework was developed by the Institute for Healthcare Improvement in Boston, Massachusetts (www.ihi.org). Available at: http://www.ihi.org/Engage/Initiatives/TripleAim/Pages /default.aspx

of demand, supply, and price. In a market, there are buyers and sellers. **Demand** is the buyer's willingness to acquire a product or service at a given price. The seller's willingness to offer the good to the buyer at an agreed-upon price is the seller's **supply**. In usual markets, the law of demand describes an inverse relationship between price and quantity demanded. As price goes up, the quantity demanded declines. This is *not* the case in health care, as there are many confounding factors that deviate from the traditional economic model. Prominent among these factors is the concept of *uncertainty* applied to health care, as discussed by Arrow, who describes consumers as being uncertain of their health status and needs at any given time.[9] This leads to uncertainty of demand and inability of healthcare providers to accurately predict how much care they must offer. In addition to uncertainty, Folland describes several additional reasons why health care does not follow the basics of supply and demand. These include insurance, asymmetry of information, large role of non-profits, competition restrictions, equity and need, and government subsidies.[10] Health care does not follow the typical rules of economics; it is unique, adding to the difficulty of managing costs and the assessment of new reimbursement models.

Health Insurance and the Elements of the Fee-For-Service, Value-Based Care Continuum

Health insurance is noted to be one source of uncertainty in health care. An understanding of its history is important but beyond the scope of this chapter. The reader is referred to Paul Starr's book, *The Social Transformation of American Medicine*,[11] for a complete review of the topic.

Health insurance is based on the principle that an insurer accepts payment of a premium from a customer and, in return, promises to pay the agreed-upon contractual medical benefits. Leiberthal describes health insurance as "a pass-through entity akin to a gas station. Just as most people rely on a gas station to store gas and then sell it to them on demand, most people may relate to health insurance as a card in their wallet to be used any time they have a demand (or need) for health care."[12] This has resulted in the development of third-party administrators (TPAs)—that is, **commercial insurance** companies—to administer the benefit payment. The functions of the insurer are summarized by Cleverley and include underwriting, utilization review, claims administration, network contracting, credentialing, accreditation, and payment negotiation.[13] The insurance company takes on the risk that they will have gathered enough premium to support payment of the claims they receive. If the claims paid at the end of the year exceed the premium revenue, the insurance company loses money and

will generally increase the premium for the following year.

Insurance companies are categorized based on the population they serve. The government provides health insurance coverage for veterans, retirees and people with chronic disabling conditions, and those who meet the economic threshold to be considered as having low income. **Medicare** is a program administered by the federal government through its Centers for Medicare and Medicaid Services (CMS) to those above the age of 65, people who are disabled by severe, chronic physical or mental conditions, and those with end-stage renal disease. Medicaid is a program administered by state governments for people whose income falls below specific federal thresholds based on the size of their household, and may include families with children, pregnant women, some of the elderly, and people with developmental disabilities. People who are old enough for **Medicare** but whose personal income is low enough to qualify for Medicaid programs are called "dual-eligible."

Commercial health insurance is the term used for insurance that is not paid for by the government and is sold by private carriers, either for-profit or not-for-profit (like United Healthcare or Blue Cross/Blue Shield). Most people are covered by commercial plans offered by their employers. In a fully insured plan, the employer pays the insurer a premium on behalf of the employee, and the insurer pays the claims and takes the risk. Larger employers are often "self-insured"; this means that the employer uses its own funds to pay the benefit claims and only hires the plan to handle paperwork associated with payment of the claims. This model, where the employer directly bears the risk for the costs of the benefits, is also known as **administrative services only** (ASO).

Regardless of the type of program, the goal is to pay all the claims at the lowest cost.

As is well known, healthcare costs continue to escalate. A variety of reimbursement methods have been developed and applied in an effort to manage to the lowest possible cost. Despite the expansion of new models, **fee-for-service** (FFS) is currently still the most common form of reimbursement. Under the fee-for-service model, healthcare providers are reimbursed for every service they perform. Each service is accompanied by a claim that is administered by the insurer; under FFS, the outcome is not taken into account in the payment.

Mayzell explains fee-for-service as follows: "our fee-for-service system reimburses on a 'per click basis'; therefore, each visit is paid whether it has the right outcome or right care."[14] Under this model, volume drives revenue; the more procedures done in the hospital or the outpatient setting, the greater the revenue. Fee-for-service has been the primary driver of escalating costs, so alternate payment models are being developed in an effort to control costs, improve the patient experience of care, and incorporate some measure of outcome associated with value—that is, achievement of the Triple Aim objectives.

Several alternate payment models have been implemented. It is important to keep in mind that there is considerable overlap among some of them, creating similarities. The models may be performance-based incentive, condition- or service-based, or be associated with accountable care programs (**FIGURE 5-2**).[15]

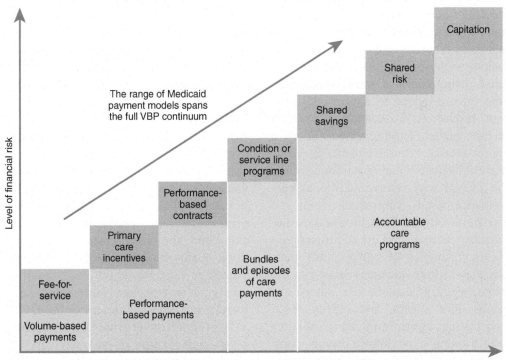

FIGURE 5-2 Range of Medicaid Payment Models.

Leitz S, McGinnis T. Medicaid Innovation Accelerator Program. October 5, 2017. Available at: https://www.medicaid.gov/state-resource-center/innovation-accelerator-program/iap-downloads/functional-areas/vbp-learning-webinar.pdf

Viewed graphically from the Medicaid Innovation Accelerator Program, the newer models contain a higher level of financial risk and require a greater degree of care, provider integration, and accountability.[15] Clearly, there are complex challenges associated with moving from the volume-based fee-for-service model to one that supports any type of value-based payment.

Performance-based reimbursement systems are based on additional elements of outcome that are defined, agreed upon by both parties, and included in the reimbursement model. An example is the primary care medical home (PCMH), also known as the **patient-centered medical home**. It is defined by the Agency for Healthcare Research and Quality (AHRQ) "as a medical home not simply as a place but as a model of the organization of primary care that delivers the core functions of primary health care."[16] The functions include high quality, safe, patient-centered, comprehensive, and coordinated care, often provided by a team of healthcare professionals. Accredited PCMHs receive higher reimbursement using a fee-for-service reimbursement. In addition to the overall higher reimbursement, the PCMH may receive additional performance-based contractual bonuses. The payer often defines the metrics that must be met to receive the additional payments. Examples of performance metrics may include outcomes related to the management of diabetes like dilated eye exams, foot checks, and kidney function testing; aspirin and statin use after a heart attack; or immunization rates. The PCMH performance-based payment model is an example of a method of value-based care reimbursement.

Condition or service-line programs, another type of value-based care reimbursement, are procedure oriented and include all costs associated with the procedure for a defined episode of care. **Bundled payments** have been implemented by CMS for hospital care in four models as Bundled Payments for Care Improvement (BPCI).[17] These are illustrated in **TABLE 5-1**, adapted from CMS's Comprehensive Care for Joint Replacement Model.[18]

In Table 5-1, Medicare Part A refers to hospital services, and Medicare Part B includes physician services. Model 1 was a discounted fixed payment for an inpatient stay. Models 2 and 3 are retrospective bundled payment models that include an acute-care stay in a hospital plus the post-acute care and all related services up to 90 days after the hospitalization. Model 4 is a payment that covers all services furnished by the hospital, physician, other practitioners during the entire stay.

In orthopedics, CMS had implemented the Comprehensive Care for Joint Replacement (CJR) program.[19] In CJR, hip and knee replacement surgeries are organized into episodes of care that begin when a patient is admitted for a surgery and end 90 days post discharge. One reimbursement includes all services including professional fees, hospital charges, home care, and the achievement of agreed-upon quality metrics. The CMS-initiated Oncology Care Model (OCM) is another emerging service line value-based payment program. CMS describes the OCM as a program to provide higher quality, better coordination of oncology care for a price less than or similar to the current fee-for-service price.[20] These payment arrangements may include the entire

TABLE 5-1	BUNDLED PAYMENT MODELS			
	Model 1: Discounted Fixed Payment for Inpatient Stay	**Model 2: Retrospective Acute Care Hospital Stay Plus Post-Acute Care**	**Model 3: Retrospective Post-Acute Care Only**	**Model 4: Prospective Acute Care Hospital Stay Only**
Episode	Selected DRGs	Selected DRGs + post-acute period	Post-acute only for selected DRGs	Selected DRGs
Services Included in the Bundle	Part A services during the stay	Part A and Part B services during the initial inpatient stay, post-acute period and readmissions	Part A and B services during post-acute period and readmissions	All Part A and B services (hospital, physician) and readmissions
Payment	Retrospective	Retrospective	Retrospective	Prospective

episode of care, chemotherapy, and provision of care coordination, while adhering to national treatment guidelines. According to the OCM Fact Sheet, the OCM model provides enhanced services including patient navigation; a 13-part care plan; access to a clinician 24 hours a day, 7 days a week; therapy consistent with national guidelines; data-driven quality improvement; and use of an electronic medical record.[21] Providers receive regular Medicare fee-for-service payments, a $160 monthly per-beneficiary fee, and a performance-based payment for the achievement of mutually agreed-upon benchmarks. CMS expects "these improvements will result in better care, smarter spending, and healthier people."[20]

Accountable care organizations (ACO) integrate various healthcare providers across the continuum to deliver care to members. ACOs currently serve defined populations from Medicare, Medicaid, and commercial health plans. In this model, an individual registers for or is assigned to an ACO. The ACO has a relationship with the payer in which they receive payment for those members. This payment may range from fee-for-service with incentive bonuses for achieving agreed-upon quality indicators to a full-risk **capitation**, whereby the ACO receives an entire monthly payment to provide care to the patient. If the ACO is able to provide care for less than the premium, it keeps all the savings, known as **upside risk**; if not, then it has to cover the remaining costs, called **downside risk**. In order to avoid the downside risk, most ACOs prefer to share the risk, with the payer assuming the downside risk. This results in a variety of **shared savings** models whereby the ACO and payer will split the leftover amount by an agreed-upon percentage. CMS has developed the Medicare Shared Savings Program (MSSP) that allows and

	BASIC Track's Glide Path				ENHANCED Track (risk/reward)
	Level A and Level B (one-sided model)	Level C (risk/reward)	Level D (risk/reward)	Level E (risk/reward)	
Shared savings (once MSR met or exceeded)	1st dollar savings at a rate up to 40% based on quality performance, not to exceed 10% of updated benchmark	1st dollar savings at a rate of up to 50% based on quality performance, not to exceed 10% of updated benchmark	1st dollar savings at a rate of up to 50% based on quality performance, not to exceed 10% of updated benchmark	1st dollar savings at a rate of up to 50% based on quality performance, not to exceed 10% of updated benchmark	No change. 1st dollar savings at a rate of up to 75% based on quality performance, not to exceed 20% of updated benchmark
Shared losses (once MLR met or exceeded)	N/A	1st dollar losses at a rate of 30%, not to exceed 2% of ACO participant revenue capped at 1% of updated benchmark	1st dollar losses at a rate of 30%, not to exceed 4% of ACO participant revenue capped at 2% of updated benchmark	1st dollar losses at a rate of 30%, not to exceed the percentage of revenue specified in the revenue-based nominal amount standard under the Quality Payment Program capped at 1 percentage point higher than the benchmark nominal risk amount (e.g., 8% of ACO participant revenue in 2019–2020, capped at 4% of updated benchmark)	No change. 1st dollar losses at a rate of 1 minus final sharing rate, with minimum shared loss rate of 40% and maximum of 75%, not to exceed 15% of updated benchmark

FIGURE 5-3　BASIC Track's Glide Path.

Centers for Medicare and Medicaid Services. Shared Savings Program Participation Options. July 1, 2019. Available at: https://s3.amazonaws.com/public-inspection.federalregister.gov/2018-17101.pdf

ACO to be accountable for cost, quality, and experience for an assigned group of Medicare enrollees. The program offers shared savings or shared loss participation tracks in levels detailed in **FIGURE 5-3**.[22]

A full discussion of the MSSP program is beyond the scope of this chapter, but one can readily see that this program requires extensive clinical, informatic, and financial infrastructure to ensure success. In 2016, Medicare launched the Next Generation ACO (NGACO) Model. The NGACO was distinguished by requiring 80% or 100% risk that included downside risk without minimum savings or loss requirements.[23] This program represented an evolution of MSSP and hypothesized that greater risk would be associated with increased savings. These ACO models incentivize the providers to create efficient, lower-cost care that meets quality and patient experience goals consistent with the Triple Aim.

Evaluating Value-Based Care Reimbursement Models

Evidence of the success of value-based care reimbursement models is mixed at best. In an October 2017 report, the National Committee for Quality Assurance (NCQA) presented the latest evidence regarding the PCMH program.[24] Summarizing the report, several studies demonstrated that the PCMH is most effective in creating cost savings with the highest risk patients. The PCMH contributed to reduced inpatient care and emergency department utilization; improved medication adherence, immunization rates, and patient satisfaction; and reduced total cost. Some studies were limited by insufficient data, did not find cost savings, and found that additional standardization of the PCMH designation criteria was needed. Many of the studies report favorable results, and some need improvement. This indicates the need for further study in the future.

Bundled payments have been used by CMS for care and cost improvement in a variety of procedures. Jubelt et al. reviewed Medicare bundled payments for some orthopedic and cardiac procedures April 2011 through December 2014. They report an average episode cost reduction decrease of $3,017 for lower extremity joint replacement, and reduction of $2,999 for cardiac procedures, but for spinal fusion the cost increased $8,291.[25] Savings were due to earlier discharges to home, and the increase in spinal fusion was due to a change in the operative technique. The results of the Medicare Comprehensive Care for Joint Replacement (CJR) was reviewed by Thirukumaran, who found that 42% of safety-net hospitals participating in CJR failed to qualify for rewards; further, safety-net hospital rewards were 39% smaller than for the non-safety-net hospitals.[26] Because safety-net hospitals provide a significant level of care to low-income, uninsured or underinsured, and vulnerable populations, their failure to qualify for rewards was thought to be due to adverse selection.

Although bundled payment is thought to be a helpful tool for cost savings and quality improvement, the population under care must be taken into consideration when using this payment strategy. CMS independently reviewed the results of the Bundled Payments for Care Improvement (BPCI) initiative: "the independent evaluation found that BPCI Models 2 and 3 reduced Medicare fee-for-service payments for the clinical episodes evaluated while maintaining the quality of care for Medicare beneficiaries. Despite these

encouraging results, Medicare experienced net losses under BPCI after taking into account reconciliation payments to participants."[27] Compared to fee-for-service, the bundled payment program did create a savings; however, when the providers were paid for all the services (including nursing homes, physical therapy, and home care) Medicare did experience a loss. Tested OCM models were reviewed by Aviki, who found that "there is limited evidence to evaluate their efficacy. Reports of outcome are lacking and are of variable quality when available, so the overall efficacy of alternative payment and delivery models in cancer remains unclear."[28] This conclusion is true for the majority of value-based programs described above as they are often challenged by implementation issues, profitability, and at times inconsistent quality.

Studies indicate that Medicare Shared Savings Program (MSSP) ACOs appear promising. McWilliams analyzed 2012 and 2013 claims of 220 MSSP ACOs. The ACO cohort reported a 1.4% savings and improved performance on some quality measures.[29] In 2016 the NGACO "providers *reduced spending* for their beneficiaries by $100.08 million (1.7%). The estimated decrease in Medicare spending of –$18.23 per beneficiary per month (PBPM) in program year 1 is similar to the decrease noted in the first two years of the Pioneer ACO model and larger than the decrease noted for MSSP ACOs in the early years."[23] Reductions were also found in spending on post-acute care and "in the number of inpatient hospital days and nonhospital evaluation and management (E&M) visits per month (1.7 and 15.6 fewer per 1,000 aligned beneficiaries, respectively) and increases in the number of annual wellness visits (by almost 12%)."[23] The current evidence suggests that value-based payment programs show promise to achieve the Triple Aim, but they are very new and will require careful study in the future to determine their place in the overall reimbursement paradigm.

Stakeholder Perspectives on Value-Based Care Models

It is important to take into account the opinion of various stakeholders when considering the transition from fee-for-service to value-based care models. The National Academy of Sciences hosted a roundtable on value in health care with expert representation from every aspect of the system. Conclusions included that "provider-level value improvement efforts depend on culture and rewards focused on outcomes; patient-level value improvement stems from quality, communication, information, and transparency. Manufacturer-level regulatory and purchasing incentives can be better oriented to value added."[30] Timothy Johnson, a pediatrician, provides a view from a family perspective: "Cost continues to be a concern for many families. Additionally, convenience, access, personal outcomes, prevention, relationships, safety, and quality may all influence decisions patients and families make about when, where, what kind, and how much health care they consume."[31] The American Academy of Family Physicians (AAFP) recommends several guiding principles as value-based care is developed[32]:

- Include patients/consumers as partners in decision making at every level of care
- Deliver person-centered care

- Design alternative payment models that benefit patients/consumers
- Drive continuous quality improvement.
- Accelerate use of person-centered health information technology
- Promote health equity for all

Stakeholders are aligned on achieving the Triple Aim; each wants the highest quality care at the best price with an optimal experience.

▶ Conclusion

Population health and the role of social determinants are discussed in detail throughout this book. Population health is concerned with the health and well-being of those being served and the non–health care–related influences on an individual's overall health. Today we spend the vast majority of our resources on the care of the sick, *not* on prevention, slowing disease progression, and creating social determinant–based initiatives.[14] A population health approach includes identification of the **social determinants of health** that are affecting the health of the individuals in question. For instance, understanding the education level of the participants in value-based care models may help craft messaging appropriate for the population. ACOs are including social determinant assessments and interdisciplinary care team interventions for their members to achieve Triple Aim outcomes. Shier reports that addressing social determinants like transportation and caregiver support reduced the number of hospital days per 1,000 patients in the population studied.[33] The Vermont Blueprint for

Health used a community health team to address social determinants and provide care coordination for targeted subgroups. They reported a reduction of 11.6% in cost, 31% in emergency department utilization, 21% lower hospitalization rates, and an estimated $2 million in annual savings per 1,000 members.[34] The future of value-based health care must include a population health approach because it aligns with the Triple Aim objectives and has been proven necessary to catalyze the transition from fee-for-service to value-based care.

Study and Discussion Questions

1. Define value.
2. Define supply and demand, and explain why health care does not follow standard economic principles.
3. Describe the Triple Aim as applied to the shift from fee-for-service to value-based payments.
4. List the types of value-based payment models.

Suggested Readings and Websites

Readings

The Social Transformation of American Medicine.[11] Essential reading for any student of health care.

Health Economics and Policy[8]. These readings by Victor Fuchs provide health economic perspectives not available elsewhere.

Population Health: An Implementation Guide to Improve Outcomes and Lower Costs.[14] Mayzell offers interesting perspectives on the many of the topic discussed.

The Economics of Health and Health Care.[10] This textbook expands on the principles of economics as applied to health care.

Websites

Centers for Medicare and Medicaid Services: https://www.cms.gov. A great place to start and in-depth review of Medicare, Medicaid, and the variety of payment models.

Centers for Medicare and Medicaid Services—Accountable Care Organizations (ACOs): https://www.cms.gov/medicare/medicare-fee-for-service-payment/aco/. All aspects of ACOs may be found here.

The Institute for Healthcare Improvement: http://www.ihi.org. IHI offers information related to all aspects of the Triple Aim.

References

1. Deloitte. *2019 Global Life Sciences Outlook.* Washington, DC: Author; 2019. Available at https://www2.deloitte.com/us/en/pages/regulatory/articles/life-sciences-regulatory-outlook.html.
2. PwC Health Research Institute. *Analysis: Medical Cost Trends.* Orlando, FL: Author; 2018. Available at https://www.ehidc.org/sites/default/files/resources/files/hri-behind-the-numbers-2019.pdf.
3. Garrison L, Towse A. Value-based pricing and reimbursement in personalized healthcare: introduction to basic health economics. *J Pers Med.* 2017 Sep; 7(3): 10. Published online 2017 Sep 4. doi: 10.3390/jpm7030010
4. World Health Organization. Frequently Asked Questions. Available at https://extranet.who.int/kobe_centre/en/who-we-are (accessed March 31, 2019).
5. Porter M. What is value in health care? *N Engl J Med.* 2017;363(26):2477–2481.
6. Berwick D, Nolan T, Whittington J. The Triple Aim: care, health, and cost. *Health Aff.* 2008;27(3):759–769.
7. Institute for Healthcare Improvement. *IHI Triple Aim Initiative.* Boston, MA:

IHI; 2008. Available at http://www.ihi
.org/Engage/Initiatives/TripleAim/Pages
/default.aspx (accessed March 1, 2019).

8. Fuchs V. Major concepts of health care economics. *Ann Intern Med.* 2015;162:380–383.

9. Arrow K. Uncertainty and the welfare economics of medical care. *Am Econ Rev.* 1963;53:941–973.

10. Folland S, Goodman A, Stano M. *The Economics of Health and Health Care* (8th ed.). New York: Routledge; 2017.

11. Starr P. *The Social Transformation of American Medicine.* New York: Basic Books; 2017.

12. Lieberthal R. *What Is Health Insurance (Good) For?* Basel, Switzerland: Springer; 2016.

13. Cleverley W, Cleverley J. *Essentials of Health Care Finance.* Burlington, MA: Jones & Bartlett Learning; 2018.

14. Mayzell G. *Population Health: An Implementation Guide to Improve Outcomes and Lower Costs.* Boca Raton, FL: CRC Press; 2016.

15. Leitz S, McGinnis T. *Medicaid Innovation Accelerator Program.* October 5, 2017. Available at https://www.medicaid.gov/state-resource -center/innovation-accelerator-program/index .html (accessed March 1, 2019).

16. Agency for Healthcare Research and Quality. *Primary Care Medical Home.* Rockville, MD: AHRQ; 2018. Available at https://pcmh.ahrq .gov/page/defining-pcmh (accessed March 1, 2019).

17. Centers for Medicare and Medicaid Services. *Bundled Payments for Care Improvement.* Baltimore, MD: CMS; 2018. Available at https://innovation.cms.gov /initiatives/bundled-payments/ (accessed March 15, 2019).

18. Centers for Medicare and Medicaid Services. *Comprehensive Care for Joint Replacement Model.* Baltimore, MD: CMS; 2019. Available at https://innovation.cms.gov/initiatives/CJR (accessed March 15, 2019).

19. Centers for Medicare and Medicaid Services. *Oncology Care Model.* Baltimore, MD: CMS; February 25, 2019. Available at https: //innovation.cms.gov/initiatives/oncology -care/ (accessed March 15, 2019).

20. Centers for Medicare and Medicaid Services. *Oncology Care Model Fact Sheet.* Baltimore, MD: CMS; 2019. Available at https://www.cms.gov /newsroom/fact-sheets/oncology-care-model (accessed March 27, 2019).

21. Centers for Medicare and Medicaid Services. *Shared Savings Program.* Baltimore, MD: CMS; December 2019. Available at https: //www.cms.gov/Medicare/Medicare-Fee -for-Service-Payment/sharedsavingsprogram /about.html (accessed March 15, 2019).

22. Centers for Medicare and Medicaid Services. *Shared Savings Program Participation Options.* Baltimore, MD: CMS; 2019. Available at https://www.cms.gov/Medicare/Medicare -Fee-for-Service-Payment /sharedsavingsprogram/Downloads/ssp-aco -participation-options.pdf.

23. Lowell K. *Next Generation Accountable Care Organization (NGACO) Model Evaluation.* Chicago, IL: National Opinion Research Center at the University of Chicago; 2018.

24. National Committee on Quality Assurance. *Benefits of NCQA Patient-Centered Medical Home Recognition.* Washington, DC: NCQA; 2017.

25. Jubelt L, Goldfield K, Blecker S, et al. Early lessons on bundled payment at an academic medical center. *J Am Acad Orthop Surg.* 2017;29(9):654–653.

26. Thirukumaran C, Glance L, Cai X, et al. Performance of safety-net hospital in year 1 of the comprehensive care for joint replacement model. *Health Aff.* 2019;38(2).

27. Centers for Medicare and Medicaid Services. Bundled Payments for Care Improvement (BPCI) Initiative, Models 2-4. Baltimore, MD: CMS; 2017. Available at https: //innovation.cms.gov/Files/reports/bpci2-4-fg -evalyrs1-3.pdf (accessed March 1, 2019).

28. Aviki E, Schleicher S, Mullangi S, Matsoukas K, Korenstein D. Alternative payment and care-delivery models in oncology: a systemic review. *Cancer.* 2018;124(16):3293–3306.

29. McWilliams J, Hatfield L, Chernew M, Landon. Early performance of accountable care organizations in Medicare. *N Engl J Med.* 2016;374:2357–2366.

30. Yong P, Olsen L, McGinnis J. *Roundtable on Value and Science Driven-Health Care.* Washington, DC: National Academies Press; 2010.

31. Johnson T. A pediatrician's perspective: value-based care, consumerism, and the practice of pediatrics: a glimpse of the future. *Pediatrics.* 2019;139(s2):s145–s149.

32. American Academy of Family Practice News Staff. Keep patient perspective prominent in value-based health care. Leawood, KS: American Academy of Family Practice. September 15, 2016. Available at https://www.aafp.org/news/practice-professional-issues/20160915transformation.html (accessed March 15, 2019).

33. Shier G, Ginsburg M, Howell J, Volland P, Golden R. Strong social support services, such as transportation and help for caregivers, can lead to lower health care use and costs. *Health Aff.* 2013;32(3):544–551.

34. Vermont Department of Health. *Vermont Blueprint for Health.* Williston, VT: Vermont Public Health; 2011.

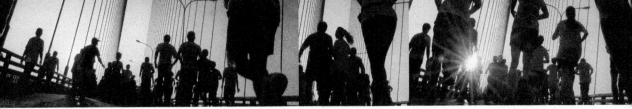

CHAPTER 6

Population Health Data and Analytics

Harm Scherpbier
Karen Walsh
Alexis Skoufalos

EXECUTIVE SUMMARY

Population health requires data to make it work—data to define target populations and identify their care needs, data to track the delivery of healthcare services to specific populations, and data to determine best practices and optimize interventions to patient groups. In this chapter, we discuss the foundation of data management that underpins an organization's population health initiatives, from data aggregation and managing data quality to the analytics programs that will focus and track care delivery to target populations and inform reimbursement.

LEARNING OBJECTIVES

1. Describe the benefits of capturing clinical data in structured form in an electronic health record (EHR).
2. Evaluate the strengths and weaknesses of clinical and administrative data for health services research and applicability in analytics.
3. Understand ways in which provider organizations can use population-level analyses for performance improvement.
4. Recognize how informatics and IT systems support patient care and outcomes.
5. Explain how big data and data science shape the healthcare system and outcomes.
6. Describe the components of population health management systems.

KEY TERMS

Analytics	Health information exchanges	Population health
Data governance	Informatics	management system
Electronic health record (EHR)	IT system	Risk stratification

▶ Population Health and the Importance of Data

Before we explore the significance of **informatics** and **analytics**, it is important to revisit the definition of population health and reconfirm its dependence on data.

Population health has been defined as the health outcomes of a group of individuals, including the distribution of such outcomes within the group.[1]

Population health has three core components:

1. Population health is a *care delivery model* focused on the health and wellness of a defined population—a group of patients in a geographic region, or attributed to a practice, or with a specific condition, or covered under a health plan.

2. This care delivery model is supported by a *reimbursement model* that aligns the incentives to maximize the health of the population at the lowest cost or utilization, over the long term. The reimbursement model often relies on shifting incentives and financial risks from the payer to the provider.

3. A *data infrastructure* supports care delivery and reimbursement—by defining and tracking the populations, targeting and managing care delivery, measuring and tracking quality and utilization measures, and determining performance of providers based on quality and utilization goals.

Data are essential to population health initiatives. Under the previous fee-for-service model, care delivery and reimbursement were simply based on transactions—the patient seeks care, and the provider delivers care and gets reimbursed. Under a population health paradigm, the provider is reimbursed for managing the care for a population—a group of patients—whether they come to visit the practice or not. Care organized under this model requires data—to identify the patients in the population, to document their clinical conditions and care needs, monitor their severity of illness, identify their care teams, document their social determinants, and track the utilization and cost of care for these patients.

This chapter deals with the data underpinnings required to support population health from several perspectives:

- The *analytical* perspective—the 30,000-foot view (primarily the health system or health plan perspective), for purposes of **risk stratification** and data analytics
- The *practice* perspective—the point of view of providers, including

attribution of patients to providers, practice and provider performance, and effectiveness and efficiency

- The *operational and care delivery* perspective—care coordination and patient engagement

Now that population health and population-based payment models have been more widely adopted, the health IT industry is developing systems to support population health initiatives, called **population health management (PHM) systems**. The key components of these systems line up exactly with the three perspectives of population health. PHM systems include these capabilities:

1. **Data Aggregation**—gathering data from multiple sources to create a full set of data on a population.
2. **Data Analysis and Risk Stratification**—creating cohorts in the overall population categorized by risk, identifying high-risk populations versus lower-risk populations.
3. **Care Management and Coordination**—systems to help coordinate care based on the level of risk in a cohort.
4. **Patient Engagement and Outreach**—capabilities to engage patients and families in their care, tailored toward their risk level and healthcare needs.

This chapter is organized to follow this sequence of PHM capabilities; they represent a logical workflow of the data. Before we can begin, however, we must review the various information systems and data sources in health care. These sources encompass clinical data from **electronic**

health records and administrative and financial data from billing systems and health plans.

Clinical Data: Electronic Health Records

The best source of clinical data is the electronic health record (EHR). Hospital EHRs are focused on acute care—that is, short episodes of ill health, often with very ill patients. Clinics, physicians' offices, and practices have EHRs focused on ambulatory care—managing patients' health and chronic conditions over time, across multiple episodes and visits.

In 2009, Congress approved the American Recovery and Reinvestment Act (ARRA), which included a stimulus plan for implementation and adoption of EHRs.[2] This plan gave financial incentives to hospitals and practices for implementing and demonstrating "meaningful use" of the EHR, through a series of metrics. To receive the incentive payments, hospitals and practices had to report their meaningful use measures to the Center for Medicare and Medicaid Services (CMS). This program created a very rapid adoption of EHRs in hospitals and even more so in physician practices:

- Prior to the meaningful use mandate imposed by ARRA, more than 50% of physician practices had paper medical records. Now, approximately 1% of practices still use a paper medical record, and most practices have some form of EHR.[3]
- Prior to meaningful use, most hospitals had limited implementation

of their EHRs, with less than 10% of hospitals requiring that physicians do their documentation and orders in the EHR. Today, most hospital physicians enter their orders and physician notes directly into the EHR, eliminating the risk of transcription or legibility errors.

- More than half of hospitals have "closed loop medication administration," meaning that patients' medication orders are entered into the EHR by physicians, validated and dispensed by pharmacists, and administered and checked by nurses through the EHR, with safety checks on allergies, dosages, and drug interactions at each point along the way.

The Analytics Division of the Healthcare Information and Management Systems Society (HIMSS) has created a tool to help organizations map and assess their level of maturity in electronic medical record (EMR) adoption. The Electronic Medical Record Adoption Model (EMRAM)[3] includes seven stages of achievement relative to EMR utilization.

Patient safety is one of the primary reasons for transitioning from paper to EHRs. EHRs are intended to improve quality of care and promote patient safety by,[4] for example:

- Only offering up valid dosages for medications and checking against over- or under-dosing
- Using order sets for common conditions and scenarios
- Making clinical documentation and notes available to all members of the care team
- Rapidly communicating test orders to the laboratory or radiology teams

- Using Clinical Decision Support to detect drug-to-drug interactions, adverse effects, or other patient safety concerns and alerting clinicians

Shifting from paper to EHRs requires major changes to the way clinicians and physicians work. Recent studies show that physicians in ambulatory practices can spend as much as 50% of their time working within the EHR—looking up information and entering their documentation.[5] They also spend 1–2 hours at the end of the workday to catch up on documentation. While most hospitals and practices successfully switched to electronic records, the transition is not yet complete, and most practices will need several cycles of optimization and improvement to regain the desired efficiencies of their healthcare providers.

The transition to EHRs was prerequisite and precursor to the transition from fee-for-service healthcare payment to value-based care or population-based care and reimbursement. EHRs provide the data infrastructure on which population health initiatives are built. Without EHRs in place, there would be no way to identify specific populations attributed to a provider, or those with chronic conditions or high levels of need; in short, it would not be possible to coordinate and manage the care for these populations. Perhaps most important, without EHRs, patients would not have the same level of access to their own data and records, which is a critical component of improving population health.

▶ Interoperability: EHRs Exchanging Data

The meaningful use mandate resulted in widespread implementation and adoption of EHRs in hospitals and ambulatory practices. However, the EHRs in place today do not easily share and exchange data; this creates islands of information in isolation, rather than the continuous flow of information necessary for effective population health. Recognizing this issue, CMS is now recasting meaningful use as "promoting interoperability" and focusing incentives to promote data sharing across providers.[2]

Some large health systems rely predominantly on a single EHR, from a single vendor, in all care settings. There is undeniable benefit to the ability for all clinicians and participants to see the same set of data for a patient and to easily communicate with each other via the EHR. However, the reality in most health systems is different. Most health systems employ multiple EHRs—for example, one brand of EHR in one or more of the acute care facilities, a different EHR in other acute care facilities, one EHR in the owned or employed practices, but a variety of EHRs in the independent but affiliated physician offices. Patients are seen in a number of settings with different EHRs, causing their clinical data to be fragmented among a number of organizations. As a result of this fragmentation, no single health provider or payer may have the full set of data for a patient. For analytical purposes, we need to bring together data from multiple organizations and multiple information sources to get a more complete and holistic view at both the patient level and the population level.

Interoperability across EHRs allows healthcare providers to share data with each other. There are several mechanisms for EHRs to exchange data, each method suitable for a particular situation.

System-to-System Interoperability via HL7-Based Interfaces

Health Level 7 (HL7) is a framework of messaging standards, created specifically for health care, to facilitate the exchange of clinical data across systems, both inside a single organization and among different organizations.[6] HL7 defines the format and layout of transactions—an admission, an order, a result, a status change—so that all health **IT systems** can easily send and receive the information in the same "language." This enables healthcare organizations to share data across systems from different vendors without the need to create an expensive custom interface. HL7-based interfaces are typically and successfully used among systems inside a single healthcare organization (point-to-point interfaces); they are less suitable for interfacing data among different organizations.

Transitions of Care Among Healthcare Organizations— C-CDA-Based Interoperability

Patients, especially those with chronic conditions, may see multiple healthcare providers across a variety of care settings (e.g., office, hospital, long-term care facility). These settings may have different EHR systems in place—and they need to send and receive patient information in a format that can be understood across all of them. The Consolidated Clinical Document Architecture (C-CDA), sometimes referred to as the Continuity of Care Record (CCD), is the format mandated by meaningful use rules for this organization-to-organization transmission of patient data.[7] By using a standard format (.xml) and standard terminologies, receiving systems know how to manage the data and store it in their organization's EMR.

C-CDA–based data exchange is important to population health initiatives in two ways. It supports and enables successful transitions of care by providing the latest patient care information to multiple participants. Since they are generated by all organizations where a patient receives care, C-CDAs can be an important source of data for population health analytics initiatives. Data from multiple sources or organizations can be compiled into a data warehouse or repository to facilitate analysis of needs and evaluation of interventions.

Application Interoperability Using FHIR

Fast Healthcare Interoperability Resources (FHIR—pronounced "fire") is the latest standard to be developed under the HL7 healthcare standards organization.[8] Unlike the transaction standards aimed at system-to-system large-scale data exchange, the FHIR standards are intended to enable very targeted and specific data exchange, specifically for small applications, running on mobile devices or as add-on applications to an EHR, to perform specific tasks. Examples of such applications are:

- A growth chart tailored to genetic disorders, requiring a patient's age, height, and weight data
- A bilirubin calculator for newborns, to decide whether a newborn baby can safely be discharged or requires follow-up care

- A population healthcare management system using FHIR to retrieve up-to-date clinical information on a patient

FHIR-based application interfaces will be particularly relevant to population health initiatives by allowing organizations to extend the capabilities of EHRs with applications from other firms. These extensions can provide population health tools to physicians, care managers, and home health providers. FHIR-based applications can also help patients and family members track their care and manage chronic conditions. These interoperability tools allow patients to use mobile phone applications to retrieve data from their providers (medication lists, recommendations), or to upload data so their providers and caregivers can access them (activity data, medication adherence, notes, or questions).

A growing library of FHIR-based applications is available online. See the Suggested Readings and Websites section at the end of this chapter for more information.

▶ Health Information Exchanges

Health Information Exchanges (HIEs) are organizations that manage and enable the exchange of health data for a particular region or state. HIEs link together healthcare organizations (hospitals, physician practices, long-term care facilities, payers, and social service agencies), typically within a concentrated region, to allow them to share their patients' health data. This data exchange helps improve patient care and can increase efficiency and reduce the cost of care by avoiding redundant testing and diagnostic procedures.

One example of healthcare organizations improving care by exchanging data through an HIE shows how Florida hospitals reduce their readmissions, and particularly readmissions to other hospitals, by exchanging data on the HIE.[9]

Some HIEs are supported by public funding at the state level or by local grants; others may be funded by the participating organizations, including payers or hospitals. Since HIEs provide shared benefit to a region, funding to sustain and grow the HIE often depends on multi-party support and commitment. To remain viable, HIEs need to demonstrate value by improving quality and directly reducing the cost of care.

HIEs are important to regional population health initiatives. They serve as an important source of data that can provide valuable insights into population care beyond the borders of a single healthcare organization.

▶ Patient-Generated Data

The largest volume of clinical data today comes from EHRs and is usually entered into and captured at the healthcare facility. However, there is a growing set of patient-generated data, which has potentially important implications for population health. Patient-generated data can include[10]:

- Data from personal health devices, health trackers, and wearable technology. These devices typically upload data to a mobile phone app; from there, sometimes the information can be uploaded into a healthcare provider's EHR. Meaningful use/promoting interoperability requirements includes EHRs to be able to incorporate patient-generated data from more than 5% of patients discharged from the hospital.

- Data from home devices (connected scales, blood pressure devices, activity sensors), not necessarily worn on the body, with the ability to send the data to a healthcare provider.

- Data entered by the patient through a portal or app and shared with healthcare providers. Examples include pain logs, food and nutrition logs, mood logs, or pregnancy logs.

Healthcare providers may have concerns about having time to receive and review patient-generated data. However, in most cases, a provider would receive an abstracted measure—for example, a monthly average daily step count or average blood pressure. Average activity measures reported via patient-generated devices may help the healthcare provider to track a patient's physical activity and serve as a motivator for the patient.[11]

▶ Payment Models and How They Depend on IT Systems

As the U.S. health system transitions from fee-for-service payment into value-based care, a number of alternative payment models (APMs) have emerged. There is a spectrum of APMs, as described and illustrated in the Health Care Payment Learning and Action Network. There are "light" APMs that are slight modifications of fee-for-service payment, with a minor or modest percent increase or decrease based on quality or utilization measures. And there are APMs that to a large extent shift the financial responsibility of the care to the provider, through capitation and monthly PMPM (per member per month) payments to the primary care provider. As the HCP-LAN documentation describes, the future state of value-based care is not a single payment model, but each practice and each health system will participate and get reimbursement through a concurrent variety of APMs—from light to full-risk, depending on the patient's plan, the patient's disease or condition, and other factors.

▶ Financial and Claims Data

Cost and utilization are a core data need for any comprehensive population health analytics project. Almost all population health analytics reports and charts include an element of utilization: cost of care, number of encounters, length of stay, and number of post-acute days.

Health Provider Organizations, through their EHRs, have access to a wealth of clinical data. The opposite is true regarding claims and financial data. Because most patients see multiple providers across multiple organizations, it is often difficult for any single healthcare provider organization to have a full picture of a patient's healthcare utilization and cost.

Payers and health plans, including Medicare and Medicaid, have a more comprehensive view of a patient's utilization and healthcare costs. The payer usually has a complete record of all encounters, all utilization, all claims, and reimbursements.

The healthcare revenue cycle is complex and convoluted, and a detailed discussion is outside the scope of this chapter. Instead, below is a brief summary of the key financial data elements and their relevance to an at-risk healthcare organization, an ACO, and a population health analytics project.

Claims

The claim is sent as a financial transaction to the payer. Sent by the healthcare provider organization to the patient's health plan, the claim will have relevant details: encounter type (emergency department visit, office visit, lab visit), diagnosis codes, and a financial variable such as paid or allowed amount for the service. The claimed amount from the hospital does not usually take into account the various contracts and arrangements with the patient's health plan, so it is usually not relevant to analytics. The "paid" or "reimbursed" amount coming from the payer is the more relevant indicator of cost and utilization.

Payment and Reimbursement

After reviewing the information contained in the claim, the payer will determine an amount to be paid and reply to the provider, as a transaction that includes the reimbursed amount. There are two complications with this reimbursement transaction. Providers don't have accurate and timely data on reimbursement until approximately 90 days after the encounter. Second, there may be several corrections and adjustments to a payment, after some back-and-forth between provider and payer. This means that even when the reimbursed amount is available, it may change, causing fluctuations in cost and utilization data until well after 90 days after the encounter. If the population of patients is large, these fluctuations won't have much impact on the overall utilization data; for smaller and more targeted populations, it is possible to see reimbursement fluctuations. Data aggregation systems need to be able to distinguish between initial reimbursement and subsequent reimbursement messages pertaining to the same encounter—and to know when to add to the payment or replace an older figure with an updated amount.

Capitation

Some providers have contracts with their payers to receive fixed monthly payments for some of their patients. This results in a monthly payment per member per month (PMPM), usually to the primary care provider, who is held responsible for the care for this patient, no matter how many encounters this patient incurs. In such cases, the provider still submits claims to the payer but would not expect to be paid for most of these encounters. Most capitation arrangements include stop-loss provisions for catastrophic healthcare needs (major trauma, cancer treatments, etc.). Capitation is a major component of value-based care. From a data perspective, it complicates the calculation and determination of a patient's cost and utilization.

All payers share financial data with providers who participate in an alternative payment model, an ACO, or any at-risk arrangement. Medicare shares claims and reimbursement data with clinical providers who are "attributed to" that organization, using the Claims and Claims Line Feed (CCLF) file.[12] The CCLF file includes all encounters for this patient, including other providers the patient may have seen, and thus gives a more comprehensive utilization picture.

Attribution

Attribution is an important concept in population health because it defines the population of patients for whom a physician is responsible. Population health databases must include attribution data to properly connect the care of a patient to the provider who would be credited with the care quality and utilization for that patient. Under any alternative payment model or capitation, the payment incentive is directed at the provider to whom the patient is attributed. This is usually the primary care physician, but it can also be the physician who provided the majority of the patient's care in a certain time period. Medicare uses an attribution algorithm based on the physician, within certain specialties, where the patient had the most encounters.[13]

Utilization Approximation by Counting Encounters and Length of Stay

Based on the complexity of the financial and claims data above, many population health analytics applications use alternative measures for utilization—such as number of ED visits, number of inpatient admissions, and average length of stay measures. These non-financial utilization measures are often more practical to identify high- and low-utilizing patients and providers.

▶ Social Determinants of Health

What is true for individuals is also true for populations. The social determinants of health (SDOH) have a significant impact on the health status of a community.[14] Bazemore refers to these social determinants as "community vital signs" or key indicators of health to a community.[15] They include economic factors, education levels, environmental pollution, food or housing insecurity, crime, and stress levels. The community vital signs study referenced above organizes the social determinants into several categories—and provides helpful links to resources where researchers can get access to data sets on these social determinants.

Some of the main domains of social determinant data, as categories of community vital signs, are race/ethnicity, education, financial resources, stress, physical activity, and social connections.[15]

In addition to publicly available resources, there are a number of private companies that package data sets on populations—from surveys, social media data, media viewing reports, and other sources. Data sets at a household or individual person level are available for a fee. For many population health analytics applications, zip code or census tract level granularity is sufficient. Together, these public and private data sets can enable the creation of detailed insight into the social factors impacting health and health care in a community.

Two cases using SDOH in a population health setting highlight how the information can be applied to promote health:

- Care Management: A study by Reed and team shows that social determinants influence the way patients respond to care management initiatives.[16] Contrary to expectations, patients in this study with higher social risk factors did not take advantage of reduced-cost medications

for their chronic illness. Insight into a population's SDOH can help care managers to tailor their programs and initiatives (e.g., provide financial support for medications, self-management education on medical conditions, or home visits) to address specific needs.

- Social Risk-Adjusting Performance Measures: Most alternative payment models offer incentives for strong performance—high-quality scores, low cost and utilization—and penalties for lower scores. Most risk adjustment today is based on utilization risk—for example, using the Johns Hopkins risk model or AP-DRGs.[17] These measures are likely impacted, to some degree, by social determinants.[18] Providers serving populations with high social risk factors may achieve lower quality scores even with the same or stronger performance, so it would be important to take that into account when devising the reimbursement model. A risk adjustment using social determinants would level the playing field and create a fairer and more equitable system of incentives and penalties for these providers.

▶ Data Aggregation

Obtaining a complete set of health data for a population requires information from multiple sources, inside and outside of the healthcare delivery system. Data aggregation is often complicated, time-consuming, and expensive—and it is not a one-time initiative; organizations must maintain and update the incoming data feeds. Start with the data already available to the organization, and identify the key pieces needed to get a good sense of the health status of the population. Prioritize the most important sources and those that are easiest to access. Data aggregation is an ongoing process, not a one-time event.

The term *extract–transform–load* (*ETL*) is often used to describe the process of data manipulation to get it from multiple sources and into a merged consolidated target database. It is pretty simple: *Extract* data from the source databases. *Transform* it to fit into the new target model. *Load* it into the aggregated database or data warehouse (or, in this case, into the PHM system). The T step, *transform*, consists of multiple adjustments, each necessary to ensure that the target database is uniform, complete, uses consistent terminology, and does not contain duplicate entries—that is, it should be as clean and up-to-date as possible. There are specific tools for ETL on the market, and many large database software systems come with ETL capabilities included.

When consolidating data from multiple organizations, one of the first steps in the transformation process is to create a unique patient or personal ID to ensure that the data for a patient from multiple sources ends up stored as one individual patient in the target database. For organizations that use a master patient index (MPI) to create a single patient ID in multiple information systems, much of this patient ID mapping is already complete. Those that assemble data from multiple sources outside their organizations will need to use a mapping algorithm. Most ETL systems have these algorithms in place, including ways for the system to escalate to a human user if there is a question as to whether records should be merged.

The next step in the data aggregation is to remove duplicate items. A patient's data may be recorded in multiple systems, so it is important to avoid double-counting clinical encounters or diagnoses. This will need to occur each time new records are added.

Mapping terms to standard terminologies is another important step in terms of data aggregation and in the preparation of data for analysis. During the meaningful use program implementation, most organizations started using standard terms in their EHRs: SNOMED (Systematized Nomenclature for Medicine)[19] codes for problems and/or ICD10 (International Classification of Diseases)[20] codes for diagnoses, Current Procedural Terminology (CPT) codes for procedures/services,[21] LOINC (Logical Observation Identifiers Names and Codes)[22] for laboratory results and other observations or test results, and RxNorm codes[23] for medications (**TABLE 6-1**).

If these codes are not already in use in the source systems, the transformation step in the ETL may need to map from the source terminology to the standard terminology used in the analytical database.

There are important reasons for standardizing codes and terms:

- Reports and queries from the analytical database would become unmanageable if there were multiple ways for "heart failure" or "serum creatinine" to be coded in the source systems. A standard code makes queries and reports simpler and easier to maintain and less prone to error.
- Many of these terminologies are built as a hierarchy, with higher-level concepts broken down into more detailed concepts; these hierarchies are useful in analysis and queries. If

TABLE 6-1 STANDARDIZED HEALTHCARE CODING TERMINOLOGIES

Name	Domain	Main Website
SNOMED Codes (Systematized Nomenclature for Medicine)	Problems	http://www.snomed.org/
ICD-10 Codes (International Classification of Diseases)	Diagnoses	https://www.who.int/classifications/icd/ICD10Volume2_en_2010.pdf
Current Procedural Terminology	Procedures/services	https://www.ama-assn.org/amaone/cpt-current-procedural-terminology
LOINC (Logical Observation Identifiers Names and Codes)	Results and observations	https://loinc.org/learn/
RxNorm	Medications	https://www.nlm.nih.gov/research/umls/rxnorm/

you're looking for all patients who use an ACE inhibitor or a beta-blocker medication, it would take a long time to list them all in your report or query. RxNorm has a code for ACE inhibitors and beta-blockers that includes all the various medications within the specific drug class. Hierarchies and groups are indispensable in reporting and analytics—and require that your data are following standard terminologies.

Population data inevitably have gaps; it is virtually impossible to obtain all data for all patients. You need to be aware of the data gaps and take them into account in all analytical results and reports. Common examples of data gaps are:

■ *Out-of-Network Data*: if a patient has multiple visits to a specialist outside of your organization, there will almost always be certain data from encounters that are out of reach.

■ *Missing or Incomplete Interfaces*: organizations that exchange data through CDAs or HIEs may not send all of their information. Not all lab results are interfaced or transmitted. The organization may withhold information on encounters with a behavioral health code. The CDA includes the bare minimum data but omits other significant clinical data.

■ *Claims Lag*: all population health databases that take in claims from one or more health plans will have to account for the delay in the claim being processed and paid by the health plan; it usually takes three months but can take longer. There's nothing that can "fix" the claims lag; it is a byproduct of the payment process. The only thing to do is to be aware and take it into account.

■ *Acute Care vs. Ambulatory Data*: acute care data (hospital admissions, ED visits) and ambulatory data (visits to doctors' offices) may not be represented equally in the database. If the main data source is hospital data in an organization with many independent physician offices, the system is likely to have more acute care data and be missing ambulatory data. To balance acute care and ambulatory care, it is important to get data feeds from hospitals and outpatient practices relevant to the patient population—possibly in collaboration with the regional HIE. Whenever there is an imbalance, be sure to take it into account in your analytical results and reports.

- *Data Quality Measures*: Overall, develop measures for data quality that can be monitored, tracked, and presented visually via a report or dashboard. Data quality is a key pillar of **data governance** within an organization.

▶ Data Quality

Regardless of the number of sources, data quality will be an ongoing concern for the organization and technology team. Even if the organization has a single EHR system, many users contribute to the data through data collection screens and documentation templates. Variability of the data will increase as additional data sources are accessed, including patients, physician practices with other EHRs, utilization and claims data, and information regarding social determinants. Data quality becomes more challenging to manage as the data set grows. Your ETL engine plays a critical role in maintaining data quality—but there are other things you can do to manage and maintain the quality of your data.

There are several data quality assurance issues to consider:

- *Completeness of Clinical Data*: Are you capturing the complete clinical data set for your patient population? If not, can you identify what's missing? For example: certain time periods (before a particular data feed became active); encounter types (inpatient and ED encounters, outpatient visits); lab results (from your organization's lab and commercial labs); claims from all payers. There are many ways in which data sets may not be complete. Data gaps must be documented and taken into account to avoid reaching false conclusions based on missing data.
- *Accuracy*: There is always a risk of inaccurate and incomplete data. Machine-generated data (e.g., lab results coming from a lab analyzer) tend to be consistent and accurate, while human-entered data (height, weight, blood pressure) may contain more inconsistencies and inaccuracies. Data should be monitored regularly and areas of inaccuracies documented.
- *Duplication*: There is greater risk of duplication in data sets where data are aggregated from multiple sources. The main reasons for duplication are the same data came from different senders (e.g., encounter claims supplied from the provider and from the payer), or the same data came from the same sender in different batches/data files (e.g., encounter data are supplied from a payer in monthly batches but the monthly batch may include corrections and modifications to previous

months). ETL data load algorithms take these into account and work to eliminate duplicate encounters and data points. Nevertheless, it is possible that some duplicate items may be overlooked.

- *Patient Matching*: With data coming from multiple sources, there could be errors in patient matching regardless of the system the organization employs (Master Patient Index or another patient-matching algorithm) to make sure that the system recognizes that data from a Mary Jones should be combined with previous data from the same Mary Jones. These errors show up in two ways: data from two patients are merged into one, or data from the same person are split between two individual patients who are really the same person. These errors are hard to find and hard to fix.

- *Attribution*: In population health, patients are assigned to practices and providers—and these attribution algorithms don't always assign the right patient to the right provider, resulting in incorrect patient panels. Usually, the provider will point out when patients are included who should not have been, but the provider will often not realize that patients who should have been included were inadvertently left out. It's important to monitor patient attribution algorithms and address issues as they arise.

- *Data Profiling*: In an effort to understand the quality of each variable, it is important to run frequencies on each column of the dataset. This will identify any "junk" in the data such as blanks or question marks.

▶ Data Governance

Organizations maintaining a large data set for analytics must create an organizational structure and data governance team to manage this important asset. The team should consist of key players in the organization, who together oversee and manage operations associated with the data asset, including data quality issues, use of data and analytics, compliance, privacy and security matters, and strategic growth.

A short definition of data governance might be: "Data governance is the exercise of decision making and authority for data-related matters." A longer definition is: "Data governance is a system of decision rights and accountabilities for information-related processes, executed according to agreed-upon models which describe who can take what actions with what information, and when, under what circumstances, using what methods."[24]

There are many possible structures and participants on a data governance team, and the exact composition of the team will be different for each organization based on its needs, capacity, and available resources. A 2015 survey by the American Health Information Management Association (AHIMA) found that nearly one-third of participants have made no headway in promoting data governance as a business imperative, and another 24% added that governance is simply not a priority for their leadership.[25] This is a legitimate concern, as data governance involves a cultural change that companies struggle to implement.

The following skill sets and responsibilities are essential for the data governance team, for any size organization[26]:

- *Business Need and Strategic Use of the Data Asset*: This individual's role is to promote and advocate for the use of the data to inform key business decisions. In a population health setting, that would include use of the data for organizational strategic decisions (mergers, acquisitions, network extensions or partnerships, clinical programs and initiatives) and tactical tracking and management of population healthcare delivery—utilization, care quality, care gaps, provider performance. In a large population health organization, this role would typically fall to the CMO, CFO, or Medical Director for Population Health. This person is the champion for the data asset.

- *Technical Staffing and Budget*: The individual filling this role would be responsible for funding and staffing the growth and management of the data asset. In large organizations, this would be the CIO. In smaller organizations, it would be the person in charge of health IT. Having this person on the data governance team ensures that the organization will invest appropriately in the data asset, by staffing and funding it corresponding to the need.

- *Technical and Analytical Expertise*: The individual is the technical expert, responsible for ensuring that tools are in place to manage the data asset and to handle the amount of data flowing in and will prioritize and manage requests for analysis and reports. This person will manage "the stack"—the layered structure of the technology managing the data: from the servers storing the data to the ETL tool managing the inflows to the visualization and dashboard tools.

- *Informatics and Analytical Skills*: The data governance team needs someone who can help drive the organization in using the data asset to solve problems and answer questions. Typically, this is a subject-matter expert (versed in clinical care, population health, value-based care) who possesses a strong background in data and analytics.

- *Compliance, Privacy, and Security*: This critical role will be filled by the Chief Information Security Officer or the Director of Compliance. This individual will be responsible for ensuring that all legal and regulatory requirements are followed in managing the security and privacy of patient data and any other regulatory needs.

▶ Risk Stratification

Population health analytics and alternative payment models revolve around identifying patients and populations who need more care than others. This process is called risk stratification—creating groups with similar "risk," in this context, meaning the likelihood that these patients will seek care, or need care, and therefore will most likely have higher utilization. A risk stratification algorithm may label patients as being in one of five risk classes—from low to medium to high. There are many ways to calculate the risk for a population, often depending on the availability of data—but all risk score calculations use prior data to predict future utilization. Therefore, calculating risk scores, or stratifying the population by risk, would fall under "predictive analytics"—the type of analytics that aims to use historical patient data to predict the future and help us manage and anticipate the care for these patients.

Most commonly used risk scores use claims data to calculate risk—from the claims, the patient demographics, diagnosis codes, types of encounters (number of ED visits), and duration of the encounters (length of inpatient stays) are all factored into the patient's risk level, which is the likelihood for needing care in the coming year, or beyond. Other risk scores may incorporate clinical data (lab results, blood pressure, height and weight, medication use) or social determinants into the risk score, and include additional data, hoping to refine the risk calculation and make more accurate predictions about the patient's anticipated need for care.

Examples of risk scores used for population health risk stratification are:

- *Hierarchical Condition Codes (HCCs)*,[27] calculated by Medicare to use past encounters and diagnosis codes to predict the severity of illness for a patient and calculate the anticipated need for care. HCCs are also used to adjust payments to providers—patients with a higher HCC score are expected to need more care and more time, and the provider will receive higher reimbursement for patients with higher HCC scores. That same HCC level can be applied to risk-stratify populations.
- *Johns Hopkins ACG system*[17] calculates a five-level risk score for each patient or member, which can

become part of a care management application, a score to calculate the case mix for a practice, and the anticipated or relative cost and utilization for a population. ACGs are calculated based on claims data only.

- *Episode Risk Groups (ERGs)* Calculates a population-based health risk assessment. ERGs predict current and future healthcare usage for individuals and groups. It predicts a member's current (retrospective) and future (prospective) need for healthcare services and associated costs.[28]
- *Milliman* is one of several commercially available proprietary risk score calculations, widely used to risk stratify a population using prior data. The MARA model[29] is used to produce category risk scores that explain the expected resource use for service components (emergency room, physician services, etc.).
- *Reference to the Social Determinant/ Cardiac disease risk score in* Health Affairs is an example of including social determinant data to improve the predictive value.[18]

Once a risk score can be assigned to each member or patient in the data set, there are several obvious applications:

- *Risk Stratification*: Subdivide the population by risk—and focus certain reports or analysis on the high-risk population only or to the group of patients who are not yet high risk but are found to be at increasing risk (often referred to as the *rising risk population*). Once identified, this population can be narrowed down by diagnosis, by provider, by care management program, and the level of care and utilization can be determined for these patients.

- *Care Management*: Stratify cohorts of patients by level of anticipated care needs, and focus care management and care coordination on specific groups of patients who will need it most. Once identified, it is important to track those patients over time and determine if care management initiatives are indeed helping the patients and reducing the need for high-acuity care (avoiding ED visits or hospital admissions).
- *Risk Adjustment of Provider Performance Data* Doctor A's patients with heart failure have more ED visits than Doctor B's patients. Is that because Dr. A doesn't manage the patients as effectively as Dr. B, or are Dr. A's patients sicker and need more care and are therefore at greater risk for going to the ED? Risk adjustment can help determine the answer by adjusting the quality and utilization measures based on the patients' average level of risk.

The ability to calculate risk scores, and adjust them regularly based on incoming data, is an important element of a population health analytics application. Whether one uses a standard or commercially available risk score calculation or creates a risk score based on an existing data set, the ability to stratify populations and cohorts by risk is a fundamental need for all population health applications.

▶ Analysis and Reporting

We have discussed the steps required to bring data from multiple sources together into a data asset ready for analysis and reporting. The data are aggregated, normalized, scrubbed, and ready for building reports and dashboards.

Analysis and reporting are the final steps in the population health data analysis cycle, and they come in various forms and deliverables. A wide variety of tools and systems are available to build the final product. In each case, your goal is to give your audience *insight*, a deeper understanding on what they can learn from the data. This can simply be a report, a spreadsheet delivered weekly or monthly, on the key performance indicators for a department or a practice.

An example of typical measures that can be used in analytics and reporting are cost and utilization data. These data can be expressed either in currency (dollars) or service units. If for any reason there is no direct access to cost information, a proxy measure can be the number of ED visits, inpatient admissions, primary care office visits, specialist visits, length of stay, or other encounter counts that reflect the level of care utilization for the population. These cost metrics or encounter counts are usually presented as a "per member" count: per member per month (PMPM), per member per year (PMPY), or as an expression of a group count per 1,000 members (/1,000). The benefit of PMPM or /1,000 measures is that they are comparable independent of the number of patients in a practice. For example, if a practice, in a given period, has 40 ED visits across a population of 250 patients, their ED visits/1,000 would be 160, which makes the number comparable and trackable across all practices.

There are a variety of reporting tools, analytical visualization tools, and dashboard applications on the market.

Examples include Tableau, Qlik, Cognos, Business Objects, Plotly, and many others. Your organization most likely already has one or more analytics and dashboard tools available. To use these tools effectively in your organization, you need to focus on two requirements: (1) Do the reports and dashboards answer the right questions? (2) Is your audience actually using the tools and dashboards available to them? In other words, are the reports and visualizations designed to answer the questions that your organization is requesting, and is there a good way to disseminate this information to the users who need it?

The process of designing reports and dashboards starts with framing the questions in full detail and specificity and then identifying the data required to answer these questions and developing the views and visualizations that give the best results and answers to the end users. This is an iterative process, requiring ongoing feedback and refinement.

The presentation of the results can take many forms, depending on the needs of the users:

- A quarterly report on the clinical performance metrics for all practices in the health system, targeted at the clinical leadership team.
- A daily list of patients scheduled for a visit with the most relevant care gaps and intervention opportunities, targeted at a practice care management team.
- An interactive dashboard on key performance measures for the organization, where users can alter the reporting parameters, such as reporting time period, patient age groups, diagnoses, practice areas, for interactive drill down into data—targeted at

business analysts with a deep understanding of the data.

- A monthly email or bulletin, targeted at physicians and nurses in the organization, giving insight and monthly updates on the key initiatives and showing them the data for the previous months.
- A daily or hourly display of a few key metrics (ED throughput or waiting times, patients at risk for readmission and in need of urgent care management), shown on monitors in key department areas, targeted at operational staff in your organization.

Different users require different methods of dissemination. Some users will log on to a dashboard and actively engage in the data analysis. Other users or audiences are better served with a regular email or even printed summary of the metrics important to them. For some users, the best format is a worklist or a chart. For others, it is a set of visualizations on a dashboard. There is no "one size fits all" delivery or dissemination, and your organization should be prepared to deliver analytics and reports in a variety of ways.

For all of these dissemination methods, it is important that you track which users are actually receiving and using the information. If you use email delivery, track how many users actually open and read the email. If you use a dashboard and visualization tool, track the number of log-ons and which users actually review the data. Also track what data are used and accessed most frequently. In an era of information overload, it is not easy to reach the right users with the right information, but that's a critical step in the analytics and reporting process.

Tracking utilization of reports and dashboards allows you to track the effectiveness of data use in your organization. In a true data-driven organization, users depend on the data to do their work at every level of the organization. If your tracking data show limited or no use of data, you would need to engage this underutilizing group of users in a conversation to improve either the content and format, or the dissemination method, or both. All workers in a population health organization need data to do their work effectively. By tracking the use of the analytics and reports, you will be able to determine which workers are using data frequently and effectively in their work and where you need to continue the cycle of analytics-based decision making to reach effective data-driven decisions.

▶ Artificial Intelligence and Machine Learning in Population Health

Davenport[30] makes the case that one of the future applications of artificial intelligence (AI) will be in analytics—which would point the way for AI applications in population health. His rationale for using AI in analytics is that in his experience, humans don't use analytical tools sufficiently to solve business problems, creating an opening for AI applications to do the work that human analysts don't do. And if we look at the use of data, and the strength of analytical teams in population health organizations, his finding seems correct: there are a lot of data available waiting to be analyzed and turned into decisions and actions.

To make AI and machine learning work in population health applications,

we need large and comprehensive data sets, which need to have both the inputs (patient data, doctor data, clinical and utilization data, social determinants) and the outputs connected to those inputs (which providers, using what methods, achieve the best combination of care quality and efficiency? What population health organizations and initiatives work and deliver strong and effective population health, and which don't? Which organizations are maximizing revenue using Alternative Payment Models and how do they do it? Those data don't exist, and until they *do* exist, we cannot rely on AI- or ML- derived recommendations. Our industry focus needs to be primarily on building the data sets that will ultimately allow us to apply AI- and ML techniques to population health data sets.

▶ Conclusion

Following are some key takeaways to support your organization's journey to data-driven population health:

- *Population health has a dependence on data and analytics*. Population health is a care delivery model focused on the health and wellness of a defined population—a group of patients in a geographic region, attributed to a practice, or with a specific condition, or covered under a health plan. This care delivery model is supported by a reimbursement model that aligns the incentives to maximize the health of the population at the lowest cost or utilization over the long term.
- *Data are an asset*. As this chapter makes clear, a strong population health initiative is built on a strong

and growing data asset. Use your own organization's data and bring them together into a data warehouse, or data asset. Then add data from other sources, through an ongoing data acquisition and data aggregation project. Aim for a strong combination of clinical data, financial and utilization data, some patient-generated data, and social determinants of health.

- *Optimize your EHR(s)*. EHRs provide the data infrastructure on which population health initiatives are built. Without EHRs in place, there would be no way to identify specific populations attributed to a provider, those with chronic conditions, or high levels of need; in short, it would not be possible to coordinate and manage the care for these populations. Perhaps most importantly, without EHRs, patients would not have the same level of access to their own data and records, which is a critical component of improving population health.
- *Create a data governance committee or capability within your organization*. The team should consist of key players in the organization, who together oversee and manage operations associated with the data asset, including master data management, data assets, use of data and analytics,

compliance, privacy and security, and strategic growth.

- *Data quality is a key component in healthcare analytics*. Data quality measures are needed to routinely report and monitor data.
- *Registries help organize data*. Create several registries in a generic format, with the ability to track populations throughout your organization. This can be patients with a chronic illness, in the more traditional use of a registry, but also patients who participate in care management programs or are enrolled in community-based health projects.
- *Implement Davenport's analytical process*. This process can be used on analytical questions of increasing complexity. Include clinical, operational, and financial or utilization metrics. Look at various patient populations.
- *Risk stratification is an important part of utilizing data in population health*. Creating groups with similar "risk"—in this context meaning the likelihood that they will seek care or need care, and therefore will most likely have higher utilization. These data are factored into the patient's risk level, which is the likelihood for needing care in the coming year or beyond.

Study and Discussion Questions

1. Why is population health management key to supporting population health initiatives?

2. Define data governance, and describe its main functions in an organization.

3. Why is the transition to electronic health records so important for population health?

4. Define risk stratification, and give some examples of how it is utilized.

Suggested Readings and Websites

Bazemore AW, Cottrell EK, Gold R, Hughes LS, Phillipos RL, Angier H, et al. "Community vital signs": incorporating geocoded social determinants into electronic records to promote patient and population health. *J Am Med Inform Assoc.* 2016;23(2):407–412.

Davenport TH, Harris J. *Competing on Analytics: The New Science of Winning.* Cambridge, MA: Harvard Business Review Press; 2017.

Davenport TH, Kim J. (2013). *Keeping Up With the Quants: Your Guide to Understanding and Using Analytics.* Cambridge, MA: Harvard Business Review Press.

Natarajan P, Frenzel JC, Smaltz DH. (2017). *Demystifying Big Data and Machine Learning for Healthcare.* Boca Raton, FL: CRC Press.

Siegel E. (2013). *Predictive Analytics: The Power to Predict Who Will Click, Buy, Lie, or Die.* New York: John Wiley & Sons.

Seiner RS. (2014). *Non-Invasive Data Governance: The Path of Least Resistance and Greatest Success.* Denville, NJ: Technics Publications.

Tufte ER. (2001). *The Visual Display of Quantitative Information* (Vol. 2). Cheshire, CT: Graphics Press.

Centers for Medicare and Medicaid Services. Risk Adjustment. Available at /medicare/health-plans/medicareadvtgspecratestats/risk-adjustors.html (accessed May 21, 2019).

Agency for Healthcare Research and Quality. Research Tools and Data. Available at https://www.ahrq.gov/research/index.html (accessed May 21, 2019).

Health Care Payment Learning and Action Network. What Is the Health Care Payment Learning & Action Network? Available at https://hcp-lan.org/ (accessed May 21, 2019).

National Quality Forum. Available at www.qualityforum.org (accessed May 21, 2019).

Fast Healthcare Interoperability Resources. SMART App Gallery. Available at https://apps.smarthealthit.org/apps/ (accessed May 21, 2019).

References

1. Kindig D, Stoddart G. What is population health? *Am J Public Health.* 2003;93(3):380–383.
2. Centers for Disease Control and Prevention. Public Health and Promoting Interoperability Programs (formerly Electronic Health Records Meaningful Use), Meaningful Use: Introduction. 2017. Available at https://www.cdc.gov/ehrmeaningfuluse/introduction.html (accessed April 3, 2019).
3. HIMSS analytics. Electronic Medical Record Adoption Model. Available at https://www.himssanalytics.org/emram (accessed April 3, 2019).
4. Singh H, Sittig DF. Measuring and improving patient safety through health information technology: The Health IT Safety Framework. *BMJ Qual Saf.* 2016:25:226–232. Available at https://qualitysafety.bmj.com/content/qhc/25/4/226.full.pdf (accessed April 3, 2019).
5. Sinsky C, Colligan L, Ling L, Prgomet M, Reynolds S, et al. Allocation of physician time in ambulatory practice: a time and motion study in 4 specialties. *Ann Intern Med.* 2016;54(11):753–760.
6. HL7 International. Introduction to HL7 Standards Health Level Seven International. 2017-2019. Ann Arbor, MI. Available at http://www.hl7.org/implement/standards/ (accessed April 3, 2019).
7. Office of the National Coordinator for Health Information Technology (ONC). Consolidated CDA Overview. Updated January 14, 2019. Washington, DC. Available at https://www.healthit.gov/topic/standards-technology/consolidated-cda-overview (accessed April 3, 2019).
8. HL7 International. FHIR Overview, Release 4.0. HL7 Foundation. December 27, 2018. Available at https://www.hl7.org/fhir/overview.html (accessed April 3, 2019).
9. Chen M, Guo S, Tan X. Does health information exchange improve patient outcomes? Empirical evidence from Florida hospitals. *Health Aff.* 2019;38(2). Available at https://doi.org/10.1377/hlthaff.2018.05447 (accessed April 3, 2019).
10. Sands DZ, Wald JS. Transforming health care delivery through consumer engagement, health

data transparency, and patient-generated health information. *IMIA Yearbook of Medical Informatics*. 2014;9:170–176.

11. Feller DJ, Burgermaster M, Levine ME, Smaldone A, Davidson PG, Albers DJ, Mamykina L. A visual analytics approach for pattern-recognition in patient-generated data. *J Am Med Inform Assoc*. 2018;25(10):1366–1374.

12. Medicare Shared Savings Program: Claim and claim line feed file data elements. Resource Version 1. January 2019. Available at https://www.cms .gov/Medicare/Medicare-Fee-for -Service-Payment/sharedsavingsprogram /Downloads/2019-CCLF-file-data-elements -resource.pdf (accessed April 3, 2019).

13. Centers for Medicare and Medicaid Services. Fact sheet: Two-step attribution for claims-based quality outcome measures and per capita cost measures included in the value modifier. Available at https: //www.cms.gov/Medicare/Medicare-Fee-for -Service-Payment/PhysicianFeedbackProgram /Downloads/2016-03-25-Attribution-Fact- Sheet.pdf (accessed April 3, 2019).

14. Hughes LS, Phillips RL Jr, DeVoe JE, Bazemore AW. Community vital signs: taking the pulse of the community while caring for patients. *J Am Board Fam Med*. 2016;29(3):419–422.

15. Bazemore AW, Cottrell EK, Gold R, Hughes LS, Phillipos RL, Angier H, et al. "Community vital signs": incorporating geocoded social determinants into electronic records to promote patient and population health. *J Am Med Inform Assoc*. 2016;23(2):407–412.

16. Reed ME, Warton EM, Kim E, Solomon MD, Karter AJ. Value-based insurance design benefit offsets reductions in medication adherence associated with switch to deductible plan. *Health Aff*. 2017;36(3):516–523.

17. The Johns Hopkins ACG System. Johns Hopkins Healthcare Solutions. Available at https://www .hopkinsacg.org/ (accessed April 3, 2019).

18. Dalton JE, Perzynski AT, Zidar DA, Rothberg MB, Coulton CJ, Milinovich AT, et al. Accuracy of cardiovascular risk prediction varies by neighborhood socioeconomic position: a retrospective cohort study. *Ann Intern Med*. 2017;167(7):456–464.

19. SNOMED International. SNOMED CT 5-step briefing. 2019. Available at http://www.snomed .org.(accessed April 3, 2019).

20. World Health Organization. International statistical classification of diseases and related health problems, 10th revision, volume 2, instruction manual. 2011. Available at https://www.who.int/classifications/icd /ICD10Volume2_en_2010.pdf (accessed April 3, 2019).

21. American Medical Association. Current Procedural Terminology (CPT). 2019. Available at https://www.ama-assnorg/amaone/cpt-current -procedural-terminology (accessed April 3, 2019).

22. Regenstrief Institute, Inc. Logical Observation Identifiers Names and Codes (LOINC) Library. 2019. Available at https://loinc.org/learn/ (accessed April 3, 2019).

23. U.S. Department of Health and Human Services; U.S. National Library of Medicine. Unified Medical Language System (UMLS). Available at https://www.nlm.nih.gov/research /umls/rxnorm/ (accessed April 3, 2019).

24. Thomas G. DGI Data Governance Framework. Data Governance Institute. 2014. Available at http://www.datagovernance.com/wp-content /uploads/2014/11/dgi_framework.pdf (accessed April 3, 2019).

25. Bresnick J. The role of healthcare data governance in big data analytics. *Health IT Analytics*, July 29, 2016. Available at https: //healthitanalytics.com/features/the-role-of -healthcare-data-governance-in-big-data -analytics (accessed April 3, 2019).

26. GovernYourData: Resources. What is data governance? Available at http://governyourdata .com/page/what-is-data-governance (accessed April 3, 2019).

27. AAPC. Hierarchical Condition Category (HCC) Model. Available at https://www.aapc.com/risk -adjustment/hcc-model.aspx (accessed April 3, 2019).

28. Optum, Inc. Symmetry Episode Risk Groups (ERG) [white paper]. Available at https://www .optum.com/resources/library/symmetry-erg .html (accessed April 3, 2019).

29. Milliman Advanced Risk Technologies. MARA 3.0—Risk scores. 2017-2019. Available at http://www.millimanriskadjustment.com/risk-scores/ (accessed April 3, 2019).

30. Davenport TH, Ronanki R. Artificial intelligence for the real world. *Harv Bus Rev.* 2018;Jan-Feb: 108–116. Available at https://hbr.org/2018/01/artificial-intelligence-for-the-real-world (accessed April 3, 2019).

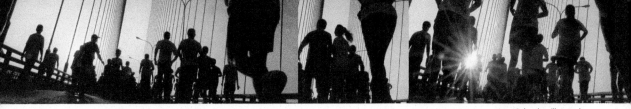

CHAPTER 7

Developing the Workforce to Enhance Population Health

Robert Sachs
Alexis Skoufalos*

EXECUTIVE SUMMARY

To be effective, a population health strategy requires a workforce capable of performing the roles that are critical to achieving the desired outcomes. The workforce that serves individuals under a population health paradigm includes, but goes well beyond, clinical care providers, support staff, administrators, and board members within a delivery network. In addition to connecting with patients and with one another, many in the workforce will need to identify and interact with the multiple community stakeholders that impact the social determinants that ultimately have a profound effect on health outcomes.

Tailored programs to introduce or improve workforce skills and competencies in population health are required to meet the critical learning needs of these diverse audiences. Training in interprofessional practice, change management, quality improvement, systems thinking, and communication are key to the success of population health interventions.

Simply working to overhaul the traditional curriculum and training of new healthcare providers, practitioners and leaders will not meet the needs of the workforce—and, more important, the needs of patients and the communities in which they live. As changes to care delivery, reimbursement paradigms, and clinical guidelines and other changes occur, the workforce needs to be capable of responding to a system that is extremely dynamic—one in which the stakeholders are required to develop and implement changes that will shift and disrupt many traditional relationships. It is critical that the right learning and development is ready and available to those who are leading that change, are working to allocate resources and personnel and to develop and manage relationships in a way that advances the goal of better care, at a better cost, and better health for everyone.

*   Thanks to Katherine Puskarz and Michael Molta for their assistance with this chapter.

▶ Introduction

A decade after the passage of the Affordable Care Act, the United States healthcare system is still in a state of disruption, and debate continues regarding the correct legislative response. Concerns over cost, quality, and access are key drivers of this turmoil. According to an analysis by Bradley Sawyer and Cynthia Cox of the Kaiser Family Foundation, "relative to the size of its wealth, the U.S. spends a disproportionate amount on health care."[1] They point out that the United States spends about twice as much per person on healthcare services as other developed countries, and spends significantly less on social service supports. Despite this high level of healthcare spending, the United States trails countries who spend less in measures of population health, including obesity, infant mortality, and life expectancy.[2]

▶ A Focus on Population Health

There have been, and continue to be, multiple efforts to address this discrepancy between spending and outcomes. Prominent among these efforts has been an ongoing shift toward paying for value rather than volume of services. The shift from volume to value has placed greater emphasis on keeping people healthy and out of the hospital.

This increased focus on population health is likely to intensify as stakeholders seek ways to use healthcare resources more effectively to improve the lifetime health and wellbeing of specific populations.[3]

Social Determinants Drive Population Health

Successful efforts at improving population health will need to address the social determinants of health. According to the Robert Wood Johnson Foundation, access to healthcare services and the quality of that care account for 20% of the health of a population (**FIGURE 7-1**). The remaining 80% is explained by social factors, including socioeconomic (income, employment, education, food insecurity), environmental (safety, housing insecurity), and behavioral factors (diet, exercise, smoking, and drug or alcohol use).[4] Kindig and Milstein

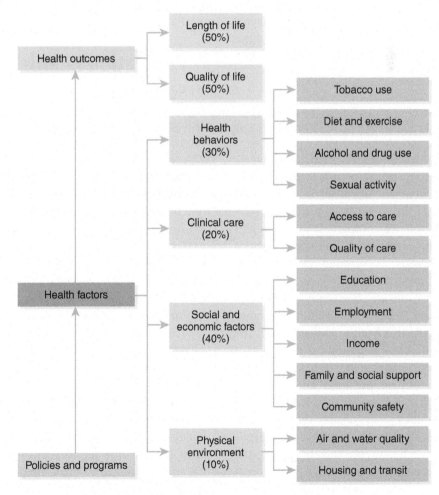

FIGURE 7-1 County Health Rankings & Roadmaps.

Reproduced from County Health Rankings & Roadmaps, http://www.countyhealthrankings.org/our-approach (accessed March 28, 2019).

suggest that efforts to address these factors examine the U.S. healthcare investment portfolio.[5] They argue that current investments are too heavily allocated to healthcare services and not enough resources address the social, economic, and environmental conditions that determine health and wellbeing. They call for a rebalancing of investments to improve population health, reduce healthcare disparities, and help build a culture of health for all Americans. This is not an easy task. Rebalancing is difficult in a healthcare delivery system consisting of multiple players that manage their investments to align with their own priorities, objectives, and perspectives.

Collaboration Is Required Across the Health Ecosystem

The health ecosystem is made up of diverse yet interdependent sectors with a shared interest in improving health outcomes and quality of life. It includes providers, payers, life science companies, public health agencies, government, and social service organizations. As argued in the book, *From Competition to Collaboration: How Leaders Cultivate Partnerships to Drive Value and Transform Health*, fragmentation across this health ecosystem and the resulting lack of alignment is a significant obstacle to rebalancing the U.S. healthcare investment portfolio and achieving demonstrable change in the health of our communities.[6] To create the balanced investment portfolio required to improve population health, the stakeholders in the health ecosystem must collaborate to create new organizational models that leverage scale, expand expertise, share risk, and support innovation.

Collaboration across this diverse set of players is a complex undertaking; it takes time and requires great skill. In trying to meet the needs of the communities and patients they mutually serve, while also balancing the interests of their respective stakeholders, health organizations will grapple with issues of reimbursement, investment, data sharing, uses of technology and, ultimately, leadership and decision-making. Despite this complexity, it is critical to develop strategies to improve the health of targeted populations.

▶ Population Health Strategy

Strategy defines how organizations will use resources to create value for customers and achieve their objectives. Because resources are finite, strategy requires choices. These choices include *who* will be served (customers), *where* resources will be focused, and *how* those resources will be used to serve the identified customers.[7] Because supporting population health requires an ecosystem perspective, organizations also need to define the *partners* they will work with to meet the defined objectives.

The *who* in a population health strategy is the target group for specific improvements in health. A population is typically defined by geography, condition or other relevant characteristics. Potential resources include time, money, facilities, staff, technology and data. *How* to serve the population includes the services and programs that will be utilized to meet the objectives and *where* those efforts are needed.

Constructing a population health strategy that effectively addresses *how* and *where* efforts will be focused requires the identification of the resources that are already available and where new resources are required. ReThink Health has developed a framework, *Negotiating a Well-Being Portfolio*, which outlines the range of activities that need to be considered in a community's health ecosystem.[8] Each of these areas represents policies, programs, and practices that address either *urgent needs* or *vital conditions*. Services in *urgent needs*, like acute care, food services, or housing insecurity, are the resources people may need to regain or restore health or wellbeing. It is also important to consider investments in *vital conditions*, like education, transportation and a living wage, that all people need to be healthy and well. ReThink also points out that any comprehensive strategy should consider including investments in arts, culture, spiritual life, and support for civil rights that support the development of the capacities of people and institutions to convey a sense of belonging and power to influence the policies, practices, and programs in the community. With this broad understanding, organizations can begin to create a comprehensive population health strategy that defines the areas requiring additional focus and investment to yield the desired results. This information also helps to identify additional partners that are required.

Having defined *who*, *where* and *how*, the strategy needs to specify the *partners* that need to be included to provide the required services or to contribute specific resources. In a best-case scenario, potential partners will all be at the table very early in the process of building the population health strategy. As additional partners are engaged and contribute their own perspectives and approaches to the discussion, the initial strategy will need to be reviewed and revised. A Community Health Needs Assessment (CHNA) can be a useful tool in pulling together these stakeholders "to identify and understand the community's health needs, and to ensure the partnership is united to pursue shared interest and vision for community health improvement."[9] In a situation in which a CHNA has not been completed, some entity needs to takes steps to identify and enlist potential partners.

Developing Workforce Support for Population Health Strategy

The success of any strategy requires that people have the skills and motivation needed to perform the necessary work and deliver the required services. Population health leaders best understand the outcomes that need to be delivered, the challenges to be faced, and the stakeholders that need to be involved. They must prioritize workforce development to ensure the organization has the people, demonstrating the capabilities, needed to deliver the population health strategy.

While individuals with expertise in areas like learning and development and recruitment can build programs to align the workforce to the strategy, they need the population health leaders to be the subject matter experts (SMEs) who inform the requirements for those programs. Population health leaders must understand workforce development in order to ask the right questions and evaluate recommended plans.

Perhaps the most important role for the leaders is as sponsors of the work. As sponsors, they must assure the necessary resources (defined as time, money and people) are available to design and deliver the appropriate workforce development solutions. Sponsorship cannot be delegated; without sponsorship, it is unlikely that workforce development efforts will be successful. The remainder of this chapter provides a blueprint that will help population health leaders to be effective SMEs and sponsors for the workforce development strategy and plan.

▶ Creating A Workforce Development Strategy and Plan

Defining the Need: Identify Critical Roles

The workforce development strategy must be tied to the organization's population health strategy and its desired outcomes. The workforce development strategy begins with the identification of roles that are critical to achieving the outcomes defined by the strategy. Defining critical roles helps the organization target development investments. Critical roles are those with the most significant impact on outcomes. If these positions are left vacant or are occupied by individuals who do not possess the right skills, the organization is not likely to realize its strategy. These could be roles that:

- Are central to creating the population health strategy
- Manage other critical positions
- Manage resources that are important to the population health strategy

- Significantly impact building and managing relationships with other organizations
- Require unique skills

The process of identifying critical roles should be broad and systematic, since critical roles can be located at multiple levels of an organization (executive, senior, middle, and front-line management as well as front-line staff) and in diverse functions. Depending on the strategy and the organization, key roles can exist in clinical, operations, sales, marketing, community relations, finance, IT, or contracting. The identification of these roles starts with the definition of the capabilities most necessary to deliver the desired results. Two examples would be: (1) the collection and analysis of data to identify population segments for health improvement and care and (2) building and managing community partnerships. Once the key capabilities are defined, the organization can systematically identify which positions are central to demonstrating those capabilities.

A population health strategy is likely to require some change in organizational capabilities. It is likely to shift the locus of care, add emphasis on enhancing health and pay more attention to social determinants. Some of the capabilities needed to address these changes may not exist in current job descriptions. In that case, job descriptions may need to be modified to reflect the new requirements or entirely new positions may need to be defined and staffed. Examples of critical population health roles are contained in the Advisory Board's library of population health-related job descriptions.[10] Among the jobs in the library are positions related to:

- **The Patient-Centered Medical Home:** Patient Care Medical Home Educator, Manager of Population Health Analytics, RN Health Coach
- **Care Management Inpatient:** Supervisor of RN Case Management, Care Manager
- **Care Management Cross-Continuum:** Care Transitions Coach, Director of Transition Management, Behavioral Health Peer Support Bridge
- **Community Health:** Community Resource Specialist, Community Education Specialist
- **Population Health/Care Transformation Leadership:** Vice President of Population Health Management
- **Telehealth:** Telehealth Coordinator, Director of E-Health for Technology Vendor

Organizations that develop population health strategies and do not directly deliver healthcare services (e.g., payers, community agencies, health science companies) will also need to identify roles that reflect their strategy and their unique contribution to population health in the broader ecosystem. And, given the need for a broad ecosystem perspective, all the stakeholders in the health ecosystem need to ensure that they have roles that focus on building relationships and working successfully across organizational boundaries and with organizations that operate in other sectors.

Defining Critical Roles and Timing

Some critical roles will be single-incumbent jobs. This is particularly true of roles at the senior levels of management. Other roles will require the organization to fill multiple jobs. The closer the role is to the front line, the more likely the role will represent multiple positions and need more people to be available.

Timing is also important and should be defined. The population health strategy will need different capabilities at different stages of the strategy design and implementation, and not all critical roles need to be staffed at the same time. The capabilities needed as the strategy is being developed are likely to be different than what will be needed once that strategy is in the process of being implemented and when it is fully operational.

Determining which critical roles are needed to advance the strategy from one stage to the next will help guide the timing and type of investment required to ensure that the right people are available at the right time. The more people required and the sooner they are needed, the more likely that it will be necessary to acquire new talent to meet some of the needs. Before this can be determined, it's important to be clear on the specific competencies required for each role.

Identifying the Competencies Required for Each Role

Competencies are the combination of knowledge, skills, and behaviors a person must demonstrate to be successful in a defined position. Competencies are gained through education, training, experience, and natural abilities. The competencies for critical roles in population health are based on the contribution of each role to achieving the outcomes defined by the strategy. For the strategy to be successful, individuals in critical roles must consistently demonstrate mastery of the competencies of each role.

The identification of competencies starts with defining outcomes. Once outcomes are clearly stated, the focus shifts to the performance that is required to achieve those outcomes. Put simply, performance is what people need to do to accomplish a specific set of outcomes. With outcomes and performance delineated, competencies can be defined by several methods, including literature review, expert panels and interviews, surveys, and study of individuals who are already demonstrating success in the role. Whatever methods are used, it is important to narrow the focus to the key results and the competencies that are most critical to achieving those results.

The Importance of Understanding Organizational Culture

When defining competencies, it is also important to consider the organizational culture that supports the strategy. Culture determines how organizations make decisions and characterizes the behaviors that are consistently demonstrated and reinforced within an organization. In other words, "it's how we do things here." Success requires a strong alignment between culture and strategy, particularly when the new strategy represents a significant shift from the existing norms.

Groysburg and colleagues provide a useful framework for thinking about culture.[11] They identified two primary dimensions that apply regardless of organization type, size, or industry:

- How people interact—highly independent to highly interdependent

- Response to change—stability to flexibility

Mapping culture against these dimensions identifies eight cultural styles that map to according to the degree they reflect the two dimensions:

1. Caring
2. Purpose
3. Learning
4. Enjoyment
5. Results
6. Authority
7. Safety
8. Order

The research by Groysburg et al. indicates that a strong culture aligned to the strategy drives organizational outcomes. The behavior of people in critical roles should reflect the cultural dimensions and styles that the organization has identified as important to achieving the desired outcomes.

Given the need for collaboration across the ecosystem and a focus on improving health in communities, it is likely that a population health strategy will seek a culture relatively strong on flexibility and interdependence and will include cultural styles of Purpose, Learning, and Caring. **Purpose** style describes an organization that is mission-driven, idealistic, and tolerant and will appreciate diversity, sustainability, and social responsibility. A **Learning** culture will be open, inventive, and willing to explore and will demonstrate improved innovation, agility, and organizational learning. Finally, a **Caring** organization will be warm, sincere, and relational, supporting teamwork, engagement, communication and trust. The competencies for critical population health roles should support these characteristics and any other cultural styles identified by the organization as important to achieving the strategy.

An Example of a Competency Model

An example of competency definition was reported by Harris, Puskarz, and Golab.[12] This model reflects the outcomes associated with population health and the culture that supports those outcomes.

Using a literature search, a scan of graduate health programs, and an expert panel, they identified six domains of knowledge and skills that population health practitioners must possess to be effective in achieving population health outcomes:

- **Health Systems**: The structure, stakeholders and processes of local, state, and national health systems
- **Legal, Regulatory, and Administrative**: Including state and federal laws, relevant regulations, and ethical standards
- **Social, Behavioral, and Environmental Factors**: The factors outside of medical care that influence health
- **Analytics**: Ability to use epidemiological, and outcomes research, sources of data, and statistical analysis
- **Process and Design**: Skills required to plan, build, and maintain an organization or intervention
- **Interpersonal**: Skills and techniques to enhance communication and collaboration between various parties

This model shows the importance of including knowledge, skills, and behaviors in the competency definition. The authors believe that a curriculum based on this framework by "drawing siloed experts into new perspectives and broadening their knowledge and skills base for successful navigation in a rapidly evolving health landscape"[12] will help build the future leaders of population health.

Identifying the Gaps

Once the critical roles (and the competencies required) have been identified and the number of individual positions represented by those roles is known, it is important to quantify the gaps between the talent available to fill those roles and the talent needed. Individuals in roles that are currently filled need to be assessed against the defined competencies. For roles that need to be created, potential feeder roles should be identified. Feeder roles require some of the important competencies but may be missing some critical elements. The incumbents in those roles are candidates for the roles that will be created and can be assessed against the requirements for those new roles. Assessing individuals against the critical role competencies will provide a picture of the number of individuals who are a potential match for the role requirements and which competency areas require some action to close the gaps.

The review of individuals currently in a key role (or those who have the potential for a key role) needs to go beyond a simple headcount. It is just as important to understand the nature of the competency gap. Gaps in knowledge require different development approaches and timelines beyond the development of skills or behaviors. In many cases the gaps will be in more than one area, requiring a combination of development approaches.

A success profile that categorizes the identified competencies can a useful tool.

A simple format distributes the competencies into four categories:

- **Knowledge**: What a high-performing individual needs to know.
- **Skills**: The tasks/activities that a high-performing individual needs to be able to perform.
- **Experience**: Successful individuals will come to the role with experience in situations where they apply and expand knowledge, and utilize, demonstrate and practice the required skills and behaviors.
- **Behaviors**: How successful performers behave.

Building on the Harris et al. model, a success profile might look like **TABLE 7-1**.

Individuals in a critical role, or candidates for one of these roles, can be evaluated with a simple 1–5 scale (1 = absent, 3 = adequate, 5 = strength) against each component of the profile. If appropriate, there are also multiple formalized tools that can be used to assess each element in the profile. Once complete, a judgement can be made about the individuals' readiness.

Identify Common Needs

Defining the needs and the gaps creates an overall picture of the workforce's readiness to move forward. Before building plans to meet the needs of specific positions, it is useful to identify themes that are common to all roles, or common to roles of specific management levels and/or functional areas. When a need in knowledge, skills, experience, or behaviors applies to multiple individuals and roles, identifying, developing, or purchasing resources to close those gaps can be implemented more efficiently. Development of experience and behavior competency areas can also realize improved efficiency and effectiveness when deployed across a group of individuals with similar needs.

Build Versus Buy

The organization needs to determine whether it is more effective to recruit the skills externally or develop the skills internally when filling critical roles. This decision must consider the cost of acquiring and onboarding external talent versus the cost of developing the internal talent, the availability of the skills internally and externally, and the viability of development interventions. The time it will take to recruit external talent, and the effort it will take for that talent to become productive, also needs to be considered.

TABLE 7-1 POPULATION HEALTH PRACTITIONER

Knowledge	Skills	Experience	Behaviors
Health systems	Analytics	Leading diverse process efforts	Collaboration
Legal, regulatory and administrative	Process & design	Participating in regional planning groups	Curiosity
Social, behavioral and environmental factors in health	Communications	Conducting research on public health	Population focus

Talent Acquisition

When talent acquisition is the appropriate strategy, the recruiting resources will define the potential talent pools and create a sourcing strategy that includes a compelling value proposition to attract the desired talent. A well-defined screening, assessment, and selection process is particularly important when the organization is filling new roles and will ensure that the best individuals move forward. Finally, an onboarding process must effectively support entry into the organization and minimize the time required for new hires to perform successfully.

Developing the Talent

A workforce development plan is not the same thing as a training plan. While training can be effective at improving knowledge and understanding, knowledge and understanding do not translate directly to performance. A comprehensive plan is required to produce the skills and behaviors needed to achieve the needed results. This plan should define a range of development approaches, including training, which matches the identified development needs.

While there are a variety of **learning and development approaches and modalities** available, these approaches can be broadly grouped into four categories:

- **Education:** The formal delivery of learning through classrooms, workshops, online courses, assigned reading, and simulations. These approaches are most effective for building knowledge and awareness that supports performance.
- **Exposure:** Coaching, mentoring, job-shadowing, communities of practice, and professional conferences can provide opportunities to observe the application of knowledge and skills and to learn from people who have successfully achieved results.
- **Experience:** Job rotations, special assignments, and projects provide opportunities to apply knowledge, use skills, and practice behaviors. Simulations and learning experiences provide opportunities for people to receive feedback and to practice and improve. They are a very powerful form of development, particularly when supported by coaching and mentoring.
- **Performance Support:** Tools that are easily accessed on demand including reference materials, internal and external information wikis, access to experts, videos, and podcasts are easy to apply and they are designed to support execution.

Defining the talent development plan starts with:

- The outcomes required for each critical role;
- The gaps between the competencies demonstrated by the available talent and the competencies required;
- The number of people who will require development; and
- The nature of the competency gaps.

The development plan must be aligned to these four points. The level of investment associated with each approach should also be considered. While the learning and development professionals have the expertise to create the most effective and cost-efficient set of development plans, it is the population health leaders who provide the input that responds to these points.

The purpose of development is to support performance that achieves outcomes. An important component of any development plan is a clearly defined approach to assessing its effectiveness, and population health leaders have a critical role in its creation. A thoughtful evaluation approach provides feedback that can be used to support and enhance the development program. The book *Six Disciplines of Breakthrough Learning* (Pollock, Jefferson, & Wick, 2015) provides a simple but powerful framework to assist in defining these measures. Their Outcomes Planning Wheel poses four important questions for creating high-impact development:

1.   What business needs will be met?
2.   What will people do better or differently as a result of the development?
3.   What or who can confirm changes? What will change and be observable?
4.   What are the specific, meaningful measures of success?

The population health leaders need to work closely with the learning professionals to ensure the answers to these questions reflect the important business objectives defined in the population health strategy.

Building the Workforce Development Plan: Another Word About Culture

Workforce development solutions are designed to equip people with the competencies they need to deliver the necessary outcomes. However, preparing people with the ability to perform does not guarantee they will consistently demonstrate those competencies. As was noted earlier, culture helps to define the individual and collective behaviors of an organization. It reinforces some behaviors and discourages others. Because culture provides reinforcement that guides and motivates behavior, it is important to identify the cultural styles that best support the population health strategy.

Having defined the desired culture, leaders need to be certain that programs and tools, including workforce development, are in place to reinforce that culture. The most critical signals of culture are sent by the behavior of leaders. Leaders cast a long shadow; it is important that they consistently reinforce values and actions that support the needed culture. Other elements that reinforce culture include organizational communications, reward, and recognition and performance management programs. All of these programs should be aligned to enable the right performance.

▶ Conclusion

To be successful, strategies must be supported by plans that identify, acquire, and deploy the resources that are critical to their success. Identifying people who are capable of performing the roles that are critical to success is one of the most important strategies that an organization needs in order to achieve its objectives. This chapter was written for leaders who create the population health strategy and are responsible for achieving its goals. They are the leaders who will ensure that the people they need to be successful are developed and in place. This chapter describes how a workforce development plan to support a population health strategy is created. Equipped with this knowledge, leaders are in a position to effectively ask for, sponsor, and contribute to a workforce development plan that supports the important work of building healthier communities.

▶ Workforce Development: An Executive Leadership Example

This section provides a brief illustration of a workforce development plan. While the focus is on the executive leadership roles, the same key elements and basic approach apply to other parts of an organization. The example begins with an introduction to Beta Health System (BHS) and its strategy. BHS is a fictitious representation of a healthcare system in the United States; it is not an actual organization.

Introducing Beta Health System

BHS is based in Aurora City, a mid-sized city in the Midwest. For the last 50 years, its mission has focused on building a healthier community for the citizens of Aurora and the surrounding area. BHS operates a large tertiary care center, two community hospitals and multiple ambulatory care sites within the greater metropolitan area. It recently opened two retail health sites and an on-site clinic at the corporate offices of the largest company in the area. In the prior year, BHS started a pilot program to test a value-based reimbursement contract with a local payer organization.

BHS recently developed a population health strategy. Leadership and the board of directors feel that this strategy supports BHS's historical mission and responds to the changing health environment. Priorities in BHS's population health strategy include:

- Effective management of chronic conditions while also seeking the long-term reduction in their incidence and in health disparities
- Facilitating, building and participating in partnerships that address social and environmental determinants of health
- Being a strong steward of community resources through collaboration, avoiding duplication of efforts and the sharing of information

BHS recognizes its strong culture has played an important role in its success and wants to be sure the organization continues to align culture with its new population health strategy.

Supporting the Culture that Supports the Strategy

BHS has utilized the culture framework developed by Groysburg et al.[11] Leadership believes that its population health strategy can build on its strong culture of **caring, purpose** and **results.** It also believes that it cannot rest on its laurels and must put additional emphasis on creating a **learning** culture. BHS has been able to balance the need to have every individual feel accountable for achieving **results** with demonstrating the teamwork and building the trust that are so important to **caring.** It will now need to take steps to ensure the innovation and agility important to a **learning** culture are reinforced. For these efforts to be successful, the leaders know that the decisions they make and the actions they take are critical to building the culture BHS needs to achieve its strategic priorities.

Identifying Critical Executive Roles, Competencies, and Competency Gaps

BHS has decided that individuals occupying all roles at the Vice President level and above must demonstrate a core set of competencies. BHS updated its existing executive competency model to enhance alignment with its population health strategy. After reviewing several population health leadership models,[12,13] the resulting competency framework includes the knowledge, skills, experience and behaviors described in **TABLE 7-2**.

Once the executive success profile was complete, all executives were given a questionnaire asking them to self-rate their level of proficiency for the knowledge, skills, experience, and behaviors described in the profile. Each executive then rated the overall executive team on each of the elements in the profile. The results were summarized and discussed with the Chief Executive and her team. This process resulted in an agreement on gaps to be addressed and the prioritization of development areas. These priorities became the basis for the BHS's executive development plan.

The Executive Development Plan

BHS developed and deployed a comprehensive executive development plan for its leaders. Elements in the plan included:

- A custom executive development program focused on the knowledge

TABLE 7-2 BETA HEALTH SYSTEM EXECUTIVE PROFILE			
Knowledge	**Skills**	**Experience**	**Behaviors**
Regional Health Ecosystem Key stakeholders: roles, capabilities and priorities	**Systems Thinking**	**Leading diverse teams in process improvement efforts**	**Envision the Future**
Health Policy National, Regional and Local	**Process & Design** **Communications**	**Participating in regional planning groups**	**Align Stakeholders** **Manage Boundaries and Obstacles**
Social, Behavioral and Environmental Factors in Health	**Systems Advocacy**	**Work with/on public health issues**	**Act and Learn** **Population focus**
Health Economics			
Regional Demographics Health Disparities			

Data from Drew Harris, Katherine Puskarz, and Caroline Golab. Population Health Management. Feb 2016. Ahead of print http://doi.org/10.1089/pop .2015.0129, Pollock RVH, Jefferson A, Wick CW. The Six Disciplines of Breakthrough Learning (3rd ed.). 2015. Hoboken, NJ: John Wiley and Sons.

and skill areas defined in the executive success profile. This intensive, face-to-face approach allows leaders to interact with and learn from each other throughout the experience. The program culminates with a learning simulation that gives participants the opportunity to create and manage a wellbeing portfolio for a hypothetical community and to track the results of those decisions over a multi-year period.

- Executive guest speakers from a range of health-related and community agencies are invited to address BHS's leadership groups. These talks broaden awareness of the diverse stakeholders that contribute to population health and focus on the purpose, strategy, programs, challenges, and successes of the speaker's organization. Selected executives are also given the opportunity to learn more by visiting some of the agencies.

- Each executive's individual development plan reflects his/her identified needs. The plan is designed to enhance skills and behaviors in the success profile. Development actions are focused on BHS's three strategic priorities of management of chronic conditions, building community partnerships, and resource stewardship. Activities range from assignments working with a community partner on a specific project, to serving on a community board, and leading or participating on an internal initiative focused on a population

health opportunity. Individual coaching focused on improving one or more of the behavioral competency areas is also included for selected individuals.

- The success of the executive development plan is measured by the implementation of improvement programs for targeted chronic conditions, and the creation of community partnerships that support the reduction of chronic conditions and/or were designed to optimize community resources.

BHS also identified a need to create a new role of Vice President for Population Health. It retained an executive search firm to help source and hire an individual who has already demonstrated success in executing a comprehensive population health strategy.

Aligning Culture

BHS knows that its culture needs to support the right behaviors. It is piloting a new technology that easily and quickly collects input from employees. This tool allows the organization to see how consistently and visibly employees see its leaders demonstrating behaviors consistent with the population health strategy. BHS also ensured that the leaders' performance plans reflect the population health approach and progress on the three identified priorities. Finally, these priorities and associated metrics are also included in the executive annual and long-term incentive programs.

Study and Discussion Questions

1. Explain the role of population health leaders in creating and implementing a workforce development strategy.
2. Explain why defining and reinforcing an organizational culture that supports population health and aligning the workforce development strategy with that culture is important.
3. How is a workforce development plan different from a training plan?

Suggested Readings and Websites

Duberman T, Sachs R. *From Competition to Collaboration: How Leaders Cultivate Partnerships to Drive Value and Transform Health.* Chicago, IL: Health Administration Press; 2018.

ReThink Health. Negotiating a well-being portfolio exercise. July 17, 2017 [Updated October 23, 2018]. Available at https://www.rethinkhealth.org.

Pollock RVH, Jefferson A, Wick CW. *The Six Disciplines of Breakthrough Learning: How to Turn Training and Development Into Business Results* (3rd ed.). Hoboken, NJ: John Wiley & Sons; 2015.

References

1. Sawyer B, Cox C. How does health spending in the US compare to other countries? Peterson-Kaiser Health Systems Tracker; February 13, 2018. Available at https://www.healthsystemtracker.org/chart-collection/health-spending-u-s-compare-countries/ (accessed March 19, 2019).

2. Papanicolas I, Woskie LR, Jha A. Health care spending in the United States and other high income countries. *JAMA.* 2018;319(10):1024–1039. Available at https://jamanetwork.com/journals/jama/fullarticle/2674671 (accessed March 19, 2019).

3. Burrill S. Health care outlook for 2019: 5 trends that could impact health plans, hospitals and patients. *Deloitte Health Care Current*; December 4, 2018. Available at https://www2.deloitte.com/us/en/pages/life-sciences-and-health-care/articles/health-care-current-december4-2018.html (accessed March 19, 2019).

4. Hussein T, Collins M. Why big health systems are investing in community health. *Harv Bus Rev.* December 6, 2016. Available at https://hbr.org/2016/12/why-big-health-systems-are-investing-in-community-health (accessed March 19, 2019).

5. Kindig DA, Milstein B. A balanced investment portfolio for equitable health and well-being is an imperative, and within reach. *Health Aff.* 2018;37(4):579–584. Available at https://www.healthaffairs.org/doi/pdf/10.1377/hlthaff.2017.1463 (accessed March 19, 2019).

6. Duberman T, Sachs R. From competition to collaboration: how leaders cultivate partnerships to drive value and transform health. Chicago, IL: Health Administration Press; 2018.

7. Pietersen W. Re-inventing strategy: using strategic learning to create and sustain breakthrough performance. Hoboken, NJ: John Wiley and Sons; 2002.

8. ReThink Health. Negotiating a well-being portfolio exercise. July 17, 2017 [Updated October 23, 2018]. Available at https://www.rethinkhealth.org/resources/negotiating-a-well-being-portfolio-exercise/ (accessed March 19, 2019).

9. AHA Center for Healthcare Governance. Learnings on governance from partnerships that improve community health. Chicago, IL: American Hospital Association; 2016. Available at http://trustees.aha.org/populationhealth/16-BRP-Learnings-on-Governance.pdf (accessed March 19, 2019).

10. Advisory Board. Population health job description library. March 26, 2018. Available at https://www.advisory.com/research/population-health-advisor/resources/2015/job-description-library?wt.ac=4member_pha_resource___pophealthjoblibrary_ (accessed March 19, 2019).

11. Groysberg B, Lee J, Price J, Cheng Y. The culture factor: the leader's guide to corporate culture. *Harv Bus Rev.* January-February 2018. Available at https://hbr.org/2018/01/the-culture-factor (accessed May 22, 2019).

12. Harris D, Puskarz K, Golab C. Population health: curriculum framework for an emerging discipline. *Popul Health Mgmt.* 2016;19(1):39–45.

13. Pollock RVH, Jefferson A, Wick CW. *The Six Disciplines of Breakthrough Learning* (3rd ed.). 2015. Hoboken, NJ: John Wiley and Sons.

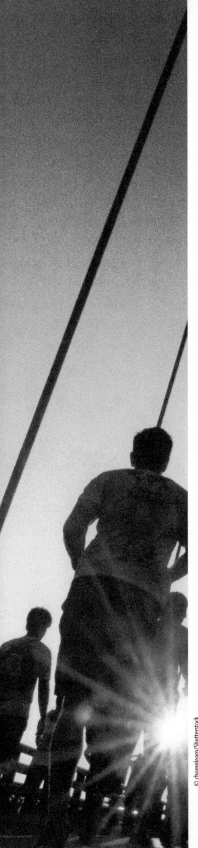

PART III

Creating Culture Change

© chomplearn/Shutterstock

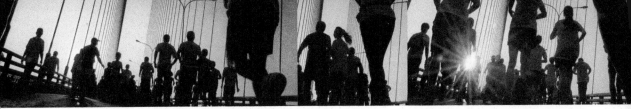

CHAPTER 8

Health Promotion and Health Behavior

Amy Leader
Preethi Selvan

EXECUTIVE SUMMARY

The field of health promotion focuses on changing health behaviors for the better. This typically involves planned, organized, and structured activities that, over time, help individuals make informed decisions about their health. The activities can be applicable to individuals in various settings and at any point in the natural history of an illness or problem but are typically designed to work with a priority population that is experiencing a higher than expected burden of risk or disease. The most successful health promotion programs are created with a theoretical model of behavior as its foundation, which not only provides a framework for implementing activities but a mechanism for evaluating their effectiveness. Initially, theoretical models focused on changing behavior of the individual, but newer theories focus on the interacting nature of factors on behavior at multiple levels of influence. As technology advances, health promotion programs are seeking to capitalize over the ability to collect real-time health behavior data. In the future, health promotion programs will continue to evolve and adapt as health populations and problems change with the times.

LEARNING OBJECTIVES

By the end of this chapter, the reader will be able to:

1. Understand how unhealthy behaviors contribute to the burden of disease in the United States.
2. Understand how health promotion programs can overcome the burden of disease in the United States by facilitating positive behavior change among individuals, communities, and society.
3. Describe prominent health behavior theories and their key concepts.
4. Appreciate the importance of rigorously evaluating health promotion programs by using evidence-based evaluation frameworks.

▶ Introduction

Health promotion has been defined as "the process of enabling people to increase control over their health and its determinants, and thereby improve their health."[1] Health promotion programs are comprised of two levels of action: providing health education and environmental actions to support the conditions for healthy living. Health education often involves facilitating new knowledge, adjusting attitudes, and acquiring new skills that could change one's behavior and ultimately one's health status. Educational strategies are typically delivered through individual or group instruction, although newer health promotion programs are using technology to deliver the messages. Mass communication through advertisements, campaigns, and other forms of media are also commonly used to deliver health education to the public. Environmental actions may include altering the physical, social, economic, or political environment around the individual to promote behavior change. This may include actions such as advocacy and legislation, resource development, social support, financial support, or organizational and community development. Working in tandem, health education and environmental actions can create opportunities for individuals to live healthy and long lives.

▶ The Role of Behavior in Morbidity and Mortality

Health, in general, is caused by factors in five domains—genetics, social circumstances, environmental exposures, behavioral patterns, and health care.[2] When it comes to reducing deaths, health care has a relatively minor role. The greatest opportunity to improve health and reduce premature mortality lies in personal behavior. It is thought that behavioral causes account for nearly 40% of all deaths in the United States (**FIGURE 8-1**).[2] In the United States, there are four **health behaviors** that account for the majority of premature death. Collectively, public health professionals refer to them as "The Big Four." They are smoking, poor diet, physical inactivity, and alcohol consumption.

Smoking

While smoking rates in the United States continue to decline, cigarette smoking remains the leading cause of preventable disease and death in the United States, accounting for more than 480,000 deaths every year, or about 1 in 5 deaths.[3] In 2017, more than 14 of every 100 U.S. adults age 18 years or older (14%) currently smoked cigarettes, translating to an estimated 34.3 million adults in the United States.[3] Smoking rates are highest among males, those with only a high school education, those of lower socioeconomic status, those with

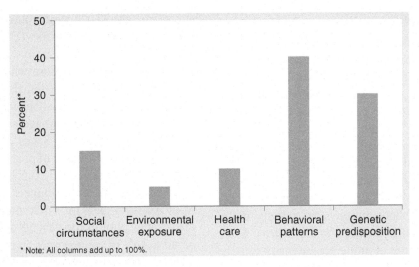

FIGURE 8-1 Determinants of Health and Their Contribution to Premature Death.

Data from Schroeder SA. We can do better: Improving the health of the American people. New England Journal of Medicine 2007; 357: 1221-1228. FIGURE 1 "Determinants of Health and Their Contribution to Premature Death." https://www.nejm.org/doi/full/10.1056/nejmsa073350

a disability or a diagnosed mental health condition, those who identify as a sexual or gender minority, and American Indian/Alaskan Natives. Current smoking rates are nearly identical for African American and Caucasian adults. Of concern to public health and medical professionals are the large number of adolescents who are trying e-cigarettes, which are a known gateway to traditional cigarette smoking, for the first time.[4]

Diet and Nutrition

Poor diet quality is a leading risk factor associated with death and disability in the United States.[5] Eating a diet rich in fruits and vegetables as part of an overall healthy diet can help protect against a number of serious and costly chronic diseases, including heart disease, type 2 diabetes, some cancers, and obesity. Fruits and vegetables also provide important vitamins and minerals that help the human body work as it should and fight off illness and disease. The 2015–2020 Dietary Guidelines for Americans recommends that adults consume 1.5–2 cups of fruits and 2–3 cups of vegetables per day.[6] Despite these recommendations, recent data show low consumption, with only 1 in 10 U.S. adults eating the recommended amount of fruits or vegetables.[7] Income-related disparities exist as well, with 7% of adults who live at or below the poverty level meeting the daily vegetable recommendation, compared to 11.4% of adults with the highest household incomes.[7] Research shows that residents of low-income, minority, and rural neighborhoods have less access to stores that sell healthy foods, including a variety of fruits and vegetables, at affordable prices.[8] Other initiatives, such as reducing sugar consumption, increasing water intake, breastfeeding infant children, and ensuring adequate micronutrient levels aim to improve dietary and nutrition status in the United States.

Physical Activity

The evidence is clear—physical activity fosters normal growth and development, can reduce the risk of various chronic diseases, and can make people feel, function, and sleep better. Some health benefits start immediately after activity, and even short bouts of physical activity are beneficial. Guidelines vary by age: children and adolescents ages 6 through 17 years should aim for 60 minutes of moderate to vigorous physical activity daily, while adults should aim for at least 150–300 minutes of moderate-intensity activity each week.[9] Guidelines also exist for older adults, women who are pregnant, adults with chronic health conditions, and those with disabilities.[9] Currently, only 26% of men, 19% of women, and 20% of adolescents report sufficient activity to meet the relevant aerobic and muscle-strengthening guidelines.[10] Sedentary behavior has received an increasing amount of attention as a public health problem because it appears to have health risks, and it is a highly prevalent behavior in the U.S. population. Data collected as part of the U.S. National Health and Nutrition Examination Survey (NHANES) indicate that children and adults spend approximately 7.7 hours per day (55% of their monitored waking time) being sedentary.[11] Thus, the potential population health impact of sedentary behavior is substantial.

Alcohol Consumption

Drinking too much alcohol can lead to numerous health and social conditions, such as high blood pressure, heart disease, stroke, liver disease, some cancers, lost productivity, family problems, and unemployment.[12] Excessive alcohol use led to approximately 88,000 deaths and 2.5 million years of potential life lost (YPLL) each year in the United States from 2006–2010, shortening the lives of those who died by an average of 30 years.[13] Further, excessive drinking was responsible for one in 10 deaths among working-age adults ages 20–64 years. In the United States, a standard drink contains 0.6 ounces of pure alcohol.[14] Generally, this equates to 12 ounces of beer, 5 ounces of wine, or 1.5 ounces of liquor. Approximately 58% of adult men report drinking alcohol in the past 30 days, compared to 46% of adult women in the United States.[15] Approximately 23% of adult men report binge drinking five times a month, averaging eight drinks per binge, while approximately 12% of adult women report binge drinking three times a month, averaging five drinks per binge.[16] Most people who report binge drinking are not alcoholics or alcohol dependent. Alcohol is the most commonly used and abused drug among youth in the United States.[17]

The Growth of Data on Health Behaviors

Contributing to the increased attention toward health behaviors in health promotion and disease prevention work is the ease in which health behavior data have become available over the past few decades. Health behavior data are collected in national, state, and local surveys. In 1984, the Centers for Disease Control and Prevention (CDC) implemented the first state-based surveillance system for health behaviors and preventive services, the Behavioral Risk Factor Surveillance System.[18] Other surveys followed in the years to come, including the Youth Risk Behavior Surveillance System,[19] the National

Survey on Drug Use and Health,[20] and the Pregnancy Risk Assessment Monitoring System.[21] Some surveys, such as Philadelphia's Southeastern PA Household Health Survey, measure health behaviors at a local level.[22] A list of national surveys that measure health behavior is in **TABLE 8-1**.

Despite strong evidence of the influence of social and behavioral factors on health, these factors are not often addressed in clinical care. Efforts are under way to include standardized measures of key social and behavioral determinants in electronic health records (EHRs) and make the data available to the appropriate professionals. In 2014, the National Academies of Science released a report entitled *Capturing Social and Behavioral Domains and Measures in Electronic Health Records*.[23] The National Academy of Medicine convened a committee to, among other things, identify core social and behavioral domains to be included in all EHRs and obstacles to adding these domains to health system EHRs. They assessed the strength of the evidence for each domain and how each one should be measured. Recommendations from the Committee are summarized in **TABLE 8-2**. The Committee acknowledged that there are several limitations to achieving this goal, including infrastructure capacities, providers' willingness to collect these data from patients, and privacy and security concerns. Nonetheless, increasing access to social and behavioral data in EHRs can lead to more effective treatment of individual patients in health care, more effective population management for healthcare systems and public health agencies, and the discovery of the pathways that link social and behavioral factors to functioning, disease processes, and mortality.

Lastly, wearable technology—electronic devices that people wear on the body to collect different types of personal biometric data (e.g., monitoring of nutrition, activity, heart rate, even blood glucose levels)—is undergoing explosive growth. According to one estimate, U.S. adults used nearly 77 million wearable devices in 2017.[24] These "wearables" are user-friendly and unobtrusive, since they are often worn as accessories. The love of wearables is driven largely by consumers wanting to eat healthier, exercise smarter, and have easier access to health care. The typical wearable device is a fitness tracker or some other smart electronic device that can be worn on the body. However, there is a wide range of types of these devices, including implantable devices and the first FDA-approved pill that can track a patient's adherence. The FDA approved the smart pill, which is an atypical antipsychotic medication used to treat schizophrenia and bipolar disorder, in 2017.[25] It represents a potential huge advance in the treatment of mental health disorders and other diseases where medication adherence has been a challenge. Future wearables focus on embedding of wearables in skin patches and clothing, such as socks that measure skin temperature in patients with diabetes to prevent foot ulcers.[26] However, this avalanche of patient data is not without a downside: an *MIT Technology Review* reports that 99.5% of newly created digital data remain unanalyzed.[27]

How Theory Informs Health Promotion and Disease Prevention

Effective public health, health promotion, and chronic disease management programs

TABLE 8-1 Major US Surveys That Measure Health Behaviors

Acronym	Name	Sponsoring Agency
ACS	American Community Survey	US Census Bureau
BRFSS	Behavioral Risk Factor Surveillance System	CDC
CPS	Current Population Survey	US Census Bureau
CSFII	Continuing Survey of Food Intakes by Individuals	US Department of Agriculture
CSHCN	National Survey of Children with Special Health Care Needs	CDC
IFPS	Infant Feeding Practice Study II	CDC
IHIS	Integrated Health Interview Series	NCHS-NHIS
HRS	Institute for Social Research Health and Retirement Study	University of Michigan, Institute for Social Research
LSOAs	Longitudinal Studies of Aging	CDC-NCHS
MEPS	Medical Expenditure Panel Survey	AHRQ
NAMCS	National Ambulatory Medical Care Survey	CDC
NAS	National Asthma Survey	CDC
NCS	National Children's Study	NIH
NCS-1	National Comorbidity Survey Replication	ICPSR
NEHIS	National Employer Health Insurance Survey	CDC
NHAMCS	National Hospital Ambulatory Medical Care Survey	CDC
NHANES	National Health and Nutrition Examination Survey	CDC
NHCS	National Health Care Surveys	CDC
NHDS	National Hospital Discharge Survey	CDC

(continues)

TABLE 8-1 Major US Surveys That Measure Health Behaviors   *(continued)*

Acronym	Name	Sponsoring Agency
NHHCS	National Home and Hospice Care Survey	CDC
NHIS	National Health Interview Survey	CDC
NIS	National Immunization Survey	CDC
NLAAS	National Latino and Asian American Study	ICPSR
NLTCS	National Long Term Care Survey	Duke University
NMFS	National Mortality Followback Survey	CDC
NMIHS	National Maternal and Infant Health Survey	CDC
NNHS	National Nursing Home Survey	CDC
NOES	National Occupational Exposure Survey	CDC
NSAS	National Survey of Ambulatory Surgery	CDC
NSCH	National Survey of Children's Health	CDC
NSDUH	National Survey on Drug Use and Health	SAMHSA, US Census Bureau
NSECH	National Survey of Early Childhood Health	CDC
NSFG	National Survey of Family Growth	CDC
PedNSS	Pediatric Nutrition Surveillance System	CDC
PNSS	Pregnancy Surveillance System	CDC
YRBSS	Youth Risk Behavior Surveillance System	CDC

Abbreviations: CDC, Centers for Disease Control and Prevention; NCHS, National Center for Health Statistics; NHIS, National Health Interview Survey; AHRQ, Agency for Healthcare Research and Quality; NIH, National Institutes of Health; ICPSR, Inter-University Consortium for Political and Social Research; SAMHSA, Substance Abuse and Mental Health Services Administration.

Mokdad A, Remmington P. Measuring health behaviors in populations. Preventing Chronic Disease 2010; 7(4): A75. Table 2: Major US Surveys that Measure Health Behaviors. Accessible at: https://www.ncbi.nlm.nih.gov/pmc/articles/PMC2901573/

TABLE 8-2 Summary of Selected and Non-Selected Domains

Candidate Set of Domains for Consideration for the Inclusion in All Electronic Heatlh Records (Chapter3)	Domains Reviewed But Not Selected (Appendix A)
Sociodemographic Domains	
▪ Sexual orientation	▪ Gender identity
▪ Race/ethnicity	
▪ Country of origin/U.S. born or non- U.S. born	
▪ Education	
▪ Employment	
▪ Financial resource strain (Food and housing insecurity)	
Psychological Domains	
▪ Health literacy	▪ Negative mood and affect (Hostility and anger, hopelessness)
▪ Stress	▪ Cognitive function in late life
▪ Negative mood and affect (Depression, anxiety)	▪ Psychological assets (Coping, positive affect, life satisfaction)
▪ Psychological assets (Conscientiousness, patient engagement/activation, optimism, self-efficacy)	
Behavioral Domains	
▪ Dietary patterns	▪ Abuse ofother substances
▪ Physical activity	▪ Sexual practices
▪ Tobacco use and exposure	▪ Exposure tofirearms
▪ Alcohol use	▪ Risk-taking behaviors (Distractive driving and helmet use)

(continues)

TABLE 8-2 Summary of Selected and Non-Selected Domains	*(continued)*
Individual-Level Social Relationships and Living Conditions Domains	
■ Social connections and social isolation	■ Social support (Emotional, instrumental, and other)
■ Exposure to violence	■ Work conditions
	■ History of incarceration
	■ Military service
	■ Community and cultural norms (Health decision making)
Neighborhood and Community Domains	
■ Neighborhood and community compositional characteristics (Socioeconomic and racial/ethnic characteristics)	■ Neighborhood and community contextual characteristics (Air pollution, allergens, other hazardous exposures, nutritious food options, transportation, parks, open spaces, health care and social services, educational and job opportunities)

Republished with permission of National Academies of Science, from Capturing Social and Behavioral Data Domains and Measures in Electronic Health Records; permission conveyed through Copyright Clearance Center, Inc.

are built on the premise of helping people make voluntary decisions about reducing their risk of illness or injury and improving their health. Interventions can improve the well-being and self-sufficiency of individuals, families, organizations, and communities. Not all health programs and initiatives are equally successful, however. Those most likely to achieve desired outcomes are based on a clear understanding of targeted health behaviors, and the environmental and social context in which they occur. Practitioners use strategic planning models to develop and manage these programs, and continually improve them through meaningful evaluation. **Health behavior**

theory can play a critical role throughout the **program planning** process.

What Is a Theory?

A theory presents a systematic way of understanding events or situations.[28] A theory is a set of concepts that explain or predict these events or situations by illustrating the relationships among variables. Theories are generalizable and must be applicable to a broad variety of situations.[29,30] They are, by nature, abstract, and do not have a specified content or topic area. They are the infrastructure that supports the activities of a novel intervention or program. Most health behavior and health promotion theories were adapted from the social and behavioral sciences but draw upon various disciplines such as psychology, sociology, anthropology, consumer behavior, and marketing.[31]

Why Use Theory in Health Promotion Practice?

Theory gives planners tools for moving beyond intuition or a "gut feeling" to designing and evaluating health promotion interventions based on understanding of behavior. Using theory as a foundation for program planning and development is consistent with the current emphasis on using evidence-based interventions in public health, behavioral medicine, and medicine. Theory provides a road map for studying problems, developing appropriate interventions, and evaluating their successes. It can inform one's thinking during all of these stages, offering insights that translate into stronger programs. Theory can also help to explain the dynamics of health behaviors, including processes for changing them, and the influences of the many forces that affect health behaviors, including social and physical environments. Most health behavior theories can be applied to diverse cultural and ethnic groups, but health practitioners must understand the characteristics of target populations (e.g., ethnicity, socioeconomic status, gender, age, and geographical location) to employ these theories correctly.

Theory can also help planners identify the most suitable target audiences, methods for fostering change, and outcomes for evaluation. Researchers and practitioners use theory to investigate answers to the questions of "why," "what," and "how" health problems should be addressed. By seeking answers to these questions, they clarify the nature of targeted health behaviors. That is, theory guides the search for reasons why people do or do not engage in certain health behaviors; it helps pinpoint what planners need to know before they develop public health programs; and it suggests how to devise program strategies that reach target audiences and have an impact.[32,33] Theory also helps to identify which indicators should be monitored and measured during **program evaluation**. For these reasons, program planning, implementation, and monitoring processes based in theory are more likely to succeed than those developed without the benefit of a theoretical perspective.

Designing Theoretically Grounded Interventions (PRECEDE-PROCEED Model)

The PRECEDE-PROCEED model is a planning model developed by Lawrence Green in the 1970s that can help health program planners design and evaluate health programs.[34] It provides a comprehensive structure for engaging stakeholders, assessing health and quality- of-life needs, and for designing, implementing, and evaluating health promotion and other public health programs. It guides planners through a process that starts with desired outcomes and then works backward in the causal chain to identify a mix of strategies for achieving those objectives. In this framework, health behavior is regarded as being influenced by both individual and environmental factors, and hence has two distinct parts. First is an "educational diagnosis"—that is, PRECEDE, an acronym for Predisposing, Reinforcing, and Enabling Constructs in Educational

Diagnosis and Evaluation. Second is an "ecological diagnosis"—PROCEED, for Policy, Regulatory, and Organizational Constructs in Educational and Environmental Development. The model consists of four planning phases, one implementation phase and three evaluation phases. A diagram of the model is in **FIGURE 8-2**. The model is multidimensional and is founded in the social/behavioral sciences, epidemiology, administration, and education.

During the first stage, *the social diagnosis*, program planners aim to gain an understanding of the social problems that affect the quality of life of the community and its members—their strengths,

weaknesses, and resources, as well as their readiness to change. This is done through various activities such as developing a planning committee, holding community forums, and conducting focus groups, surveys, and/or interviews. The second stage, *the epidemiological, behavioral, and environmental diagnosis*, focuses on the assessment through data collection and analysis of the underlying social, behavioral and environmental factors linked to a particular health issue. From here, program planners can work to identify the modifiable factors that could be the focus of an intervention in the *educational and ecological diagnosis*. The fourth phase, *the administrative and*

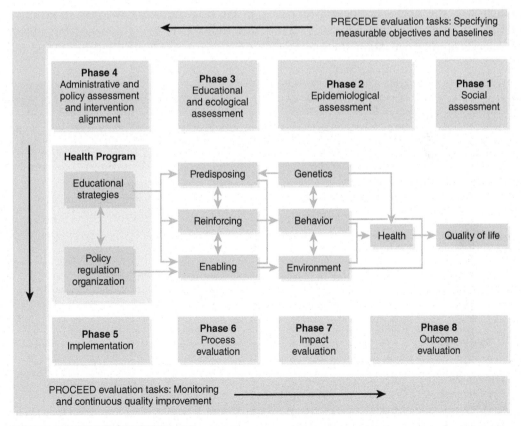

FIGURE 8-2 PRECEDE-PROCEED Model.

Reproduced from Lawrence Green, Marshall Kreuter, *Health Program Planning: An Educational and Ecological Approach*, Volumes 1-2, McGraw-Hill Education, 2005.

policy assessment, focuses on the administrative and organizational concerns that must be addressed prior to program implementation. After completing the comprehensive assessment, planners can move to the next phase, *implementation*, where they conduct the activities of the intervention. The final three phases—process, impact, and outcome evaluation—focus on assessing the short-, medium-, and long-term impacts of the intervention. To date, there are more than 1,000 publications using the PRECEDE-PROCEED framework for program planning and evaluation purposes.

Major Theories in Public Health and Interventions in Practice

Much like the Socio Ecological Model (SEM), theories have applications at various levels of influence. Some theories that operate at the individual level aim to change individual characteristics that influence behavior, such as knowledge, attitudes, beliefs, and personality traits. Theories that operate at the interpersonal level aim to influence interpersonal processes and primary groups, including family, friends, and peers. Some theories operate at the community level, aiming to influence institutional factors, community factors, or public policies. An overview of the levels of influence of theories can be found in **TABLE 8-3**.

Health Belief Model

The Health Belief Model (HBM) was one of the first theories of health behavior and remains one of the most widely recognized in the field. Initially developed to identify determinants of being screened for tuberculosis in the 1950s,[35] it has been used to

TABLE 8-3 LEVEL OF INFLUENCE OF THEORIES

Change Strategies	Examples of Strategies	Ecological Level	Useful Theories
Change People's Behavior	▪ Educational sessions ▪ Interactive kiosks ▪ Social marketing campaigns	Individual	▪ Stages of Change/ Transtheoretical Model[40] ▪ Precaution Adoption Process ▪ Health Belief Model[36] ▪ Theory of Planned Behavior[38]
	▪ Mentoring programs ▪ Lay health advising	Interpersonal	▪ Social Cognitive Theory[42]
Change the Environment	▪ Media advocacy campaigns ▪ Advocating changes to company policy	Community	▪ Communication Theory ▪ Diffusion of Innovations ▪ Community Organizing

Glanz, K. & Rimer, B.K. (2005). Theory at a glance: A guide for health promotion practice. National Cancer Institute. National Institutes of Health. US Department of Health and Human Services. NIH Pub. No. 05-3896. Washington, DC: NIH.

address a wide range of topics related to prevention such as cancer screening tests, HIV testing, vaccination, and injury prevention.[32] The HBM theorizes that people's beliefs about whether they are at risk for a problem and their perceptions of the benefits and barriers to taking action influence their readiness to take action.[28,32,36] Core constructs of the HBM are perceived susceptibility (the degree in which one feels vulnerable to a situation or health problem); perceived severity (the degree to which one thinks that the situation or health problem has serious consequences); perceived benefits (the positive outcomes a person believes will result from the action); perceived barriers (the negative outcomes a person believes will results from the action); self-efficacy (a person's belief in his or her ability to take action); and cues to action (an external event that motivates a person to act). A conceptual model of the HBM is displayed in **FIGURE 8-3**.

The Health Belief Model in Action

The HBM has been used widely in practice for more than 40 years. Numerous strengths to the theory exist, including its easy-to-understand framework and its applicability to a broad range of preventive health behaviors. However, critics of the theory often mention its oversimplification of a complex issue and its lack of including factors beyond the individual in considering or predicting behavior change. Noting the strengths and weaknesses, it is not surprising that the HBM has had successes and challenges when used in everyday practice. A systematic review of the HBM used to explore factors influencing cervical cancer screening among immigrant and ethnic minorities included 55 studies in its analysis.[37] The researchers found both common and unique factors that were held across the Asian, Hispanic, Middle Eastern, African American, and Native American populations. For example, a lack of knowledge about cervical cancer was contributing to a deficit in perceived susceptibility among all five populations, but issues of embarrassment as a barrier to screening were only evident among the Asian and Hispanic populations. Understanding nuances in beliefs about a particular health topic will

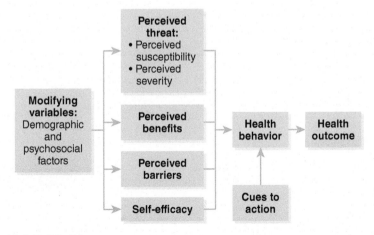

FIGURE 8-3 Health Belief Model.

Modified from Becker MH and & Maiman, LA. Sociobehavioral determinants of compliance with health and medical care recommendations. *Medical Care* 1975; 134(1): 10–24. Figure 1, p. 12.

allow public health professionals to create culturally tailored, theoretically grounded interventions using the HBM.

The Theory of Reasoned Action/ Planned Behavior

The Theory of Planned Behavior (TPB) and its predecessor, the Theory of Reasoned Action (TRA), explore the relationship between behavior and beliefs, attitudes, and intentions.[38] Both the TPB and the TRA assume behavioral intention is the most important determinant of behavior. According to the TRA, behavioral intention is influenced by a person's *attitude* toward performing a behavior and by beliefs about whether individuals who are important to the person approve or disapprove of the behavior (*subjective norm*). The subjective norm is a combination of a person's beliefs about what other people in his or her social group will think about the behavior, combined with his or her motivation to comply with those individuals. The TPB is a reformulated version of the TRA and includes

the construct *perceived behavioral control*, to account for times when a person has strong intentions to perform a behavior but the act of doing so is outside of their control. A conceptual model of the TRA/TBP is displayed in **FIGURE 8-4**.

The Theory of Planned Behavior in Action

Both the TRA and the TPB have strengths and weaknesses to their approach. The hallmark of both theories is that attitudes are the strongest predictors of behavior, which has largely been seen in the literature. However, the theories assume that behavior is the result of a linear, rational thinking process that does not account for all of the decisions that people base on "gut reaction" or emotional appeals. The theories also assume that intentions lead to behavior, which may not always be the case. A systematic review of dietary interventions for adolescents based on the TRA or TPB analyzed 11 interventions for their effectiveness, approach, and

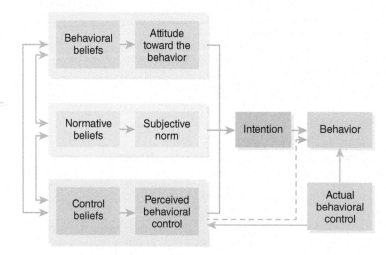

FIGURE 8-4 Theory of Reasoned Action/Theory of Planned Behavior.
© Icek Aisen, 2002.

measurement.[39] Nine of the 11 interventions resulted in positive dietary behavior change, usually measured as an increase in fruit and vegetable consumption. All of the interventions occurred in school-based settings. The interventions were conducted in countries all around the world, a testament to the reach of the theories in health promotion research and practice.

Transtheoretical Model

Both the HBM and the TRA/TPB can be considered "point in time" theories—predicting a behavior that happens once, like being vaccinated or tested for HIV. But many behaviors, particularly lifestyle behaviors, occur daily or because of a more complex process in decision making. Consider the behavior of beginning a new exercise routine, such as training for a marathon. A person may initially be completely unprepared and unsure of how to train for such an endeavor, and progress to buying new training clothes and sneakers, to finding a group of friends to train with, to running routinely each week, to successfully completing the marathon. This is more of a process of decisions and actions than a single action. The Transtheoretical Model (TTM) best accounts for changing behaviors where multiple steps are involved, such that a person can move forward or regress in his or her behavior change over time.[40] According to the TTM, there are six stages to describe the overall process of behavior change: Precontemplation (Stage 1, a person does not intend to take action); Contemplation (Stage 2, a person is thinking about taking action sometime in the near future); Preparation (Stage 3, a person is ready to take action); Action (Stage 4, a person has recently taken action toward change); Maintenance (Stage 5, a person who has been taking action for quite some time); and Termination (Stage 6, a person has completed the process of behavior change). A conceptual model of the TTM is displayed in **FIGURE 8-5**. Helping people move from one stage to the next are processes of change, which are guidelines for how to approach a behavior change recommendation. The underlying premise of the TTM is that people in different stages of readiness to adopt a new behavior will need different types of support (processes of change); hence, interventions using TTM are somewhat tailored to each stage of readiness.

Transtheoretical Model in Action

The TTM is often praised for its ability to recognize that not all people are ready to change their behavior at the same time and that people's readiness to change

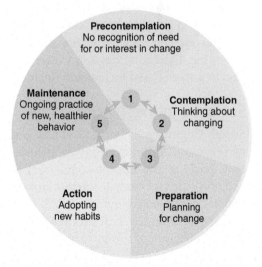

FIGURE 8-5 Transtheoretical Model.

Modified from Prochaska, JO & Di Clemente CC Transtheoretical therapy: toward a more integrative model of change. *Psychotherapy: Theory, Research and Practice,* 1975; 19(3): 276–288. Figure 2, p. 283.

often occurs as a process over time. Furthermore, the TTM rightfully accounts for people's ability to go forward and backward in behavior change. Behavior change is rarely a straight line forward, and the TTM nicely incorporates that aspect into its theoretical foundation. On the flip side, some critics have noted that the theory can be burdensome to use in practice. In order to design an intervention that meets someone's level of readiness, one has to know (i.e., assess) where that individual is on the continuum of readiness. A Cochrane Review examination of stage-based interventions for smoking cessation included 41 randomized controlled trials covering more than 33,000 smokers.[41] The review found that providing intervention support to people who wanted to quit smoking, whether in a stage-based format or non-stage-based format, was an effective method for cessation. However, in the four studies that directly compared whether providing the intervention in a stage-based format was superior to a non-staged-based format, there was no difference in effectiveness. The review concluded that the value of providing a smoking cessation intervention in a stage-based format was unclear.

Social Cognitive Theory

Social Cognitive Theory (SCT) is one of the most common behavior theories that exists at the interpersonal level. It explores the reciprocal interactions of people, health behaviors, and their environments[42]—namely, that people's behavior is a reflection of the environment they are in and the social cues around them. It is based on the foundation of operant conditioning—that people learn from the positive or negative experiences resulting

from a behavior. A child learns to not touch a hot stove after burning her hand while previously touching the hot stove. The original formulation of the theory, named Social Learning Theory, introduced the new idea of vicarious learning—that people learn merely from watching others. A child learns to not touch a hot stove because she saw her brother get burned when he touched the stove. It was renamed Social Cognitive Theory in the 1980s to better reflect situations when individuals consciously behave within their environment. According to SCT, changing one's behavior is a function of the following factors: individual characteristics, such as a person's self-efficacy that he or she can perform a behavior or the extent to which he or she can deal with the emotions involved in behavior change, and environmental factors, such as the ability for someone to directly observe the behavior change in question or the positive or negative feedback that someone gets from others for changing a behavior. Many argue that the concept of self-efficacy is the pivotal construct in SCT. A conceptual model of SCT is in **FIGURE 8-6**.

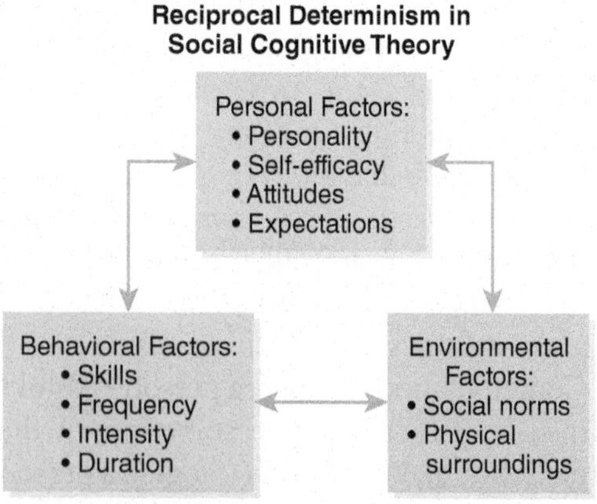

FIGURE 8-6 Social Cognitive Theory.

Social Cognitive Theory in Action

SCT has seen many successes in the literature but is not without its critics. Successes include the development of many concepts we use across the behavioral science and health promotion field: vicarious learning, self-efficacy, and outcome expectations. Self-efficacy has received far more attention that the other constructs, such that some interventions claim to be grounded in SCT when, in fact, they are merely grounded in self-efficacy. Critiques include the complex nature of the theory and the lack of cohesiveness between the constructs. A meta-analysis of 44 interventions (with 55 distinct tests of SCT models) to increase physical activity in the general population revealed that only 22 of the 55 models used all of the major SCT constructs; the remaining models were combinations of constructs.[43] Overall, SCT explained almost one-third of the variance in physical activity, which is a moderate effect size for a theory to explain a behavior. Of the major constructs in SCT, self-efficacy and goal setting were the most likely to be associated with changes in physical activity. However, the authors noted that intervention quality—accurately using the theory as it was intended—was quite low across the studies, limiting the generalizability of the findings.

Which Theory to Use?

No single theory dominates health education and promotion, nor should it; the problems, behaviors, populations, cultures, and contexts of public health practice are broad and varied. Some theories focus on individuals as the unit of change. Others examine change within families, institutions, communities, or cultures. Adequately addressing an issue may require more than one theory, and no single theory is suitable for all cases. Choosing a theory that will be the most successful at improving the population at risk should not involve selecting the most common theory, the theory mentioned in a recent journal article, or the one you are most comfortable using. Instead, the process should start with a firm understanding of the situation: the population of interest, the topic of concern, and the type of behavior to be addressed. Because different theoretical frameworks are appropriate and practical for different situations, selecting a theory that "fits" should be a careful, deliberate process.

The Future of Health Promotion Interventions

Recently, interventionists have suggested that theoretical integration may be a viable way to improve our understanding of how to change behavior. Many of the theories described in this chapter have overlapping constructs that we may be able to reduce complexity through streamlining theories and reducing redundant constructs. For example, self-efficacy in SCT shares considerable overlap with perceived behavioral control in TPB; outcome expectations in SCT is similar to one of the processes of change in TTM. If feasible, an integrative model of behavior change could reduce some confusion in the field about which theory is most applicable to a given public health problem. A second idea for streamlining health promotion interventions is to bundle certain behaviors together, in multiple behavior change interventions. Recognizing that many chronic conditions have similar health risk behaviors, an intervention to reduce cardiovascular disease could incorporate elements of dietary change, physical activity, and smoking cessation. However, there is a balance between aggregating similar behaviors while not overburdening participants with too many changes at one time. Future research in this field seeks to determine the optimal number of behaviors, the timing of the behavior changes, and the most appropriate theoretical model to accommodate multiple health **behavior interventions**.

Evaluating Theory-Based Programs in Public Health Practice

Health promotion programs aim to prevent or control disease, injury, disability, and death. Over time, as this task has become more complex, interventions have become more complex. Increasingly, public health programs address large problems, the solutions to which must engage large numbers of community members and organizations. In addition, the context in which public health programs operate is very important. Programs that work well in some settings work poorly in others because of changes in fiscal, socioeconomic, demographic, interpersonal, and interorganizational factors. At the same time, demands for accountability and success from policymakers and other stakeholders have increased the pressure of interventionists to do well. Understanding program effectiveness means paying attention to documenting and measuring the implementation of the program and its success in achieving intended outcomes and

using such information to be accountable to key stakeholders. Next, we describe two prominent mechanisms for evaluating the impact of a program or intervention.

The CDC Framework for Program Evaluation

The Centers for Disease Control and Prevention developed a framework that is widely used among health promotion professionals.[44] The six steps, connected and interdependent, are ordered in how one might approach an evaluation (**FIGURE 8-7**). The first step is to *engage stakeholders*: those would be people involved in operating the program, those being served by the program, and those who will be end users of the evaluation. Stakeholders must be engaged in the inquiry to ensure that their perspectives are understood. The next step is to *describe the program*: a description should include the rationale for the program, its expected outcomes, the activities involved,

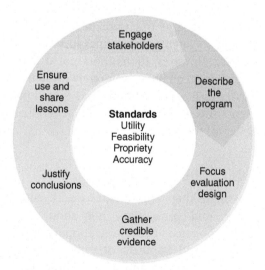

FIGURE 8-7 CDC's Framework for Evaluation.

Centers for Disease Control and Prevention. Framework for program evaluation in public health. *MMWR* 1999;48 (No. RR-11).

resources utilized, and the environment surrounding the program. The third step is to *focus the evaluation design*: this includes deciding on appropriate research questions, the evaluation design, the methods and procedures for collecting data, and roles and responsibilities for all those involved. The fourth step is to *gather credible evidence*: this focuses on the quality, quantity, and logistics of collecting data for the evaluation. The fifth step is to *justify conclusions*: Stakeholders must agree that conclusions are justified before they will use the evaluation results with confidence. The final step is to *ensure use and share lessons learned*: Deliberate effort is needed to ensure that the evaluation processes and findings are used and disseminated appropriately. This includes creating and adhering to a dissemination plan that reaches all stakeholders and allowing feedback from stakeholders about the findings of the evaluation.

The RE-AIM Model

The RE-AIM tool, introduced in the late 1990s, is a valuable tool for implementation scientists, health promotion professionals, and practitioners.[45] It can be applied to assist with the translation of research to practice and to estimate the public health impact of programs and interventions. RE-AIM is an acronym for five aspects of an evaluation: Reach, Effectiveness, Adoption, Implementation, and Maintenance. The tool has been used to address topics such as aging, cancer screening, dietary change, physical activity, medication adherence, health policy, environmental change, chronic illness self-management, well-child care, eHealth, worksite health promotion, women's health, smoking cessation, quality improvement, weight loss, diabetes prevention, childhood obesity, and practice-based research. An overview of the RE-AIM tool is in **TABLE 8-4**.

Reach is the absolute number, proportion, and representativeness of individuals who are willing to participate in a given initiative. Effectiveness is the impact of an intervention on outcomes, including potential negative effects, quality of life, and economic outcomes. Adoption is the absolute number, proportion, and representativeness of settings and intervention agents who are willing to initiate a program. Implementation refers to the intervention agents' fidelity to the various elements of an intervention's protocol. This includes consistency of delivery as intended and the time and cost of the intervention. Maintenance is the extent to which a program or policy becomes institutionalized or part of the routine organizational practices and policies. Maintenance also has referents at the individual level. At the individual level, it is defined as the long-term effects of a program on outcomes six or more months after the most recent intervention contact.

▶ Conclusion

Effective health promotion programs help people live healthy and fulfilled lives. Interventions that are successful can improve the well-being and self-sufficiency of individuals, families, organizations, and communities. Much is known about how to design theoretically grounded interventions that are targeted to certain populations; the most common health behavior theories are described in this chapter. The challenge is to create interventions that are appropriate, meaningful, and engaging

TABLE 8-4 A DESCRIPTION OF THE RE-AIM MODEL

Dimension	
Reach	Number, percentage, and representativeness of eligible patients who participated in the intervention ■ Is the intervention reaching the target population? ■ Is the intervention reaching those most in need?
Effectiveness	Intervention's effects on targeted outcomes ■ Does the intervention accomplish its goals?
Adoption	Number, percentage, and representativeness of participating settings and providers ■ To what extent are those targeted to deliver the intervention participating?
Implementation	The extent to which the intervention was consistently implemented by staff members
Maintenance	The extent to which the intervention becomes part of routine organizational practices and maintains effectiveness

Kessler RS, Purcell EP, Glasgow RE, Klesges LM, Benkeser RM, Peek CJ., What does it mean to "employ" the RE-AIM model? Evaluation and the Health Professions 2013;36(1):44-66 by SAGE Publications Inc.Reprinted by Permission of SAGE Publications, Inc.

to the population, to maximize success in the short and long term. As technology advances, there are more ways to collect behavior data, engage patients, and monitor health status. Frameworks to evaluate health promotion interventions exist to elucidate their impact on individuals, communities, and societies.

Study and Discussion Questions

1. What is the goal of the field of study of health promotion?
2. What are the core components of health promotion programs?
3. What are the most prominent health behaviors that contribute to the burden of morbidity and mortality in the United States?
4. What is theory? Why are theories useful in health promotion planning?
5. Choose one behavioral theory described in this chapter, and describe how it could be used to support a behavioral intervention.
6. Name one framework for evaluating health promotion interventions, and describe the core components of the framework.

Suggested Readings and Websites

The National Cancer Institute's Theory at a Glance (2nd ed.). 2005. Available at https://cancercontrol .cancer.gov/brp/research/theories_project/theory.pdf (accessed May 23, 2019).

Partnering4Health. National Implementation and Dissemination for Chronic Disease Prevention Initiative. Available at https://partnering4health.org (accessed May 23, 2019).

Centers for Disease Control and Prevention. National Center for Chronic Disease Prevention and Health Promotion. Available at https://www.cdc.gov/chronicdisease/index.htm (accessed May 23, 2019).

U.S. Department of Health and Human Services, Office of Disease Prevention and Health Promotion. Available at www.health.gov (accessed May 23, 2019).

Centers for Disease Control and Prevention. Framework for Program Evaluation. Available at https://www.cdc.gov/eval/framework/index.htm (accessed May 23, 2019).

RE-AIM Model. www.re-aim.org (accessed May 23, 2019).

References

1. World Health Organization. Ottawa Charter for Health Promotion. Adopted November 21, 1986. Available at https://www.who.int/healthpromotion/conferences/previous/ottawa/en/index.html (accessed on February 19, 2019).

2. McGinnis JM, Foege WH. Actual causes of death in the United States. *JAMA.* 1993;270:2207–2212.

3. Centers for Disease Control and Prevention. Current cigarette smoking among adults in the United States. Available at https://www.cdc.gov/tobacco/data_statistics/fact_sheets/adult_data/cig_smoking/index.htm (accessed on February 19, 2019).

4. Centers for Disease Control and Prevention. Quick facts on the risks of e-cigarettes for kids, teens, and young adults. Available at https://www.cdc.gov/tobacco/basic_information/e-cigarettes/Quick-Facts-on-the-Risks-of-E-cigarettes-for-Kids-Teens-and-Young-Adults.html (accessed on February 19, 2019).

5. Murray CJ, Atkinson C, Bhalla K, Birbeck G, Burstein R, Chou D, et al. The state of US health, 1990-2010: burden of diseases, injuries, and risk factors. *JAMA.* 2013;310(6):591–608.

6. U.S. Department of Health and Human Services and U.S. Department of Agriculture. 2015–2020 Dietary Guidelines for Americans (8th ed.). Available at https://health.gov/dietaryguidelines/2015/guidelines/ (accessed on February 19, 2019).

7. Lee-Kwan SH, Moore LV, Blanck HM, Harris DM, Galuska D. Disparities in state-specific adult fruit and vegetable consumption — United States, 2015. *MMWR Morb Mortal Wkly Rep.* 2017;66:1241–1247.

8. Larson NI, Story MT, Nelson MC. Neighborhood environments: disparities in access to healthy foods in the U.S. *Am J Preventive Medicine.* 2009;36(1):74–81.

9. U.S. Department of Health and Human Services. Physical Activity Guidelines for Americans. 2nd Edition. Available at https://health.gov/paguidelines/second-edition/pdf/Physical_Activity_Guidelines_2nd_edition.pdf (accessed on February 19, 2019).

10. Blackwell DL, Clarke TC. State variation in meeting the 2008 federal guidelines for both aerobic and muscle-strengthening activities through leisure-time physical activity among adults aged 18–64: United States 2010–2015. *National Health Statistics Reports*; no. 112. Hyattsville, MD: National Center for Health Statistics; 2018.

11. Ekelund U, Steene-Johannessen J, Brown WJ, Fagerland MW, Owen N, Powell KE, et al. Does physical activity attenuate, or even eliminate, the detrimental association of sitting time with mortality? A harmonised meta-analysis of data from more than 1 million men and women. *Lancet.* 2016;388(10051):1302–1310.

12. World Health Organization. *Global status report on alcohol and health, 2018.* Available at https://www.who.int/substance_abuse/publications/global_alcohol_report/gsr_2018/en/ (accessed on February 19, 2019).

13. Stahre M, Roeber J, Kanny D, Brewer RD, Zhang X. Contribution of excessive alcohol consumption to deaths and years of potential

life lost in the United States. *Prev Chronic Dis.* 2014;11:E109.

14. National Institute on Alcohol Abuse and Alcoholism. *What is a standard drink?* Available at https://www.niaaa.nih.gov/alcohol-health /overview-alcohol-consumption/what -standard-drink (accessed on February 19, 2019).

15. Esser MB, Hedden SL, Kanny D, Brewer RD, Gfroerer JC, Naimi TS. Prevalence of alcohol dependence among US adult drinkers, 2009– 2011. *Prev Chronic Dis.* 2014;11:140329.

16. Centers for Disease Control and Prevention. *Fact Sheets: Binge Drinking.* Available at https://www .cdc.gov/alcohol/fact-sheets/binge-drinking. htm (accessed on February 19, 2019).

17. U.S. Department of Health and Human Services. *The Surgeon General's Call to Action to Prevent and Reduce Underage Drinking.* Washington, DC: U.S. Department of Health and Human Services, Office of the Surgeon General, 2007.

18. Centers for Disease Control and Prevention. *Behavioral Risk Factor Surveillance System.* Data available at https://www.cdc.gov/brfss/index .html (accessed on February 19, 2019).

19. Centers for Disease Control and Prevention. *Youth Risk Behavior Surveillance System.* Data available at https://www .cdc.gov/healthyyouth/data/yrbs/index .htm (accessed on February 19, 2019).

20. Substance Abuse and Mental Health Services. *National Survey on Drug Use and Health.* Data available at https://nsduhweb.rti.org/respweb/ homepage.cfm (accessed on February 19, 2019).

21. Centers for Disease Control and Prevention. *Pregnancy Risk Assessment Monitoring System.* Data available at https://www.cdc.gov/prams /index.htm (accessed on February 19, 2019).

22. Public Health Management Corporation. *Community Health Database.* Available at http://www.chdbdata.org (accessed on February 19, 2019).

23. Institute of Medicine. *Capturing Social and Behavioral Domains in Electronic Health Records: Phase 1.* Washington, DC: The National Academies Press;2014.

24. Gartner. *Worldwide Wearable Device Sales to Grow 26 Percent in 2019.* November 29, 2018. Available at https://www.gartner.com /en/newsroom/press-releases/2018-11-29

-gartner-says-worldwide-wearable-device -sales-to-grow- (accessed on February 19, 2019).

25. U.S. Food and Drug Administration. FDA approves pill with sensor that digitally tracks if patients have ingested their medication. November 13, 2017. Available at https: //www.fda.gov/newsevents/newsroom/press announcements/ucm584933.htm (accessed on February 19, 2019).

26. Segura Anaya LH, Alsadoon A, Costadopoulos N, Prasad PWC. Ethical implications of user perceptions of wearable devices. *Sci Eng Ethics.* 2018 Feb;24(1):1–28.

27. Regalado A. Big data gets personal. *MIT Technol Rev.* July-Aug 2013. Available at http://www .technologyreview.com/news/514346/the-data -made-me-do-it/ (accessed on February 19, 2019).

28. Glanz K, Rimer BK. *Theory at a Glance: A Guide to Health Promotion Practice.* NIH Publication 97-3896. Bethesda, MD: National Cancer Institute; 1995.

29. Glanz K, Lewis FM, Rimer BK, eds. *Health Behavior and Health Education: Theory, Research, and Practice.* San Francisco: Jossey-Bass; 1990.

30. Glanz K, Lewis FM, Rimer BK, eds. *Health Behavior and Health Education: Theory, Research, and Practice* (2nd ed.). San Francisco: Jossey-Bass; 1996.

31. DiClemente RJ, Crosby RA, Kegler MC, eds. *Emerging Theories in Health Promotion Practice and Research.* San Francisco: Jossey-Bass; 2002.

32. Glanz K, Rimer BK, Viswanath K, eds. *Health Behavior and Health Education: Theory, Research, and Practice* (4th ed.). San Francisco: Jossey-Bass; 2008.

33. Hochbaum GM, Sorenson JR, Lorig K. Theory in health education practice. *Health Educ Q.* 1992;19:295–313.

34. Green LW. Toward cost–benefit evaluations of health education: some concepts, methods, and examples. *Health Educ Monogr.* 1974; 2(Suppl. 2):34–64.

35. Hochbaum GM. *Public Participation in Medical Screening Programs: A Socio-psychological Study.* Washington, DC: U.S. Department of Health, Education, and Welfare; 1958.

36. Rosenstock IM. The health belief model and preventive health behavior. *Health Educ Monog.* 1974;2(4):354–386.

37. Johnson CE, Mues KE, Mayne SL, Kiblawi AN. Cervical cancer screening among immigrants and ethnic minorities: a systematic review using the Health Belief Model. *J Low Genit Tract Dis.* 2008 Jul;12(3):232–241.

38. Ajzen I. The theory of planned behavior. *Org Behav Human Decis Process.* 1991;50(2):179–211.

39. Hackman CL, Knowlden AP. Theory of reasoned action and theory of planned behavior-based dietary interventions in adolescents and young adults: a systematic review. *Adolesc Health Med Therap.* 2014;5:101–114.

40. Prochaska JO, DiClemente CC. Stages and processes of self-change of smoking: toward an integrative model of change. *J Consult Clin Psychol.* 1983;51(3):390–395.

41. Cahill K, Lancaster T, Green N. Stage-based interventions for smoking cessation (review). *Cochrane Database Syst Rev.* 2010;11: CD004492.

42. Bandura A. *Social Foundations of Thought and Action: A Social Cognitive Theory.* Englewood Cliffs, NJ: Prentice Hall; 1986.

43. Young MD, Plotnikoff RC, Collins CE, Callister R, Morgan PJ. Social cognitive theory and physical activity: a systematic review and meta-analysis. *Obes Rev.* 2014;15:983–995.

44. Centers for Disease Control and Prevention. *A Framework for Program Evaluation.* Available at https://www.cdc.gov/eval/framework/index .htm (accessed on February 19, 2019).

45. Kessler RS, Purcell EP, Glasgow RE, Klesges LM, Benkeser RM, Peek CJ. What does it mean to "employ" the RE-AIM model? *Eval Health Prof.* 2013;36(1):44–66.

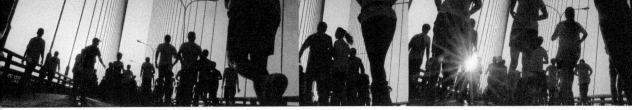

CHAPTER 9

Consumer Engagement and Technology

Joseph F. Coughlin
Adam Felts

EXECUTIVE SUMMARY

Information technologies have empowered consumers to engage in a variety of health management activities far outside the purview of health professionals. Internet-enabled devices, media platforms, and services have the potential to influence health-related decisions and behaviors. Fitbit and other wearable individual trackers apply "nudges" designed to encourage fitness activity. Facebook allows its users to signal health behaviors to their peers, thereby influencing their behavior. Instagram employs novel marketing techniques using personal stories, photo, and video to influence consumer decision making. Blue Apron indirectly teaches its customers norms of nutrition such as portion size and sodium quantity.

Some of these influences can be beneficial. Others, such as the spread of pseudoscience by anti-vaccination groups on social media platforms, can be harmful. Consumers must balance personal autonomy and judgment with the potential benefits of a technology-enabled life. Healthcare professionals can adopt methods to leverage new consumer technologies to improve health literacy and care, such as by utilizing patient-generated data in their practices or by learning to communicate health-related information effectively through new forms of media.

LEARNING OBJECTIVES

By the end of this chapter, the reader will be able to:

1. Identify a range of commonly used consumer technologies that may influence health behaviors.
2. Describe theoretical models and explanations of human behaviors.
3. Explore prospective models of application of consumer-facing technologies in the healthcare field.

▶ Introduction

The proliferation of information technology in the 21st century has significantly changed the culture of health and wellness in the United States. Culture can be defined as the roles, rituals, and rules that delineate human behavior. Information technology has altered the role of individuals-as-patients by providing them with access to tools that aid and influence the management of health. Modern patients daily encounter a considerable quantity of information, independent of that provided by healthcare professionals, related to health, wellness, and care. Smartwatches track exercise and activity; social media warns about the spread of a dangerous virus; perhaps the local grocery store ranks its products by their nutritional value. Patients may belong to specialized Facebook groups regarding a particular health issue of interest (e.g., caregivers of older parents with type 2 diabetes). Many use WebMD to determine whether their symptoms warrant a visit to a physician or emergency department.

Due to everyday phenomena like these, the relationship between patients and their physicians should be viewed as profoundly different from what it was 30 or even 15 years ago. In the era prior to the Internet, patients possessed comparatively limited knowledge, had minimal health technology at their personal disposal, and obtained information and direction primarily from a physician. A key part of the physician's role, accordingly, was as the keeper of health knowledge and controller of technology. Today, such powers are increasingly in the patient's hands, and this transfer of power has transformed the relationship between doctor and patient. That transformation can be illustrated, to begin with, by one simple piece of data: the primary first source of health information for Americans is not their personal physician, but the Internet[1]—although this finding represents only one element of the change. Today, it may be more accurate to refer to the patient as the *healthcare consumer*, with the chief feature of consumers being that they are always shopping around.

One effect of this new dynamic is that the consumer is more conscientious and informed about health, with tools at hand that allow for self-monitoring and self-management. Consumers can look up information, interact with people like them, contact their healthcare providers, and even monitor their own physical metrics at minimal cost. At the same time, however, this democratization of resources can lead to the development of harmful cultural norms and proliferate spurious information, such as in the case of the spread of misinformation around the risk of childhood vaccinations.[2] Uncontrolled effects such as these are the reason why the development of information technology should not be seen merely as an augmentation of the powers of health professionals but as a more fundamental change in the cultural characteristics of the individual-as-patient.

To obtain a better picture of the healthcare consumer as being in thrall to a variety of different informational and motivational sources, we suggest the adoption of an **ecological model of health behavior**. An ecological model attempts to grasp the influence of the totality of the environment on human behavior, delineates the elements of that environment, and theorizes ways in which those components complement or oppose each other in shaping an individual's decision making.[3]

In order to furnish a wider view of this ecology, this chapter will investigate three overlapping spheres that have changed the culture of health in the United States: personal technology, social media, and retail. We will examine each of these spheres in turn before looking briefly at how they converge in the case of the caregiver–care recipient relationship.

▶ Sphere 1: Personal Technologies

Wearables and the Internet of Things (IOT)

The 2018 model of the Apple Watch can perform an electrocardiogram, allowing it to detect heart abnormalities in its users when they are far away from the doctor's office. The advancement of the Apple Watch to detect heart problems may be a step toward what has been referred to as "the Holy Grail" of healthcare monitoring: measuring blood pressure.[4] If Apple were to succeed, its smartwatch would have practical utility for the 75 million Americans who suffer from hypertension. As a technology that users tend to wear most of the time, the watch would be able to monitor blood pressure continuously, overcoming the problem of patients needing to remember to check their blood pressure. Moreover, the blood pressure data could be transmitted instantly and automatically to a doctor. The ability of doctors to identify cardiovascular problems before they become emergencies and perform proactive interventions could be greatly facilitated by such an innovation. However, the ability of patients to procure their blood pressure reading on demand may give rise to unforeseen complexities. How would such an innovation change patients' relationship with their own health? How would it change their relationship with their doctor? How might it impact physician practices?

Imagine a doctor who is the provider for a family of intelligent, affluent, and deeply conscientious patients. These family members own of an array of technologies that monitor and collect their health data. Out of the great depths of their conscientiousness, they want to send all those data directly to their doctor: waves of information about heart rate, physical activity, diet, sleep patterns, weight, and blood sugar. "Let us know if something looks off, or what we can do better," the head of the family requests.

Now imagine you are the doctor. Would you be able to fulfill their request? Would it be worth trying? Is this family a group of model patients? Or are they a problem for how you conduct your practice?

Studies of physicians show a mixed set of attitudes toward incorporating patient-generated data into their medical practice. One study found an even split between physicians who considered it their job to receive, review, and discuss patient-related data and those who did not.[5] The same study also asked whether patient-generated data from a smart device has a beneficial effect on the physician–patient relationship. Sixty-eight percent agreed that it would be beneficial, leaving about one-third of physicians saying that it wouldn't.

Perhaps the most meaningful statistic from the study was that 65% of the providers had not received any training regarding how to receive, review, assess, or discuss patient-generated health data with their patients. Even physicians who are willing to bring new health information technology into their practices may not know how to do so effectively. There may also be a gulf between the ideas of patients and those of physicians as to what kinds of data are useful for health management.[6] Physicians acknowledge the potential benefits of patient-generated data in providing care but express concerns about the increased workload that will come with having to manage more patient information.[7] Physicians may need to innovate their practices in such a way that they can absorb a new and constant stream of patient information. That might mean a new subset of medical education; it may even require a new kind of medical

professional dedicated to the reading and analysis of patient data.[8] It is a physician's fantasy to be able to diagnose a patient at the very moment of appearance of symptoms; as that fantasy moves closer to reality, it may change the way medicine is practiced in a fundamental way.

Nudges and Social Comparisons

With or without the physician as a factor, digital devices already play a role in how patients manage their health. One way that they do so is through **nudges**, which are prompts and reinforcements that encourage but don't mandate people to make certain decisions. A nudge is a common phenomenon that is probably most prevalent in the field of advertising. When a person walks into a bookstore and is met with a glossy new hardcover release stacked up front and center, a nudge is being applied. When Amazon.com provides a selection of products a person might like, it is nudging that customer. Nudges fall under a field coined by Richard H. Thaler and Cass R. Sunstein as **choice architecture**, which refers to the organization of the context in which people make decisions.[9]

Companies nudge people to purchase their products and services almost constantly, but entities like governments and employers deploy nudging in subtler ways. For example, a 2006 law encourages employers to no longer ask new hires if they want to invest a portion of their salary in a 401K savings plan; instead, most employers ask whether employees want to *decline* to put their money in, thereby making saving for retirement the default option. Nobody is forced to save, but they are nudged toward doing so. The result of this policy shift has been a doubling of 401K participation rates.[10]

One benefit of nudges is that they may avoid the political and ethical problems involved in compelling individuals to adopt behaviors. For example, the Office of Disease Prevention and Health Promotion recommends a 90% flu vaccination rate among healthcare workers. Healthcare workers agree on the importance of being vaccinated, but they tend to oppose vaccination mandates being written into policy and have protested against the institution of such mandates. Substituting nudges for mandates allows for the encouragement of positive behavior and the overcoming of biases rather than compelling subjects toward certain actions and inviting conflict.[11]

Nudges have historically been delivered to consumers from outside entities— businesses, governments, or employers. Today, however, it is increasingly common for individuals to nudge themselves. Nearly everyone in the United States owns one of the most powerful behavior-altering tools ever invented: the smartphone. Such a device has the potential to influence behavior in a variety of ways. One basic tool that phones have is the "bedtime" feature. This simple function allows the user to program the phone with a notification for when to go to bed in order to achieve a full night's sleep. For whatever reason, modern human beings struggle to go to bed on their own, and failure to get enough sleep can have a significant impact on health. The academic literature on smartphone use and sleep has largely been on the numerous ways that they might interfere with human sleep behavior.[12] Far less research has gone into the potential positive utility such devices

could have in *improving* sleep habits, if they were used differently.

Some smart devices provide nudges by design. Consider the Fitbit, an electronic device worn on the wrist that tracks daily levels of physical activity. A central feature of the Fitbit is that it automatically provides the user a 10,000-daily-step goal. The device tracks how many steps the user has taken throughout the day and can be set to give reminders for hourly step quotas. When 10,000 steps are reached, the digital display provides the user with a miniature fireworks show. These forms of encouragement have been shown to have positive effects on the fitness behavior of its users. They appear to be more effective than more paternalistic forms of nudges such as text message reminders.[13]

The ability to track and record one's activities numerically, whether that's sleep, exercise, or even mindfulness, can facilitate a powerful psychological phenomenon: **social comparisons**. Another study of the Fitbit as a behavioral influence paired the device with a Twitter support group so that participants could encourage each other, provide advice, and share their progress.[14] The other side of cooperation is competition, which also can push individuals toward better behavior. A 2016 study of social comparisons and financial behavior looked at how the amount of money people save might be influenced by the behavior they observe in their peers. To demonstrate this, study participants were first asked to allocate an imaginary sum of money to different expenses, including savings. Once that activity was complete, they were shown how they compared with others who had taken the survey. They were automatically given a normative label such as "poor saver," "fair saver," "good saver," and "supersaver." The participants were then asked whether they wanted to perform the money allocation exercise again. They weren't required to do the exercise a second time, nor were they given any incentive to do so. The money they were allocating was imaginary. Yet a remarkable number of participants who were classified as fair and poor savers chose to do the task over again, merely so that they could rank better on the "saver" scale.[15]

It is important to also observe the destructive influence that social comparisons can have on positive norms of health and health behaviors. One example can be found in cultural perceptions of healthy body weight. Far more goes into norms of what constitutes a "good" body weight than the recommendations of the medical profession. For example, one study demonstrated that college-aged women felt more dissatisfied with their bodies when they spent time exercising in proximity to a highly fit peer. Rather than feeling encouraged to work to improve their health by comparing themselves to another, they were more likely to shorten their exercise routines in the face of the negative comparison.[16] Peer comparisons have the potential to positively impact health behavior, but in some cases, they can warp perceptions to a degree that individuals lose sight of what's best for them.

▶ Sphere 2: Social Media and Trust

The behavioral phenomena we are highlighting in this chapter are not peculiar to modernity; however, technology has worked to accentuate them. This is particularly the case for the topic of this section: what sources individuals turn to for health information and advice. The physician has never had a monopoly over a patient's search for information, always having to compete with folk remedies, old wives' tales, urban legends, word on the street, and plain guessing. By the time a patient goes to the doctor with a problem, he or she may have already tried a battery of solutions. The physician may not have been the patient's first source of advice but the object of last resort.

Where do people go today to find health information outside of the doctor's office? A resource that consumers rely on relatively infrequently is "traditional" media—books, articles, and television. An immutable source is friends, family, and colleagues—people who are close to us and who are like us. But the most frequently used source is the Internet.

This brings us to the intersection between **behavioral psychology** and information technology. Social networks have always been a prime source of advice and information. With the advent of online **social media**, those networks are now much larger, more diverse, and more immediately accessible. As a platform that seems to encompass every conceivable human interest and that is used by nearly everyone in the United States, social media is an important phenomenon to understand as a modern influence on health behavior. A review of studies on the role of social media as a facilitator of health information describes the variety of ways that the medium works to connect consumers with knowledge:

YouTube has been used by the general public to share health information on medications, symptoms, and diagnoses and by patients to share personal cancer stories. Blog sites create a space where individuals can access tailored resources and provide health professionals with an opportunity to share information with patients and members of the public. Facebook is employed by the general public, patients, carers, and health professionals to share their experience of disease management, exploration, and diagnosis. Asthma groups are using MySpace to share health information, in particular their personal stories and experiences.[17]

Social media can amplify and better disperse useful information, as in the case of the Zika outbreak in South America. Users of Instagram employed the platform to warn others about Zika transmission and advise modes of prevention against the virus. However, the information these users posted was inaccurate, incomplete, or misleading 60% of the time, and half of the studied posts included expressions of fear or negativity, illustrating the potential for social media not only to spread useful information but also to sow uncertainty and panic.

One example of this dangerous side of social media lies in vaccination adherence. Facebook has been heavily linked to the spread of the anti-vaccine movement, a disparate collection of individuals who believe that vaccinations cause autism and other severe health issues. The role of Facebook in propagating this idea cannot be exactly specified, but anti-vaccine pages have been common on the website, and the networks that exist on it have been used to push out anti-vaccine stories and viewpoints to those who are outside of the movement.[18] Facebook has recognized that these practices have had a negative impact on immunization rates and, as of March 2019, has taken steps to ensure that users receive information from authoritative sources.[19]

Part of the language of the anti-vaccine movement involves **trust**. The government and media, the movement claims, play an active role in suppressing information about the harmfulness of vaccines. Government and the mass media are among the least trusted institutions in the United States;[20] the very fact that these institutions are *against* the movement is held up as evidence that the movement is right to question vaccine safety. This distrust in expertise shows how the position of physicians as authorities can work *against* their ability to encourage positive behaviors.

Is it possible for health professionals to turn social media into a public good by engaging consumers? A meta-analysis of social media campaigns designed to encourage positive health behaviors suggests that social media *could* be a useful tool to modify population health behaviors, with many interventions showing modest effects.[21] But we will observe shortly that the strategies health professionals typically employ on these platforms may not be the best examples to follow.

The Internet is a powerful tool to influence behavior, but it is important to point out that in-person interaction is nearly always more meaningful—and more capable of building trust—than virtual connection and outreach. One way of seeing this in data is the fact that respondents say that "friends and family" are far more trustworthy than "Facebook posts," notwithstanding the fact that the Facebook posts they see predominantly come from their friends and family. Another indirect way of illustrating the power of personal over impersonal is the distinction in trust people make between "doctors" and "my doctor" (doctors are highly untrustworthy, but *my* doctor, whose name I know and face I recognize, is highly trustworthy).[22]

One implication of these findings for practicing physicians lies in how they establish and use channels of communication with patients. Digital messaging and telemedicine have become increasingly popular as means of increasing efficiency and cutting costs. They might also be ways of pushing the doctor's voice above the cacophony of other informational sources that patients are exposed to. But if one result of these developments is a decrease in interpersonal interaction between doctor and patient, then it may in fact grow *harder* for physicians' voices to cut through the thick wave of information that patients are exposed to from all different sources.

"Influencers" and the Growing Wellness Industry

We share and receive information about our health, not only for functional reasons but also for aspirational ones. Health and **wellness** have grown into a value system in the United States. It's not only that consumers want to be healthy enough to do the things they like to do—they want to be *as healthy as they possibly can be*, elevating health to a good in and of itself. Improving health is not merely an instrumental good but a pursuit of its own.

A strange source of influence in how people think about health and wellness is Instagram. An important distinguishing feature of Instagram (and to a lesser extent, YouTube and Twitter) as a social media platform is that it allows its users to connect with prominent cultural figures—athletes, actors, politicians, writers, models, and so on—in what appears to be the same way they connect with the people they know in real life. The platform makes no distinction between the famous people that users "follow" and those they know in their lives, and many celebrities use Instagram as a mode of personal expression in equal measure as a means of self-promotion and image management. The result is that Instagram functions as a powerful tool for reaching consumers. Companies pay celebrities to promote their products via the celebrity's Instagram account. The celebrities endorse them not in the mode of a paid personality reading from a script but as a regular person who happens to be an avid user of the product.

To increase their influence and relatability, celebrities use Instagram to show themselves as simultaneously representing the ordinary and approachable and the ideal and unattainable. One way they accomplish this is by allowing their followers to observe their dietary and exercise habits. The consumer can witness the lifestyle and health behaviors of famous individuals—and perhaps attempt to adopt them.

The common colloquialism for powerful social media users is **influencers**—someone who can shape the behavior of thousands of people simply by expressing a preference. One famous showcasing of the power these influencers possess was when pop singer Taylor Swift exhorted her Instagram followers to vote in the 2018 United States midterm elections. After Swift's post, voter registrations among Americans age 18–24 rose to unprecedented levels.[23] Research has shown that influencers meaningfully sway social media users' behaviors regarding nutrition and food choices, with some consumers even reporting that social media influencers are the *most* significant source of information on their dietary choices.[24] One study demonstrated that health promotion organizations tend to operate in their communications on social media in the same terms as in more formal mediums—that is, "serious in tone and often rely[ing] on statistics and facts to communicate their intended message." If measured in terms of user engagement, this style of communication is less effective than the informal, interpersonal style used by influencers.[25]

Influencers can align with other trends and fads to help create cultural movements that promote better health. For example, CrossFit, a seemingly unremarkable exercise regimen, has grown into a national phenomenon partly because of the tendency of its adherents to proselytize on social media.[26] Religious theorists have described CrossFit gyms as sites of spiritual bonding and transformation that increasingly are coming to replace churches in modern American life.[27]

Exercise is an important health behavior, but it serves many other purposes beyond health management: social, cultural, psychological, instrumental, even spiritual. The bleeding over of health into myriad other areas of human life can encourage beneficial practices, but it can also have strange consequences for how consumers perceive and enact health behavior. Consider the wellness industry. "Wellness" is a nebulous term with multiple meanings. It can merely be synonymous with the idea of health-as-pursuit that we have been examining. But it also refers to an ecosystem of businesses that use the language of health care to sell remedies with empirically unproven benefits, things like healing crystals, powders, and supplements.[28] These are not remedies so much as totems and rituals; they are the latest development in the strange relationship between medicine and sorcery that has existed throughout history.[29]

Social media and the influence of celebrities have their own role to play in the wellness industry. For example, one of the most successful wellness brands in the world is called Goop, a company founded by American actress Gwyneth Paltrow. The brand was built from an online newsletter, ostensibly curated by Paltrow herself, that recommended products the actress liked. It is now a $250 million company.[30]

The cult of wellness is mostly harmless, except in those cases in which it muddies the adherent's ability to distinguish between medicine and sorcery—between rational information and emotional information. The anti-vaccination movement, arguably, is an outgrowth of the belief that the ritual and emotive elements that surround medical treatment are more important than the medicines themselves. The fearsomeness of the needle, the crying of the child, the cold sterility of the doctor's office become what matter, not the empirical evidence showing the effects of vaccines in eradicating diseases and saving lives.

Everyone worships something, observed American writer David Foster Wallace, whether that something is a church, CrossFit, a celebrity icon, the process of scientific inquiry, or an arrangement of crystals. To an outsider, the act of worshipping always appears foreign. The only objective criterion we can impose in evaluating one form of worship over another is whether it enriches us or harms us.

▶ Sphere 3: Retail and Business

The heightened role of the consumer in making health decisions has placed some erstwhile non-healthcare companies into the position of dispensing health advice and products. Best Buy is a consumer electronics company that is probably best recognized by its "Geek Squad" technical support service. At its founding, Best Buy's flagship products were televisions and desktop computers. But as wearable technologies become more popular as health management tools, Best Buy is growing not only into an electronics retail entity but increasingly into a healthcare company. In 2018, Best Buy acquired GreatCall, a company that sells health and safety technologies to older adults.[31] The company has also been hiring away experts and professionals from the healthcare sector to bolster a new division called Best Buy Health.[32] One significant aspect of this development is that the Best Buy retail space—its stores, website, and customer support representatives—can now be viewed as fitting into the consumer-healthcare ecology. A Best Buy store employee may not have any formal healthcare training but nonetheless may be involved in the recommendation and sale

of products that are used, at least in part, in the monitoring and managing of health.

Best Buy is not the only retail company whose business intersects with population health. Food and grocery retailers also fall into the consumer-health ecology, which has increasingly shaped their businesses. To promote better health behaviors and to satisfy consumer preferences, some grocery companies actively structure the choice architecture of their stores. This structuring can involve very simple forms of reorganization, like putting a certain product on the eye-level shelf in the grocery store, or it can involve an extensive delivery of information to a consumer about a product or set of products in order to motivate better decision making. Hannaford's grocery stores, for example, use a "Guiding Stars" system that rates foods based on their nutritional value. "Guiding Stars is not intended to tell you what to buy," Hannaford's website explains, "but rather point you toward foods that have more nutritional value while having less added and artificial substances." The use of color-coded labeling to denote the nutritional content of foods has been shown to positively impact consumer behavior in the grocery aisle in terms of health decision making.[33]

Whole Foods CEO John Mackey has designed Whole Foods grocery stores with the mission of "curating" nutrition by being selective as to which foods they stock, educating their employees to be nutrition advisors, and stocking their checkout aisle shelves with magazines on nutrition and well-being.[34] Not only upscale retailers like Whole Foods but also small food stores in underserved locations have improved consumer choices through the manipulation of choice architecture.[35]

Talking about food labeling and grocery store layouts may seem far afield of our subject—health communication technology—but these sorts of small innovations are their own kind of technological advancement. Within the realm in which they present themselves, they may have more power to influence consumer health choices than the advice of physicians and public health professionals, not because packages and colorful signs are more trustworthy or persuasive than the professional in the white coat, but because they are present at the crucial moment of decision.

Grocery stores like Whole Foods and Hannaford's have developed decision architectures that provide consumers with more information and signals to assist in making decisions. Other nutrition delivery services take the opposite approach, offering to make dietary choices on the consumer's behalf to keep him or her from making bad decisions. This is the way of meal-delivery diet programs like the Jenny Craig Weight Loss Program and Nutrisystem. By having all three daily meals mailed to their door, adherents to these programs have their nutrition prescribed to them, effectively controlling their portions and keeping them from straying toward unhealthy foods. It is what one could call an authoritarian decision architecture, in which the consumer gives away freedom in the expectation of being cared for. Particularly for individuals who must keep to a specific diet in order to treat a chronic health condition, the prescription and delivery of meals can serve as a more effective means of ensuring adherence to a diet plan than putting the decision in the hands of the consumer.[36]

Delivery meal plans are very much a creation of the 20th century; a 21st-century iteration of the concept is Blue Apron, which also delivers foods straight to the consumer's door, although for ends other than promoting weight loss. Blue Apron delivers apportioned ingredients of a selected recipe instead of pre-prepared meals, involving the consumer in the technical process of cooking but taking away the chore of selecting, buying, and measuring out the ingredients. Blue Apron does not advertise itself as a diet plan or as a way for consumers to make healthier choices, but by delegating exactly what its customers eat for their meals, the company puts forward an implicit norm of what humans ought to eat and how much they should eat. Blue Apron can function as training wheels for aspiring home cooks, taking away some of the friction of decision making while still helping the user to grow comfortable and confident in the kitchen. When users "graduate" from Blue Apron to cook on their own, they may bring some of the "lessons" they have learned from the service, whether they are good or bad lessons, along with them. To give one example, the sodium content of Blue Apron's meals is higher than what nutritional guidelines recommend.[37] A consumer can learn this easily by reading the nutrition facts that are printed with each Blue Apron recipe, but the stronger normative influence is likely to be the small package of salt that comes from the Blue Apron box.

▶ The Case of Caregiving

Many of the phenomena we have examined so far have particular relevance for the aging population. Older adults have more chronic conditions and health needs generally than younger individuals. The upcoming generation of older Americans, the Baby Boomers, are generally more proactive and conscious about health and well-being than their predecessors.[38] In contrast to their parents, the Baby Boomers also spent their formative years and their working lives in the company of personal technologies. The health of the next cohort of older adults will be profoundly shaped by new technologies.

What's more, the children of the Baby Boomers have grown up steeped in the technologies that have been highlighted throughout this chapter: smartphones, **wearables**, and convenience services like Blue Apron. As their parents age, and they grow into the role of caring for them, they are bound to employ these tools to help with the responsibility of caregiving. Caregiving is a strenuous and demanding role, and any tools that prove to make it easier will be valuable in reducing the challenges associated with an aging society.

Many tasks having to do with caregiving are informational in character, especially for caregivers who do not live in the same dwelling as their care recipient. Many common caregiving tasks may be facilitated by technology. A pill reminder system, either in the form of a smartphone app or a smart pill bottle, may help to improve medication adherence. A smart home monitoring system may help caregivers ensure that their recipients are safe and in a secure environment. A care recipient who likes to cook but has trouble going out into the neighborhood could have groceries delivered through Blue Apron. Wearables can be used to provide remote updates to a caregiver about a recipient's health metrics. According to one report, the technologies of greatest interest to caregivers are those that assist in checking in with or monitoring a loved one.[39] These tools are sold primarily by technology retailers, not by healthcare professionals.

The framework of actors involved in the care of a dependent adult can be complicated. As we have discussed, the physician often does not stand on the front line of influencing the patient's health decision making, and this observation is particularly salient in the case of caregiving. For the care recipient, the physician as prescriber and advice giver is always mediated by the caregiver. In addition to the caregiver is the care recipient as an agent—replete with preferences, values, and personal knowledge.

The success of health information technology in the facilitation of caregiving depends on all stakeholders involved being willing adopters and users. Both the caregiver and the care recipient must be on board, for example, with the idea of the recipient's activities and metrics being monitored. The care recipient must be willing to accept a loss of **autonomy**—above that of already being dependent on another person for care—in allowing devices, cameras, and nudges into the home and daily life. Research on the attitudes of older adults and aging advocates toward monitoring technology shows a mix of preferences and concerns about privacy, autonomy, and trust. Some respondents are horrified by the idea of being technologically cared for; others are far more receptive to the idea, seeing health as a first-order good worth protecting.

▶ Conclusion

It is a fair question as to whether the benefits to health these tools may provide are worth the losses of personal freedom.[40] This is a question that lies at the heart of all personal technologies that assist in the management of health, wellness, and care, not only for older consumers but for everyone. We are all, to varying degrees, care recipients. In a world of such intense technological flourishing, we will be continually faced with the choice between having the freedom to choose and act for ourselves or handing some part of our agency over to an entity that we believe can manage our care better than we can. We should not make such a decision casually.

Study and Discussion Questions

1. Given that wearable devices produce many better health outcomes for their users, which stakeholders should be responsible for paying for them (e.g., insurance companies, the user)? Will issues of affordability limit access to technology-driven health care?
2. What infrastructural changes could the current healthcare system explore to better take advantage of patient-generated data?
3. Think of a health-behavior issue that could be addressed through the application of nudges or another approach to behavioral change.
4. How do issues of privacy and personal autonomy relate to the use of personal technology and behavioral science as tools for health management?
5. How can healthcare professionals utilize social media to more effectively deliver health information to consumers?

Suggested Readings

Coughlin J. *The Longevity Economy*. New York: Public Affairs, an imprint of Perseus Books, LLC, a subsidiary of Hachette Book Group, Inc.; 2017.

Cugelman B, Thelwall M, Dawes P. Online interventions for social marketing health behavior change campaigns: a meta-analysis of psychological architectures and adherence factors. *J Med Internet Res.* 2011;13(1):e17. DOI:10.2196/jmir.1367

Kvedar J. *The New Mobile Age: How Technology Will Extend the Healthspan and Optimize the Lifespan*. Seattle, WA: Amazon Digital Services LLC-Kdp Print Us; 2017.

Sallis JF, Owen N, Edwin EB. Ecological models of health behavior. In Glanz K, Rimer BK, Viswanath K, eds. *Health Behavior and Health Education: Theory, Research and Practice* (4th ed.). San Francisco: Jossey-Bass; 2008:465–485.

Thaler R, Sunstein C. *Nudge: Improving Decisions About Health, Wealth, and Happiness*. New Haven, CT: Yale University Press; 2008.

References

1. Jacobs W, Amuta AO, Jeon KC, Alvares C. Health information seeking in the digital age: an analysis of health information seeking behavior among US adults. *Cogent Social Sci.* 2017;3(1). DOI: 10.1080/23311886.2017.1302785

2. Kata A. A postmodern Pandora's box: anti-vaccination misinformation on the Internet. *Vaccine.* 2010;28(7):1709–1716.

3. Sallis JF, Owen N, Edwin EB. Ecological models of health behavior. In Glanz K, Rimer BK, Viswanath K, eds. *Health Behavior and Health Education: Theory, Research and Practice* (4th ed.). San Francisco: Jossey-Bass; 2008:465–485.

4. Farr C. How Apple could turn the Apple watch into a blood pressure monitor. CNBC, October 2, 2018. Available at https://www.cnbc.com/2018/10/02/apple-watch-could-measure-blood-pressure.html (accessed January 17, 2019).

5. Psyhojos MA. Aging, empathy, and the Internet of Things: a measure of physician readiness to treat older adults [master's thesis]. Cambridge, MA: Massachusetts Institute of Technology; June 2017. Available at http://hdl.handle.net/1721.1/111222 (accessed January 17, 2019).

6. Zhu H, Colgan J, Reddy M, Choe EK. (2017). Sharing patient-generated data in clinical practices: an interview study. *AMIA Annu Symp Proc.* 2017 Feb 10;2016:1303–1312.

7. Huba N, Zhang Y. Designing patient-centered personal health records (PHRs): health care professionals' perspective on patient-generated data. *J Med Syst.* 2012;36(6):3893–3905. DOI:10.1007/s10916-012-9861-z.

8. Murdoch TB, Detsky AS. The inevitable application of big data to health care. *JAMA.* 2013;309(13):1351–1352. DOI:10.1001/jama.2013.393.

9. Thaler R, Sunstein C. *Nudge: Improving Decisions About Health, Wealth, and Happiness.* New Haven, CT: Yale University Press; 2008.

10. Salisbury I. Meet Richard Thaler, the man who just won the Nobel Prize for helping you save for retirement. *Time,* October 9, 2017. Available at http://time.com/money/4974462/thaler-nobel-economist-retirement-savings-nudge/ (accessed January 18, 2018).

11. Dubov A, Phung C. Nudges or mandates? The ethics of mandatory flu vaccination. *Vaccine.* 2015;33(22): 2530–2535.

12. Demirci K, Akgonul M, Akinpar A. Relationship of smartphone use severity with sleep quality, depression, and anxiety in university students. *J Behav Addict.* 2015 Jun;4(2):85–92. DOI: 10.1556/2006.4.2015.010.

13. Wang JB, Cadmus-Bertram LA, Natarajan L, White MM, Madanat H, Nichols JF, et al. Wearable sensor/device (Fitbit One) and SMS text-messaging prompts to increase physical activity in overweight and obese adults: a randomized controlled trial. *Telemed e-Health.* 2015;21(10). Available at https://www.liebertpub.com/doi/pdfplus/10.1089/tmj.2014.0176 (accessed January 17, 2019).

14. Chung AE, Skinner AC, Hasty SE, Perrin EM. Tweeting to health: a novel mHealth intervention using Fitbits and Twitter to foster healthy lifestyles. *Clin Pediatr (Phila).* 2016;56(1):26–32. DOI:10.1177/0009922816653385.

15. Raue M, D'Ambrosio LA, Coughlin JF. Savings competition: social comparison as motivation to save. Poster presented at the annual meeting of the Society for Judgment and Decision Making (SJDM). Boston, MA: November. 18–21, 2016.

16. Wasilenko KA, Kulik JA, Wanic RA. Effects of social comparisons with peers on women's body satisfaction and exercise behavior. *International Journal of Eating Disorders.* 2007 Dec;40(8):740–745. DOI:10.1002/eat.20433.

17. Modified from Chou WY, Hunt YM, Beckjord EB, Moser RP, Hesse BW. Social media use in the United States: implications for health communication. *J Med Internet Res.* 2009;11(4):e48. DOI:10.2196/jmir.1249.

18. Gebelhoff R. The anti-vaccine movement shows why Facebook is broken. *Washington Post.* January 9, 2018. Available at https://www.washingtonpost.com/blogs/post-partisan/wp/2018/01/09/the-anti-vaccine-movement-shows-why-facebook-is-broken/?utm_term=.da89083f08cc (accessed January 17, 2019).

19. Caron C. Facebook announces plan to curb vaccine misinformation. *New York Times.* March 7, 2019. Available at: https://www.nytimes.com/2019/03/07/technology/facebook-anti-vaccine-misinformation.html (accessed August 28, 2019)

20. Edelman.com. 2018 Edelman Trust Barometer Global Report. January 21, 2018. Available at https://www.edelman.com/sites/g/files/aatuss191/files/2018-10/2018_Edelman_Trust_Barometer_Global_Report_FEB.pdf (accessed January 17, 2019).

21. Cugelman B, Thelwall M, Dawes P. Online interventions for social marketing health

behavior change campaigns: a meta-analysis of psychological architectures and adherence factors. *J Med Internet Res*. 2011;13(1):e17. DOI:10.2196/jmir.1367.

22. Blendon RJ, Benson JM, Hero JO. Public trust in physicians — U.S. medicine in international perspective. *N Engl J Med*. 2014;371:1570–1572. DOI: 10.1056/NEJMp1407373.

23. Haag M. Voter registrations spike as deadlines loom. Taylor Swift had something to do with it. *New York Times*. October 9, 2018. Available at https://www.nytimes.com/2018/10/09/us/politics/taylor-swift-voter-registration.html (accessed January 17, 2019).

24. Byrne E, Kearney J, MacEvilly C. The role of influencer marketing and social influencers in public health. *Proc Nutr Soc*. 2017;76(OCE3):E103. DOI:10.1017/S0029665117001768.

25. Klassen KM, Borleis ES, Brennan L, Reid M, McCaffrey TA, Lim MS. What people "like": analysis of social media strategies used by food industry brands, lifestyle brands, and health. *J Med Internet Res*. 2018;20(6):e10227. DOI:10.2196/10227.

26. Heywood L. The CrossFit sensorium: visuality, affect and immersive sport. *Paragraph*. 2015;38(1):20–36. Available at https://doi.org/10.3366/para.2015.0144.

27. Beck J. The church of CrossFit. *The Atlantic*. June 24, 2017. Available at https://www.theatlantic.com/health/archive/2017/06/the-church-of-crossfit/531501/ (accessed January 17, 2019).

28. Kickbusch M, Payne L. Twenty-first century health promotion: the public health revolution meets the wellness revolution. *Health Promot Int*. 2003;18(4). DOI: 10.1093/heapro/dag418.

29. Gunter J. Worshipping the false idols of wellness. *New York Times*. August 1, 2018. Available at https://www.nytimes.com/2018/08/01/style/wellness-industrial-complex.html (accessed January 17, 2019).

30. Brodesser-Acker T. How Goop's haters made Gwyneth Paltrow's company worth $250 million. *New York Times*. July 25, 2018. Available at https://www.nytimes.com/2018/07/25/magazine/big-business-gwyneth-paltrow-wellness.html (accessed January 17, 2019).

31. Howland D. What's behind Best Buy's $800M foray into healthcare services? *RetailDive*. August 22, 2018. Available at https://www.retaildive.com/news/whats-behind-best-buys-800m-foray-into-healthcare-services/530603/ (accessed January 18, 2019).

32. Crosby J. Best Buy bones up on health care biz. *Star Tribune*. December 28, 2018. Available at http://www.startribune.com/best-buy-bones-up-on-health-care-biz/503634392/ (accessed January 18, 2019).

33. Thorndike AN, Sonnenberg L, Riis J, Barraclough S, Levy DE. A 2-phase labeling and choice architecture intervention to improve healthy food and beverage choices. *Am J Public Health*. 2012;102(3):527–533.

34. Paumgarten N. Food fighter. *The New Yorker*. January 4, 2010. Available at https://www.newyorker.com/magazine/2010/01/04/food-fighter (accessed January 17, 2019).

35. Gittelsohn J, Rowan M, Gadhoke P. Interventions in small food stores to change the food environment, improve diet, and reduce risk of chronic disease. *Prev Chronic Dis*. 2012;9:E59. Available at https://www.ncbi.nlm.nih.gov/pubmed/22338599. August 1, 2012 (accessed January 17, 2019).

36. Metz JA, Kris-Etherton PM, Morris CD, Mustad VA, Stern JS, Oparil S, et al. Dietary compliance and cardiovascular risk reduction with a prepared meal plan compared with a self-selected diet. *Am J Clin Nutr*. 1997;66(2):373–385. Available at https://doi.org/10.1093/ajcn/66.2.373 (accessed March 24, 2019).

37. Jones BL. A review of Blue Apron by a registered dietician. *Healthy Bachelorette*. January 13, 2016. Available at https://thehealthybachelorette.com/2016/01/13/a-review-of-blue-apron-by-a-registered-dietitian/ (accessed March 24, 2019).

38. Kahana E, Kahana B. Baby boomers' expectations of health and medicine. *Virtual Mentor*, 2014;16(5):380–384. DOI:10.1001/virtualmentor.2014.16.05.msoc2-1405.

39. AARP. Caregivers and technology: what they want and need. April 2016. Available at https://www.aarp.org/content/dam/aarp/home-and-family/personal-technology/2016/04/Caregivers-and-Technology-AARP.pdf (accessed January 17, 2018).

40. Coughlin JF, D'Ambrosio LA, Reimer B, Pratt MR. Older adult perceptions of smart home technologies: implications for research, policy and market innovations in healthcare. In: 2007 29th Annual International Conference of the IEEE Engineering in Medicine and Biology Society. 2007:1810-1815. DOI:10.1109 /IEMBS.2007.4352665 (accessed March 24, 2019).

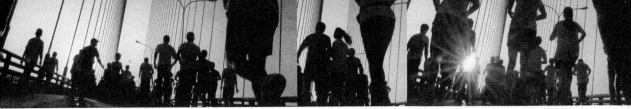

CHAPTER 10

Accountability for Outcomes

Matthew Stiefel

EXECUTIVE SUMMARY

This chapter is organized into three main sections that describe the purpose, methodology, and measures associated with accountability for outcomes. The first section describes the three main purposes of measurement—improvement, accountability, and research—and the different approaches to measurement based on the purpose. The measurement for improvement section describes the Model for Improvement, complementary improvement science tools, and other scientific methods for improvement in health care. Beyond specific methods, it also includes a discussion of the adaptive side of improvement and the psychology of change. The section on measurement for accountability is organized around the Donabedian "structure/process/outcome" model, wherein *structure* describes the context in which care is delivered, *process* denotes the transactions within the system, and *outcomes* refer to the effects of care on the health status of patients and populations. Historically accountability measurement has focused on process, but there is growing interest and application of outcome measures for accountability. The section on measurement for research discusses the differences in how the environment is treated between improvement science and research, the distinctions between efficacy and effectiveness research, and within effectiveness research, the distinction between comparative effectiveness and cost-effectiveness.

The second section on accountability for outcomes acknowledges health care's historically limited contribution to population health but growing interest in addressing the upstream behavioral, social, and environmental determinants of health, as well as the downstream outcomes of health and well-being. With this expanded role comes greater need for collaboration with other stakeholders, including individuals and families, professional societies, purchasers, regulators, social services, and the broader communities in general.

The third section on measurement for outcomes is organized around the Institute for Healthcare Improvement's Triple Aim framework: improving population health, per capita cost, and the care experience. It covers measurement of each of the three aims and discusses how they can be combined to assess overall value, as well as discussion of proposed additional aims, such as provider satisfaction and equity.

The chapter concludes with the observation that despite rapid advances in research and improvement science, enormous gaps remain between what we know about what works best in health care and how it is actually provided and provides current and future healthcare leaders with frameworks and resources to address these gaps.

LEARNING OBJECTIVES

By the end of this chapter, the reader will be able to:

1. Distinguish among the three main purposes of measurement: improvement, accountability, and research and the different approaches to measurement based on the purpose.
2. Learn about the role of health care in accountability for outcomes, and the need for multi-stakeholder collaboration.
3. Learn about the "Triple Aim" outcomes of population health, care experience, and cost and how to measure them.

KEY TERMS

Big data
Comparative effectiveness
    research (CER)
Cost effectiveness
Driver diagram
Effectiveness
Efficacy

Efficiency
Healthy life expectancy
Model for Improvement
Plan, do, study, act (PDSA)
    cycle
Predictive analytics
Qualitative research

Quality-adjusted life-years
    (QALYs)
Return on investment (ROI)
Run chart
Triple Aim
Value

▶ Purposes of Measurement: The "Why"

Improvement, accountability, and research are the three main purposes of measurement.[1] Approaches to measurement differ according to purpose. In measurement for improvement, the general strategy is to measure just enough to learn. This approach is characterized by limited data and small, sequential samples. Hypotheses are flexible and apt to change as learning takes place. Trend data are typically analyzed, and the data are used by those doing the improvement. Measurement for accountability focuses on reporting, oversight, comparison, choice, reassurance, or motivation for change. It is not about hypothesis testing but rather about evaluation of current performance. It is important to make adjustments to reduce bias in comparisons through approaches such as severity indexing, and equally important to collect all available, relevant data so that the analysis is significant and credible. Measurement for research seeks to discover new knowledge that may have broad application, where the standard of evidence is beyond doubt. In the research context, tests are carefully blinded and controlled, and the experimental design seeks to eliminate bias. Hypotheses are fixed, with a single, large test that typically employs traditional statistical techniques.

Because the purpose of measurement should determine the methods, mismatching purposes and methods can have adverse consequences. For example, applying traditional research methods in an improvement setting can slow down the learning process and, more importantly, set the bar for statistical significance too high to detect potentially useful changes. Alternatively, applying improvement methods to research questions can lead to inappropriate generalization of findings. However, the boundaries between the

methods are not fixed, and there are times when it makes sense to blend methods for greater effectiveness and efficiency. While there are three main purposes of measurement, there are many differences in the methods used for each purpose, as shown in **TABLE 10-1**.

TABLE 10-1 THE THREE PURPOSES OF MEASUREMENT

Aspect	Improvement	Accountability	Research
Aim	Improvement of care	Comparison, choice, reassurance, spur for change	New knowledge
Methods			
Test observability	Test observable	No test, evaluate current performance	Test blinded or controlled
Bias	Fixed hypothesis Accept consistent bias	Measure and adjust to reduce bias	Design to eliminate bias
Sample size	"Just enough" data, small sequential samples	Obtain 100% of available, relevant data	"Just in case" data
Flexibility of hypothesis	Hypothesis flexible, changes as learning takes place	No hypothesis	Fixed hypothesis
Testing strategy	Sequential tests	No tests	One large test
Determining if a change is an improvement	Run charts or Shewhart control charts	No change	Hypothesis, statistical tests (t test, F test, chi-square), p values
Confidentiality of the data	Data used only by those involved with improvement	Data available for public consumption	Research subjects' identities protected

Data from Solberg L, Mosser G, McDonald S. The three faces of performance measurement: improvement, accountability, and research. *Jt Comm J Qual Improv.* 1997;23(3):13–147. Provost L, Murray S. *The Data Guide: Learning from Data to Improve Health Care.* Austin, TX: Associates in Process Improvement; 2007.

Measurement for Improvement

The Model for Improvement

Measurement for improvement is built on a rich tradition of quality improvement measurement methods dating back to the early 1900s and was led by the pioneering work of Deming, Shewhart, and Juran. Developed by Associates in Process Improvement, in collaboration with the Institute for Healthcare Improvement (IHI), the **Model for Improvement** incorporates many of the tools and techniques introduced by these pioneers.[2] It is a simple but powerful tool for accelerating improvement. The Model for Improvement consists of two parts. The first part focuses on three basic questions used to frame the improvement journey:

1. What are we trying to accomplish?
2. How do we know that a change is an improvement?
3. What change can we make that will result in an improvement?

The second part consists of continual **plan, do, study, act (PDSA) cycles** to test and implement changes in real-world settings. A clear goal statement is essential to answer the first question concerning what we are trying to accomplish. A useful technique for developing goal statements is to make them SMART: *specific, measurable, attainable, realistic,* and *timebound.*

The tools of statistical process control were developed to answer the question of whether a change is an improvement. In general, the process involves plotting data over time and applying tests to determine whether there has been a change in the underlying results of a process. The first step is to gather data on performance. The data

collection tool need not be sophisticated but should include basic information about the process and outcomes, as well as observations about barriers or new ideas to test. The data should then be plotted in a **run chart** (i.e., a trend graph that includes a median line). Simple rules are used to analyze the data in a run chart to determine special cause variation as opposed to common cause variation, or chance. These rules are illustrated in **FIGURE 10-1**.

The control chart is a more sophisticated version of a run chart and is used to detect special-cause variation. This chart adds upper and lower control limits to a run chart and includes rules about the behavior of the data in relation to the control limits to determine whether a process is in control. After the run or control charts are developed, it is important to prominently display them for review by all those involved in the process and to include the charts in the improvement process.

Armed with the tools to determine improvement, the next logical step is to identify process changes that will result in an improvement. The PDSA cycle is a time-tested framework for generating and testing ideas for improvement. The *plan* step involves developing objectives, predictions, and plans to carry out the cycle. The *do* step involves carrying out the plan and documenting data and observations. The *study* step involves analyzing the data, comparing results to predictions, and summarizing what was learned. The *act* step involves determining the changes to be made in the next cycle, after which the cycle repeats. A key feature of the Model for Improvement is the rapid and repeated use of the PDSA cycle. In significant contrast to measurement for research, PDSA cycles might be measured in days or even hours.

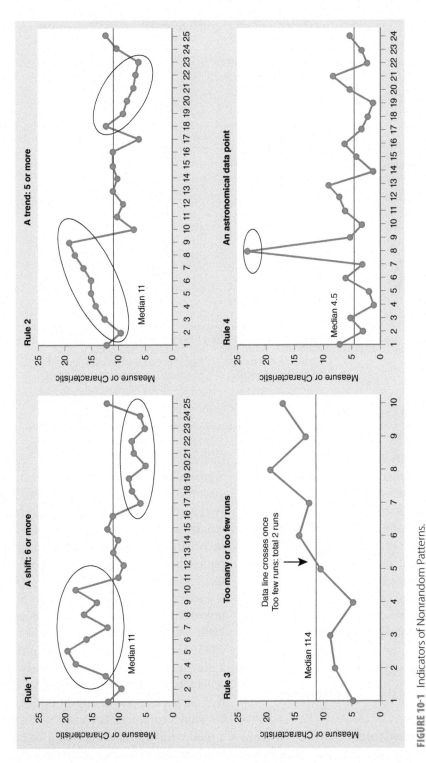

FIGURE 10-1 Indicators of Nonrandom Patterns.

Reproduced from Provost L, Murray S. *The Data Guide: Learning from Data to Improve Health Care*. Austin, TX: Associates in Process Improvement; 2007:3–10.

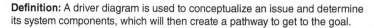

Definition: A driver diagram is used to conceptualize an issue and determine its system components, which will then create a pathway to get to the goal.

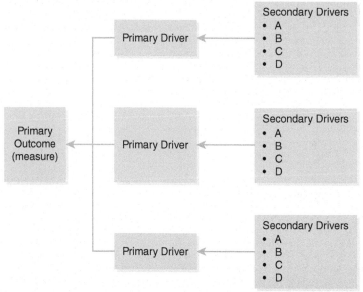

Primary drivers are system components, which will contribute to moving the primary outcome.

Secondary drivers are elements of the associated primary driver. They can be used to create projects or change packages that will affect the primary driver.

FIGURE 10-2 Driver Diagram Template.

Reproduced from Institute for Healthcare Improvement, Stiefel M, Nolan K. *A Guide to Measuring the Triple Aim: Population Health, Experience of Care, and Per Capita Cost.* IHI Innovation Series white paper. Cambridge, MA: Institute for Healthcare Improvement; 2012. (Available on www.IHI.org.)

The **driver diagram** developed by the IHI is another useful tool for designing changes that will result in an improvement. This diagram organizes the theory of improvement for a specific project, visually connecting the outcome or aim, key drivers, design changes, and measures. Typical key drivers include performance of a component of the system, an operating rule or value, or some element of system structure. A driver diagram template is shown in **FIGURE 10-2**.

Complementary Improvement Science Tools: Lean and Lean Six Sigma

Related improvement science methods adapted for use in health care from manufacturing include Lean and Lean Six Sigma. Lean manufacturing or lean production, often called simply "lean," is a systematic method for waste minimization within a manufacturing system without sacrificing productivity. This management philosophy was derived primarily from the Toyota Production System.[3] Six Sigma is a set of techniques and tools for process improvement introduced by Motorola in 1986 and adapted by General Electric in 1995.[4] The widely accepted definition of a Six Sigma process is an extremely high-reliability process that produces 3.4 defective parts per million opportunities. Lean Six Sigma combines Lean and Six Sigma in a methodology that relies on a collaborative team effort to improve performance by systematically removing waste and reducing variation.[5] The relationship between the Model for Improvement and Lean is addressed in an IHI white paper.[6] It notes that because they are complementary ways of approaching improvement, it is not necessary to choose one over the other as a guide to action.

Other Scientific Methods for Improvement in Health Care

In addition to improvement science, related scientific disciplines provide valuable tools to complement those of improvement science, including qualitative and ethnographic methods, information science, and **predictive analytics**.

Qualitative and Ethnographic Methods. **Qualitative research** is a scientific method of observation in social sciences to gather non-numerical data that can complement quantitative data by providing richer context and background. Qualitative and ethnographic methods, including video ethnography, can be effective tools to keep patients and caregivers at the center of quality improvement.[7-9] When embedded within an established quality improvement framework, video ethnography can be an effective tool for innovating new solutions, improving existing processes, and spreading knowledge about how best to meet patient needs. Frontline practitioners can practice video ethnography without expensive technology or extensive training, and the videos can powerfully convey the voice of the patient through storytelling.

Information Science. The explosion of "**big data**" in health care has the potential to dramatically change the scale and pace of improvement.[10] Big data is an evolving term that refers to the exploding volume, velocity and variety of data available together with novel methods for making sense of the data beyond traditional analytic methods.[11] Applications enabled by big data in health care include wearable devices that keep track and share in real time health-related data such as exercise and physiology; expanded diagnostic services that give patients greater access to professional care; expanded predictive analytics (see below); precision medicine through customization of therapies to individuals; and platforms to facilitate the use of big data for research.[12-15]

Predictive Analytics. Predictive analytics are a related powerful set of tools for performance improvement, growing in importance and relevance given the increased availability of big data. In general, this approach relies on mathematical algorithms to predict the probability of an outcome. The ultimate goal of using a predictive model is to deliver tailored interventions and resources to a specific population segment based on their specific needs.

The traditional approach to population care management has been to intervene with those individuals who historically have the worst outcomes or the highest utilization. This threshold approach assumes that members with poor outcomes this year are the most likely to have poor outcomes next year. The problem with this assumption is that those with the highest utilization in the general population are likely to have *lower* utilization in the next period, even in the absence of any intervention, because (1) the natural progression of an acute condition or the effect of treatment tends to cause people to get better over time unless they have a progressively deteriorating condition, and (2) the statistical phenomenon of regression toward the mean causes outliers in one period to move closer to the mean in the next period due to stochastic or random variation. The predictive modeling approach addresses this problem by looking retrospectively at patterns to apply to current data and forecast future patterns.

The main challenge with predictive modeling is *impactibility*, or the identification of those with the highest probability of benefit from an intervention. In a predictive model identifying high-cost individuals, the cost trajectory can be influenced only for a subset. Therefore, it is necessary to also predict high-cost individuals whose cost trajectories can be reduced using evidence-based and cost-effective interventions. Nationally recognized guidelines for care can assist in establishing these action plans.

Beyond Specific Methods for Improvement

Improvement science has provided health care with the technical skills to understand variation, study systems, build learning, and determine the best evidence-based interventions ("what") and implementation strategies ("how") to achieve the desired outcomes. Yet healthcare organizations worldwide still struggle with the adaptive side of change, which relates to unleashing the power of people ("who") and their motivations ("why") to advance improvement. The IHI has developed a "psychology of change" framework and related tools and methods to address the "who" and the "how," including the following five domains of practice: unleash intrinsic motivation, coproduce in authentic relationship, distribute power, codesign people-driven change, and adapt in action.[16]

In response to widespread demand for an improved healthcare system, the Institute of Medicine (now National Academy of Medicine [NAM]) developed a report in 2013 entitled "Best Care at Lower Cost: The Path to Continuously Learning Health Care in America," exploring healthcare challenges and recommending ways to create a continuously learning healthcare system.[17] Characteristics of a learning healthcare system include real-time access to knowledge; digital capture of the care experience; engaged, empowered patients; incentives aligned for value; full transparency; a leadership-instilled culture of learning; and supportive system competencies, including feedback loops for continuous learning and system improvement.

Measurement for Accountability

As noted above, measurement for accountability focuses on reporting, oversight, comparison, choice, reassurance, or motivation for change. The Donabedian model, developed in 1966, remains the dominant framework for accountability measurement.[18] According to the model, information about quality of care can be drawn from three categories: structure, process, and outcomes. *Structure* describes the context in which care is delivered, including hospital buildings, staff, financing, and equipment. *Process* denotes the transactions between patients and providers throughout the delivery of health care. *Outcomes* refer to the effects of health care on the health status of patients and populations.

Historically, the predominant accountability measures in health care have been process measures, including clinical processes, care experience, and financial performance. However, there is a growing interest in outcome accountability measures (see section on Triple Aim measurement). For example, the National Quality Forum (NQF) established the Prevention and Population Health Standing Committee in 2016 to broaden its perspective beyond traditional clinical measures to include a focus on healthy lifestyle behaviors and community interventions that improve health and well-being, as well as social and economic conditions.[19] The Centers for Medicare and Medicaid Services (CMS), as part of its Star rating and payment incentive system developed in 2008 for Medicare Advantage plans, included health outcome measures from the Medicare Health Outcomes Survey in its performance measurement set.[20] The International Consortium for Health Outcomes Measurement (ICHOM) was founded in 2012 with the purpose to transform healthcare systems worldwide by measuring and reporting patient outcomes in a standardized way through performance registries.[21]

There are also a growing number of scorecards at the local community, county, state, and national levels that provide ratings or rankings related to population health, such as the County Health Rankings,[22] America's Health Rankings,[23] and Healthiest Communities Rankings.[24] In addition, the National Committee for Vital and Health Statistics developed a measurement framework for community health and well-being in 2017.[25]

Measurement for Research

An important distinction between measurement for improvement and measurement for research is how the environment is treated in investigating causation. In general, epidemiologic research seeks to establish causation *in spite of* the practice environment by controlling for environmental influences, while improvement science seeks to establish causation *because of* change in the environment.[26] Improvement science acknowledges that the process of providing care has as much to do with patient outcomes as the care itself, and there is growing interest in the complementarity of improvement and research methods.[27]

One important, high-level topic for decision support is the distinction between efficacy and effectiveness research. Both are focused on whether a particular intervention works. The term **efficacy** refers to whether an intervention can work under ideal conditions. The pragmatic question of whether an intervention works in routine clinical care is addressed by the term **effectiveness**. Clinical trials are examples of efficacy research. They are designed to isolate the effect of a particular intervention by controlling, to the extent possible, for other factors of potential influence. In real life, these factors *do* intervene and influence the effectiveness of the intervention (e.g., patients enrolled in clinical trials usually have no health problems other than the ones under investigation, and compliance is carefully controlled). In contrast, patients treated in routine clinical practices often have multiple conditions and may fail to follow medical advice. The questions addressed by efficacy research and effectiveness research are both meaningful and complementary, but it is important to be clear about which question is being addressed in a particular research study.

Comparative effectiveness and **cost-effectiveness** are two related and important types of health services research.

The NAM defines **comparative effectiveness research** (CER) as:

> ... the generation and synthesis of evidence that compares the benefits and harms of alternative methods to prevent, diagnose, treat, and monitor a clinical condition or to improve the delivery of care. The purpose of CER is to assist consumers, clinicians, purchasers, and policy makers to make informed decisions that will improve health care at both the individual and population levels.[20]

Cost-effectiveness research views economic considerations in relation to effectiveness. It is a construct closely related to efficiency, measuring the cost of a program or intervention associated with a given level of effectiveness. In health services research, **quality-adjusted life years**, or QALYs, is the measure of individual health most commonly used in cost-effectiveness analysis. The QALY is the individual health building block of the population health measure of healthy life expectancy. It is defined as a year of life lived in less-than-perfect health compared to a year of life in perfect health (e.g., a year lived with acid reflux may be equated to half a year in perfect health). Healthcare regulatory agencies in many countries (e.g., the National Institute for Health and Clinical Excellence in the United Kingdom) use cost-effectiveness analysis explicitly in their evaluations of new drugs and technologies. In the context of the Triple Aim value framework, cost-effectiveness can also be seen as a combination of two elements of the Triple Aim: cost and health.

A full review of research methods for health services and population health research is beyond the scope of this chapter. See Suggested Readings and Websites at the end of this chapter for resources on health services research methods.

▶ Accountability for Outcomes: The "How"

As noted above, health care's contribution to population health is relatively small when compared to the contributions of behavioral, social, environmental, and genetic determinants. However, this is more of a descriptive than a normative view, and healthcare organizations are reaching upstream to address the behavioral, social and environmental determinants and reaching downstream to measure health and well-being outcomes that matter to people. As healthcare organizations embrace this expanded role, the question of relative accountabilities for outcomes becomes important, and the need for multi-stakeholder collaboration for outcomes becomes essential.

There is growing international momentum among healthcare organizations moving upstream to address the behavioral, social, and environmental determinants of health. It is not new for healthcare systems to address the proximal upstream behavioral determinants of health, such as tobacco use, alcohol use, diet, and exercise. Incentives for addressing primary prevention and behavioral risk factors have always existed for health maintenance organizations, and the focus has increased recently for other types of healthcare organizations in the movement from payment for volume (fee for service) to payment for value, and the promotion of accountable care organizations.[28,29]

Recognition is also growing at national policy levels of the benefits that accrue from greater integration of health care with social services to address the upstream determinants of health. Several countries, including Finland, Scotland, and England, have consolidated, or "joined up," their health care and social services budgets.[30-32] In 2016, the U.S. Department of Health and Human Services announced the Accountable Health Communities Model, which focuses on linking clinical and community-based services that address a range of social needs, including transportation and housing.[33] In addition, governments at many levels are increasingly focusing on the health impact of policies formulated in sectors other than health, often referred to as "health in all policies."[34,35] There have also been calls to extend this idea to "well-being in all policies" to broaden the frame beyond health and health care and more fully engage other sectors.[36] Many healthcare organizations are also moving to address the upstream determinants of health, and evidence of the positive impact on improving outcomes and reducing disparities is beginning to emerge.[37] In 2017, 19 states required Medicaid managed care plans to screen for and/or provide referrals for social needs, and a survey of Medicaid managed care plans found that almost all responding plans reported activities to address social determinants of health.[38]

There are multiple levels of accountability for population health, including individuals and families, the healthcare delivery system, professional societies, purchasers, regulators, and communities.

Individuals and families have substantial but not complete accountability for their own health, since factors outside their control, such as genetics and social or environmental circumstances, also have powerful influence. In 2000, the U.S. Centers for Disease Control and Prevention (CDC) estimated that tobacco use, unhealthy dietary practices, physical inactivity, and excess consumption of alcoholic beverages accounted for approximately 40% of all deaths in the United States.[39] As these behaviors occur in clusters, they also are related to approximately 80% of chronic diseases and, as such, are associated with almost 75% of all medical care expenditures in the United States.[40]

Given these statistics, there is growing recognition within the healthcare system of the importance of partnering with patients and families to take joint accountability for their health. It has become a standard of care based on the recognition that patients and families are essential allies for quality and safety—not only in direct care interactions but also in quality improvement, safety initiatives, education of health professionals, research, facility design, and policy development.[41]

Within healthcare delivery, there is an incentive for performance measurement to align with measures that are required for regulatory or certification requirements. Internal healthcare system accountability measures cover multiple levels, including clinical interactions, operations, and mission/strategy. These measures are often the same measures as reported externally.

Professional societies in health care also have an important role in accountability measurement. Leading professional societies include the American Medical Association (AMA) and American Hospital Association (AHA), as well as professional societies for each of the major medical professions. For example, in 2000, the AMA convened the Physician Consortium for Performance Improvement (PCPI) as a physician-led program to develop performance measures that addressed a significant gap in the measurement landscape. PCPI has developed hundreds of quality measures for use by CMS, states, and private health plan payment models.[42]

Purchasers also have a vested interest in healthcare system performance. In general, purchasers rely on publicly reported regulatory and accreditation measures, but in some cases, large national purchasers or collaboratives have developed their own reporting requirements. Purchasers have promoted the concept of "value-driven" health care and have developed pay-for-performance systems that reward value, in the domains of health information technology, quality, price, and incentives.[43] The Leapfrog Group, a national non-profit group founded in 2000 by large employers and other purchasers, has been a leading advocate for value-based purchasing.[44]

The primary regulatory and accreditation organizations for health care include the CMS, The Joint Commission (TJC), the National Committee for Quality Assurance (NCQA), and the NQF. CMS is not only a regulatory organization but is also the largest purchaser of healthcare services in the United States, and its reporting requirements are extensive.[45] CMS coordinates its accountability reporting system with TJC, NCQA, and NQF. TJC, an independent, non-profit organization founded in 1951, accredits and certifies healthcare organizations and programs in the United States, including hospitals and healthcare organizations that provide ambulatory and office-based surgery and behavioral health, home health care, laboratory, and nursing care center services.[46] TJC accreditation and certification are voluntary. NCQA, founded in the early 1990s, is also an independent, non-profit organization that manages voluntary accreditation programs for individual physicians, health plans, and medical groups. Health plans seek accreditation and measure performance through the administration and submission of the Healthcare Effectiveness Data and Information Set (HEDIS) and Consumer Assessment of Healthcare Providers and Systems (CAHPS) survey.[47] NQF is another independent, non-profit organization, founded in 1999, which conducts a consensus-based quality measure endorsement process that brings together diverse healthcare stakeholders from the public and private sector to foster quality improvement. Under contract to the federal government, NQF convenes a consensus body to recommend measures for specific federal programs. The federal government, states, and private-sector organizations use NQF's endorsed measures, which must meet rigorous criteria, to evaluate performance and share information with patients and their families.[48]

The role of communities in public health is fundamental and well established. The traditional role of public health has been understood by many to be the critical functions of state and local public health departments such as preventing epidemics, containing environmental hazards, and encouraging healthy behaviors. Population health advocates argue that the frame for population health is broader, including the outcomes, distribution, and determinants of health in a population. However, in a report on "The Future of the Public's Health in the 21st Century," the NAM reaches beyond the narrow governmental view of public health and calls for significant movement in "building a new generation of intersectoral partnerships that draw on the perspectives and resources of diverse communities and actively engage them in health action."[49]

The distinction between public health and population health deserves attention since the terms sometimes have been incorrectly used interchangeably. Although the two disciplines are related, there are important differences between the two. *Public health* refers to the policies and actions we undertake as a society to create the conditions that allow people to be healthy. *Population health* builds on the foundation of public health to explore the conditions that influence health outcomes and measure their impact.[50]

▶ **Outcomes Measurement: The "What"**

Triple Aim Measurement Framework

The IHI's **Triple Aim** provides a useful framework for health care measurement.[51] It focuses on three main components—improving population health, per capita cost, and the care experience. This section covers measurement of each of the three aims and discusses how they can be combined to assess overall value.

Population Health Measurement Framework

Many frameworks and models have been developed to illustrate the relationships among the determinants and outcomes of population health. The model shown in **FIGURE 10-3** is based on one originally published by Evans and Stoddart. In their landmark 1990 publication,[52] they expanded the relationship between health care and disease by describing broader determinants of health, including genetics, physical and social environment, and behavior. They also broadened the concept of health beyond the absence of disease to include well-being and prosperity.

The model elaborates on the causal pathways and relationships described by Evans and Stoddart and provides a framework for measurement by distinguishing between determinants (upstream and individual factors) and outcomes. Within outcomes, the model distinguishes between intermediate outcomes and health outcomes (states of health).

Following the original Evans and Stoddart model, Kindig and Stoddart later added the important dimension of the *distribution* of health in a population to differentiate it from individual health.[53] McGinnis and colleagues then estimated the relative effects of the various determinants of health described by Evans and Stoddart.[54] These effects are shown in **FIGURE 10-4**.

A provocative conclusion of their analysis is health care's relatively small contribution to population health when compared to the contributions of behavioral, environmental, and genetic determinants. Kindig later operationalized this framework in a measurement system, ranking the counties in Wisconsin on both the determinants and outcomes of population health, as shown in **FIGURE 10-5**.[55]

The contributions of the healthcare delivery system shown in the model (i.e., prevention, health promotion, and medical care) are discussed as part of the frameworks for the care experience and cost elements of the Triple Aim.

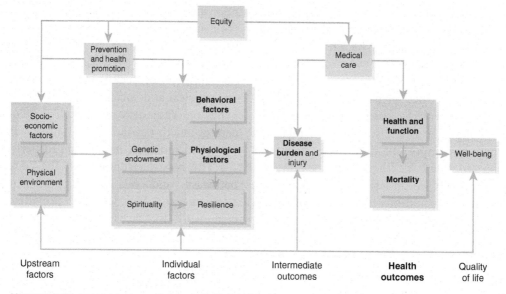

Measures in the measurement menu below are highlighted in **bold**

FIGURE 10-3 Population Health.

Reproduced from Stiefel M, Nolan K. A Guide to Measuring the Triple Aim: Population Health, Experience of Care, and Per Capita Cost. IHI Innovation Series white paper. Cambridge, MA: Institute for Healthcare Improvement; 2012. (Available on www.IHI.org.)

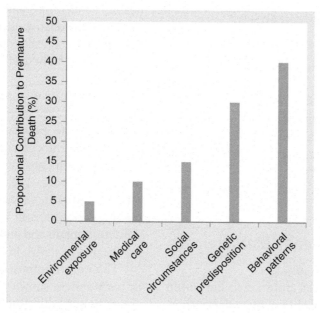

FIGURE 10-4 Determinants of Health.

Data from McGinnis JM, Williams-Russo P, Knickman JR. The case for more promotion. *Health Aff. (Millwood)* 2002;21:78–93.

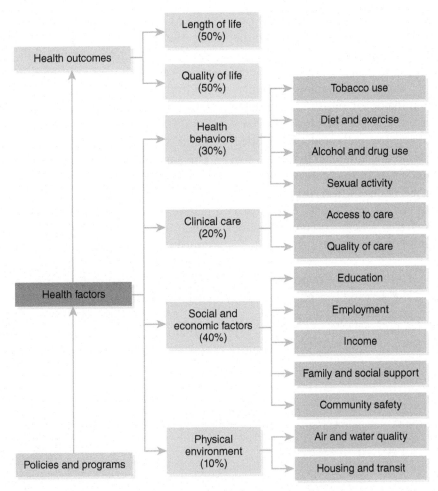

FIGURE 10-5 Determinants and Outcomes of Population Health in the United States by State.

Reproduced from County Health Rankings & Roadmaps, http://www.countyhealthrankings.org/our-approach (accessed March 28, 2019).

Care Experience Measurement Framework

The six aims for health care articulated by the NAM in its landmark report, *Crossing the Quality Chasm* (i.e., care that is safe, effective, patient centered, timely, equitable, and efficient), are useful as a framework for measuring the determinants of the care experience and providing decision support for those managing the health status of populations.[56] When used as a population strategic outcome measure, the six aims should be considered

as a bundle (i.e., most if not all should be included as the measure of care experience rather than using just one or two). Together with an overall measure of patient experience, these aims are helpful in constructing a driver diagram for the care experience, as shown in Figure 10-2.

Cost Measurement Framework

The concept of cost measurement is more straightforward than is the measurement of population health and care experience, because there are common monetary units with built-in exchange rates that easily can be rolled up or drilled down. However, the practice of cost measurement is complicated by a number of factors. Like population health, per capita cost requires a population denominator for measurement; however, most of the U.S. healthcare delivery and financing data are stored and analyzed separately, making it difficult to identify the population served by the delivery system. In addition, it is unclear which costs to include and from whose perspective. **FIGURE 10-6** provides a framework for cost measurement that includes three lenses on cost:

1. The supply lens of providers
2. The demand lens of consumers, purchasers, and the general public
3. The intermediary lens of health plans and insurers

The different lenses assist in understanding the costs being measured. Provider costs can be disaggregated into various types of health care as shown. It is useful to further disaggregate provider costs into volume and unit cost (e.g., hospital days and cost per day) to better understand sources of variation and change. The sum of provider costs and overhead and margins equals the total costs of care. These costs are paid by a combination of payments from health plans and insurers, public and private payer self-funding, and consumer out-of-pocket payments. These payments and their associated overhead and margins constitute the premium costs paid by public and private payers (e.g., Medicare and Medicaid, employers and union trusts, and individual consumers). Medicare Advantage health plans are managed care plans for Medicare

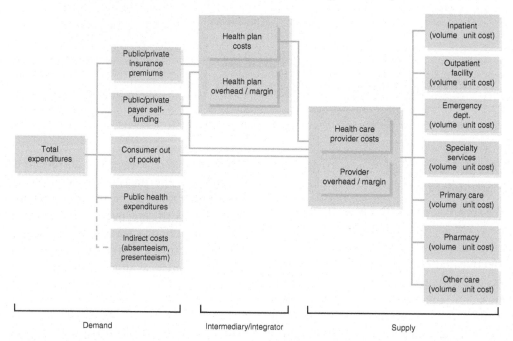

FIGURE 10-6 Per Capita Cost.

beneficiaries. Payments are based on a monthly fee per enrollee (capitation), as opposed to traditional Medicare where providers bill a fee for each medical service provided (fee-for-service). Public and private payers also purchase care directly from providers through self-funding; however, these payments are often administered by insurers through third-party administrator services.

From a broad public policy perspective, total costs include public health expenditures as well as direct healthcare costs. Finally, employers increasingly recognize that the indirect costs of poor health (e.g., absenteeism, loss of productivity) may exceed direct healthcare expenditures and must be taken into account when assessing the value of their health promotion and healthcare programs.

The cost of care has been used as a proxy for illness burden. Although this can be directionally correct, great care must be taken when comparing costs between areas or organizations because there is significant variation in utilization of services and unit costs from one to another.[57]

Overall Value Measurement Framework

Value and return on investment are important decision support metrics to those purchasing health care for a population. A common definition of **value** is "worth, utility, or importance in comparison with something else."[10] This definition highlights an important characteristic of value—that it is relative. Value is more than finding something desirable. It requires a determination of what would be given up in exchange for something. For market goods, value is

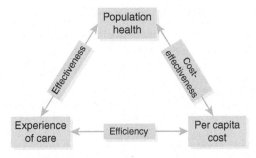

FIGURE 10-7 Overall Value.

indicated by the amount of money a person is willing to pay. The ultimate test of value is choice—people "vote with their feet" if given an opportunity. Another key characteristic of value is that it is subjective. There is no one, right answer, and different stakeholders have different perspectives on value.

Taken together, the three parts of the Triple Aim provide a useful framework for measuring *value* in health care, as shown in **FIGURE 10-7**. Value can be conceptualized as the optimization of the Triple Aim, recognizing that different stakeholders may weigh the three parts differently. Cost measurement in isolation has little utility; to be useful, it must be combined with measures of the other parts of the Triple Aim.

The combination of cost and care experience enables measurement of **efficiency**, a term that has been both hotly debated and loosely defined in recent years. The American Quality Alliance (AQA), formerly known as the Ambulatory Care Quality Alliance, has developed a useful definition of efficiency in health care that was subsequently endorsed by the NQF: "Efficiency of care is a measure of the relationship of the cost of care associated with a specific level of performance measured with respect to the other five NAM aims of quality."[11] Similarly, the combination of health outcomes with the care received enables measurement of *effectiveness* of care, or *comparative effectiveness* of alternative treatments. Combining all three parts of the Triple Aim enables measurement of *cost effectiveness*, or overall value.

Although all three aims are important, purchasers place a priority on cost, consumers focus on health outcomes and the care experience (and cost, because they bear an increasing responsibility for costs), and clinicians emphasize the quality of care and service provided. For health plans, the challenge is to develop products that balance these aims to be able to compete successfully in the marketplace.

Another concept related to value, **return on investment** (ROI) for health care is especially important from the purchaser's perspective. ROI describes the size of a return relative to an investment. The ROI measure has some important limitations in that projects with the same ROI can have very different total savings. For any two projects,

the one with the lower ROI may actually have the higher total savings. This issue is particularly important to purchasers evaluating disease management programs. For example, a program costing $1 million and returning $3 million in savings has a 3:1 ROI and $2 million in net savings. In contrast, a program costing $10 million and returning $20 million in savings has a 2:1 ROI and $10 million in net savings. Of course, budget constraints are relevant, but the program with the lower ROI in this case produces $8 million more in savings. For this reason, the Population Health Alliance recommends net savings over ROI in the evaluation of disease management programs.[58]

Triple Aim Measurement Guide

A menu of population outcome measures, developed for the IHI Triple Aim Collaborative with consideration given to the measurement frameworks outlined in the previous section, is shown in **TABLE 10-2**.[59]

TABLE 10-2 POTENTIAL POPULATION HEALTH OUTCOME MEASURES

Dimension of the IHI Triple Aim Outcome Measures

Health outcomes:
- Mortality: Years of potential life lost, life expectancy, standardized mortality ratio

- Health and functional status: Single-question assessment (e.g., from CDC HRQOL-4) or multidomain assessment (e.g., VR-12, PROMIS Global-10)

- Healthy life expectancy (HLE): Combines life expectancy and health status into a single measure, reflecting remaining years of life in good health

Disease burden:
- Incidence (yearly rate of onset, average age of onset) and prevalence of major chronic conditions

This menu is based on a combination of the analytic framework presented earlier and the practical experience of participating organizations in the IHI Triple Aim Collaborative. The selection of measures depends in part on data availability, resource constraints, and overall objectives.

The menu of measures for population health follows the analytic framework, including the logical flow from behavioral and physiologic factors to disease burden to health outcomes.[60] Measures of behavioral and physiologic factors and disease burden are included because they are direct causes of health outcomes and are generally more available than true outcome measures of quantity and quality of life. However, as noted above, there is increasing interest in and availability of these outcome measures. For example, life expectancy data are available by county in the United States, with efforts under way to report at sub-county levels.[61] In addition, patient-reported health and functional status outcomes are becoming standard outcome measures. The Patient-Centered Outcomes Research Institute (PCORI) works to improve healthcare decision making, care delivery, and health outcomes by focusing on patients' desired health outcomes.[62] The advancement of subjective measures is also supported by the NIH Patient-Reported Outcomes Measurement Information System (PROMIS), which promotes the use of these measures in clinical research and practice.[63] The Medicare Health Outcomes Survey has been used by the Medicare program since 1998 to monitor performance for Medicare managed care programs.[64] The goal is to gather valid, reliable, and clinically meaningful health-status data from the Medicare Advantage (MA) program to use in quality improvement activities, pay for performance, program oversight, public reporting, and to improve health.

The ultimate outcome measures for population health (i.e., length and quality of life) can be combined to create a measure of **healthy life expectancy**. This has become a standard for assessing health outcomes for many countries.[65,66] A wide variety of measures are used in practice in countries around the world for the quality of life component of healthy life expectancy measures, including disease status, functional status, self-reported health, and well-being.[67-70] Healthy life expectancy was recently reported for all states in the United States, along with an analysis of trends and influencing factors, using the same clinical disability measure as used by the World Health Organization for countries around the world, called "disability-adjusted life-years."[71,72] One significant advantage of such composite measures is that they enable analysis of the relative contributions of mortality and morbidity to the overall measure. For example, cancer and heart disease are typically listed as the most important population health problems when viewed through the single lens of mortality. However, using the composite outcome measure, non-fatal conditions such as arthritis and chronic pain have much greater influence. For example, a recent Canadian study estimated that chronic pain had four times the impact on healthy life expectancy than either cancer or heart disease.[73]

There has been increasing interest lately in moving beyond a measure of health to the broader construct of well-being to measure quality of life, positioning health as both a component of and contributor to overall well-being.[74] This broader frame underscores the importance of health care collaboration with other sectors to achieve shared well-being goals for communities and society.

Although there is no standard definition of well-being, most definitions include an element related to over-all life evaluation, including meaning and purpose, and an affective element related to emotional well-being, including happiness and sadness. For example, the Organisation for Economic Co-operation and Development (OECD) defines subjective well-being as: "good mental states, including all of the various evaluations, positive and negative, that people make of their lives and the affective reactions of people to their experiences."[75] The Gallup-Sharecare "Well-Being Index" is the world's largest data set on well-being, with ongoing assessment in the United States and other countries around the world.[76]

There are two important perspectives on the experience of care: (1) the perspective of the individual who interacts with the healthcare system (i.e., patient experience surveys) and (2) the perspective of the healthcare system focused on designing a high-quality experience for its patients as defined by the NAM's six aims. Patient surveys are a good source to determine the individual perspective. The measurement menu includes two commonly used assessments: the CAHPS family of surveys and the "How's Your Health?" survey.[77,78] Some health systems utilize an overall measure of "likelihood to recommend" as an indirect measure of care quality.

The main accountability measures for healthcare quality based on the NAM's Six Aims come from the regulatory and accreditation organizations discussed above: CMS, TJC, NCQA, and NQF.

Total cost per member of the population per month (PMPM) is the desirable measure for cost. Sources for per capita cost measurement include the relative resource use measures from the NCQA's HEDIS and the Dartmouth Atlas.[79,80]

A healthcare system that doesn't serve a defined population is not able to use population-based measures. In that case, organizations often use a high-cost services measure (e.g., inpatient utilization and costs). Because these services account for a substantial share of healthcare expenditures, such a measure is a good surrogate measure for cost. In addition, episode-based costing is more commonly used today. The unit of analysis—the episode of care—is defined as "a series of temporally contiguous health care services related to the treatment of a given spell of illness or provided in response to a specific request by the patient or other relevant entity."[81]

The Quadruple Aim

Since the introduction of the Triple Aim, many organizations and individuals have suggested the addition of a fourth aspect to create the "Quadruple Aim." The most common addition is an aim around improving the work life of providers, often referred to as "joy in work."[82] Others have added health equity, and the Military Health System has added the dimension of military readiness.[83] IHI, the original developer of the Triple Aim, has expressed support for other organizations prioritizing such worthy efforts, but has recommended that the following points be kept in mind:

- Remember that the Triple Aim, at its core, is about improving the lives of patients.
- There is still much work to do in pursuit of the Triple Aim, and don't lose that focus in measurement and in setting priorities.
- Both joy in work and equity are essential to achieve the Triple Aim.[84]

▶ Conclusion

The tools and methods used in population health are dictated by the kinds of decisions needing support. Decisions in the areas of improvement, accountability, and research require different types of decision support, and the distinctions have been highlighted in this chapter for clarity. However, the boundaries are not as distinct in practice, and it is important to consider how they fit together in an integrated analytic and evaluation system.

Local improvement efforts frequently reach a point at which a large investment or change is required for widespread implementation. At that point, more tightly controlled research methods may be required to enhance confidence in the investment decision. As clinical information systems and electronic medical records become more widespread, there is increasing opportunity to thoughtfully design data systems that can be used for all three purposes of process improvement, external reporting, and research. Expanding knowledge in health informatics and healthcare delivery means that clinical decision support increasingly will be built into the electronic process with embedded clinical guidelines and alerts. With such an integrated decision-support infrastructure, it is possible to envision improvement projects generating ideas for research, research findings more quickly implemented in practice, and reporting requirements fulfilled through automated extractions from electronic data systems. Data could seamlessly roll up to the board of directors and external reporting agencies for accountability, down to frontline teams for improvement, and over to research teams to generate new knowledge and insights.

Despite rapid advances in research and improvement science, enormous gaps remain between what we know about what works best in health care and how it is actually provided. In the United States, the magnitude of these gaps has been documented in several major reports from the NAM, including "Crossing the Quality Chasm: To Err Is Human," and "Unequal Treatment: Confronting Racial and Ethnic Disparities in Health Care."[85-87] Similar problems have been noted globally in both advanced economies and in countries with limited resources. Improvement in health and outcomes has been agonizingly slow, but increasing global evidence and experience suggest that progress can be accelerated through a scientific approach to quality improvement.

This chapter has provided an overview of the purposes for measurement in population health (the "why"), accountability for outcomes (the "how"), and measurement of outcomes (the "what"). It has also provided frameworks, practical tools, and examples in each of these areas to enable current and future population health leaders to address the profound challenges of improving the level and distribution of health and well-being in our communities.

Study and Discussion Questions

1. What are the three main purposes of population health measurement?
2. What are the three basic questions in the Model for Improvement?
3. What are the three elements of the Donabedian model for evaluating health care quality?

4. How does efficacy research differ from effectiveness research in health services?
5. What are the key determinants of population health?
6. Who are the key stakeholders of accountability for population health?
7. What are the three elements of the Triple Aim?
8. What are three perspectives on cost that are included in a cost measurement framework?

Suggested Readings and Websites
Suggested readings

Vital Directions for Health and Health Care. https://nam.edu/wp-content/uploads/2018/02/Vital-Directions-for-Health-and-Health-Care-Final-Publication-022718.pdf

National Quality Forum ABCs of Measurement. https://www.qualityforum.org/Measuring_Performance/ABCs_of_Measurement.aspx

Scoville R, Little K. *Comparing Lean and Quality Improvement.* IHI white paper. Cambridge, MA: Institute for Healthcare Improvement; 2014.

Websites

NCQA Release New Standards Category for Population Health Management. https://www.ncqa.org/news/ncqa-release-new-standards-category-population-health-management/

NCQA Population Health Program Accreditation. https://www.ncqa.org/programs/health-plans/population-health-program-accreditation/

References

1. Solberg LI, Mosser G, McDonald S. The three faces of performance measurement: improvement, accountability, and research. *Jt Comm Qual Improv.* 1997;23(3):135–147.
2. Langley GJ, Moen RD, Nolan KM, Nolan TW, Norman CL, Provost LP. *The Improvement Guide: A Practical Approach to Enhancing Organizational Performance.* San Francisco, CA: Jossey-Bass; 2009.
3. Holweg M. The genealogy of lean production. *J Operations Mgt.* 2007;25(2):420–437. DOI: 10.1016/j.jom.2006.04.001.
4. Pyzdek T, Keller PA. *The Six Sigma Handbook* (5th ed.). McGraw-Hill Education; 2018.
5. George ML, Rowlands D, Kastle B. What is Lean Six Sigma? New York: McGraw-Hill; 2004.
6. Scoville R, Little K. *Comparing Lean and Quality Improvement.* IHI white paper. Cambridge, MA: Institute for Healthcare Improvement; 2014. Available from http://www.ihi.org/resources/Pages/IHIWhitePapers/ComparingLeanandQualityImprovement.aspx (accessed September 1, 2018).
7. Rashid M, Caine V, Goez H. The encounters and challenges of ethnography as a methodology in health research. *Int J Qual Methods.* 2015;14(5). DOI: 10.1177/1609406915621421.
8. Neuwirth EB, Bellows J, Jackson AH, Price PM. How Kaiser Permanente uses video ethnography of patients for quality improvement, such as in shaping better care transitions. *Health Aff.* 2012;31(6). DOI: 10.1377/hlthaff.2012.0134.
9. Kaiser Permanente. Getting started in video ethnography. Available from http://kpcmi.org/ethnography/video-ethnography-tool-kit.pdf (accessed September 1, 2018).
10. New England Journal of Medicine Catalyst. Healthcare big data and the promise of value-based care. New England Journal of Medicine [cited September 1, 2018]. Available from https://catalyst.nejm.org/big-data-healthcare (accessed May 31, 2019).
11. De Mauro A, Greco M, Grimaldi M. A formal definition of big data based on its essential features. *Library Rev.* 2016;65(3):122–135. DOI: 10.1108/LR-06-2015-0061.

12. UK Biobank. Biobank. Available from http://www.ukbiobank.ac.uk (accessed September 1, 2018).

13. Innovative Medicines Initiative Joint Undertaking. European Medical Information Framework. Available from http://www.emif.eu (accessed September 1, 2018).

14. Innovative Medicines Initiative Joint Undertaking. Open PHACTS. Available from https://www.openphacts.org (accessed September 1, 2018).

15. National Institutes of Health. *About BD2K.* Available from https://datascience.nih.gov/bd2k/about (accessed September 1, 2018).

16. Institute for Healthcare Improvement. Use the psychology of change to lead safety transformation. 2018. Available from http://www.ihi.org/communities/blogs/use-the-psychology-of-change-to-lead-safety-transformation (accessed September 1, 2018).

17. Institute of Medicine. 2013. *Best care at lower cost: The path to continuously learning health care in America.* Washington, DC: The National Academies Press. DOI: 10.17226/13444.

18. Donabedian, A. The quality of care: how can it be assessed? *JAMA.* 1988;260(12):1743–1748. DOI: 10.1001/jama.1988.03410120089033.

19. National Quality Forum. Prevention and Population Health. Available from http://www.qualityforum.org/ProjectDescription.aspx?projectID=86178 (accessed September 1, 2018).

20. McKinsey & Company. Assessing the Medicare advantage star ratings. Available from https://www.mckinsey.com/industries/healthcare-systems-and-services/our-insights/assessing-the-medicare-advantage-stars-ratings (accessed September 1, 2018).

21. International Consortium for Health Outcomes Measurement. What is ICHOM? http://www.ichom.org (accessed September 1, 2018).

22. University of Wisconsin Population Health Institute. County Health Rankings & Roadmaps 2018. Available from www.countyhealthrankings.org (accessed September 1, 2018).

23. United Health Foundation. America's health rankings. Available from https://www.americashealthrankings.org (accessed September 1, 2018).

24. U.S. News & World Report. Healthiest communities rankings. Available from https://www.usnews.com/news/healthiest-communities/rankings (accessed September 1, 2018).

25. U.S. Department of Health and Human Services. NCVHS measurement framework for community health and well-being, V4. Available from https://ncvhs.hhs.gov/wp-content/uploads/2018/03/NCVHS-Measurement-Framework-V4-Jan-12-2017-for-posting-FINAL.pdf (accessed September 1, 2018).

26. HiQuiPs. QI Series Part 3 Differentiating quality improvement and clinical epidemiology. Available from https://canadiem.org/qi-clinical-epidemiology (accessed September 1, 2018).

27. Institute for Healthcare Improvement. Building a learning health care system. Available from http://app.ihi.org/FacultyDocuments/Events/Event-2354/Presentation-10006/Document-7652/Lloyd_Provost.pdf (accessed September 1, 2018).

28. Miller HD. From volume to value: better ways to pay for health care. *Health Aff.* 2009 Sep/Oct;28(5). DOI: 10.1377/hlthaff.28.5.1418.

29. Centers for Medicare and Medicaid Services. Accountable care organizations. Available from https://www.cms.gov/Medicare/Medicare-Fee-for-Service-Payment/ACO/index.html (accessed September 1, 2018).

30. National Institute for Health and Welfare. History. Available from https://thl.fi/en/web/thlfi-en/about-us/what-is-thl-/history (accessed September 1, 2018).

31. The Scottish Government. Joining up health and social care. Available from http://news.scotland.gov.uk/News/Joining-up-health-and-social-care-9c7.aspx (accessed January 21, 2016).

32. Bate A. Health and social care integration [Internet]. House of Commons Library Briefing Paper Number 2902; 2017 [cited September 1, 2018]. Available from http://researchbriefings.files.parliament.uk/documents/CBP-7902/CBP-7902.pdf (accessed May 31, 2019).

33. Centers for Medicare & Medicaid Services. Accountable health communities model announced. Available from http://stateofreform.com/news/federal/cms/2016/01/accountable-health-communities-model-announced (accessed September 1, 2018).

34. Puska P. Health in all policies — from what to how. *Eur J Public Health.* 2014;24(1):1. DOI: 10.1093/eurpub/ckt133.

35. Leppo KE, Ollila E, Peña S, Wismar M, Cook S. Health in all policies: seizing opportunities, implementing policies [Internet]. United Nations Research Institute for Social Development. 2013 [cited September 1, 2018]. Available from http://www.unrisd.org/80256B3C005BCCF9/search/5416E4680AD46606C1257B730038FAC1 (accessed May 31, 2019).

36. Kottke TE, Stiefel M, Pronk NP. "Well-being in all policies": Promoting cross-sectoral collaboration to improve people's lives. *Prev Chronic Dis.* 2016;13:160155. DOI: 10.5888/pcd13.160155.

37. Williams DR, Costa MV, Odunlami AO, Mohammed SA. Moving upstream: how interventions that address the social determinants of health can improve health and reduce disparities. *J Public Health Manag Pract.* 2008 Nov;14(Suppl):S8–17. DOI: 10.1097/01.PHH.0000338382.36695.42.

38. Artiga S, Hinton E. Beyond health care: the role of social determinants in promoting health and health equity. Henry J. Kaiser Family Foundation issue brief. Kaiser Permanente; 2018. Available from https://www.kff.org/disparities-policy/issue-brief/beyond-health-care-the-role-of-social-determinants-in-promoting-health-and-health-equity/ (accessed September 1, 2018).

39. Mokdad AH, Marks JS, Stroup DF, Gerberding JL. Actual causes of death in the United States, 2000. *JAMA.* 2004;291:1238–1245. DOI: 10.1001/jama.291.10.1238.

40. Pronk N. An optimal lifestyle metric: Four simple behaviors that affect health, cost, and productivity. *ACSMs Health Fit J.* 2012;16(3):39–43. DOI: 10.1249/01.FIT/0000414748.25945.58.

41. Institute for Patient- and Family-Centered Care. PFCC Best Practices: Patient- and Family-Centered Care. Bethesda (MD); [cited September 1, 2018]. Available from http://www.ipfcc.org/about/pfcc.html (accessed May 31, 2019).

42. PCPI. Welcome to PCPI. Available from https://www.thepcpi.org/ (accessed September 1, 2018).

43. Carlos RC. Value-driven health care: the purchase perspective. *J Am Coll Radiol.* 2008 Jun;5(6):719–726. DOI: 10.1016/j.jacr.2008.02.002.

44. The Leapfrog Group. Available from http://www.leapfroggroup.org/ (accessed September 1, 2018).

45. Centers for Medicare and Medicaid Services. *Regulations and Guidance.* Available from https://www.cms.gov/Regulations-and-Guidance/Regulations-and-Guidance.html (accessed September 1, 2018).

46. The Joint Commission. About The Joint Commission. Available from https://www.jointcommission.org/about_us/about_the_joint_commission_main.aspx (accessed September 1, 2018).

47. National Committee for Quality Assurance. Available from https://www.ncqa.org (accessed September 1, 2018).

48. National Quality Forum. Available from http://www.qualityforum.org/Home.aspx (accessed September 1, 2018).

49. Institute of Medicine. *The future of the public's health in the 21st century.* Washington, DC: The National Academies Press; 2003. DOI: 10.17226/10548.

50. Faulk LH. What is population health and how does it compare to public health? *Health Catalyst,* July 30, 2014. Available from https://www.healthcatalyst.com/what-is-population-health/.

51. Berwick DM, Nolan TW, Whittington J. The Triple Aim: care, health, and cost. *Health Aff.* 2008;27(3):759–769.

52. Evans RG, Stoddart GL. Producing health, consuming health care. *Soc Sci Med.* 1990;31(12):1347–1363.

53. Kindig D, Stoddart G. What is population health? *Am J Public Health.* 2003;93(3):380–383.

54. McGinnis JM, Williams-Russo P, Knickman JR. The case for more active policy attention to health promotion. *Health Aff.* 2002;21(2):78–93.

55. University of Wisconsin Population Health Institute. County Health Rankings & Roadmaps 2018. Available from www.countyhealthrankings.org (accessed September 1, 2018).

56. Institute of Medicine. *Crossing the Quality Chasm: A New Health System for the 21st Century.* Washington, DC: National Academies Press; 2001.

57. Marder B, Carls GS, Ehrlich E. et al. *Geographic Variation in Spending and Utilization Among the Commercially Insured.* Thomson Reuters white paper, July 27, 2011. Available from http://archive.rgj.com/assets/pdf/J7178046812.PDF (accessed October 31, 2014).

58. DMAA: The Care Continuum Alliance. *DMAA Outcomes Guidelines Report*. Washington, DC: DMAA: The Care Continuum Alliance; 2008.

59. Stiefel M, Nolan K. *A guide to measuring the Triple Aim: population health, experience of care, and per capita cost*. IHI Innovation Series white paper. Cambridge, MA: Institute for Healthcare Improvement; 2012. Available from http://www.ihi.org/resources/Pages/IHIWhitePapers/AGuidetoMeasuringTripleAim.aspx (accessed October 31, 2014).

60. Stiefel MC, Perla RJ, Zell BL. A health bottom line: Healthy life expectancy as an outcome measure for health improvement efforts. *Milbank Q.* 2010;88(1):30–53. DOI: 10.1111/j.1468-0009.2010.00588.x.

61. Boothe VL, Fierro LA, Laurent A. et al. Sub-county life expectancy: a tool to improve community health and advance health equity. *Prev Chronic Dis.* 2018;15:170–187. DOI: 10.5888/pcd15.170187.

62. Patient-Centered Outcomes Research Institute. Available from https://www.pcori.org/ (accessed September 1, 2018).

63. Patient-reported outcomes measurement information system (PROMIS). Program snapshot. Available from https://commonfund.nih.gov/promis/index (accessed September 1, 2018).

64. Centers for Medicare & Medicaid Services. *Health Outcomes Survey*. Available from https://www.cms.gov/Research-Statistics-Data-and-Systems/Research/HOS/ (accessed September 1, 2018).

65. European Commission. Public health. Available from https://ec.europa.eu/health/home_en (accessed September 1, 2018).

66. Stiefel MC, Perla RJ, Zell BL. A health bottom line: healthy life expectancy as an outcome measure for health improvement efforts. *Milbank Q.* 2010;88(1):30–53. DOI: 10.1111/j.1468-0009.2010.00588.x.

67. Eurostat: Statistics explained. *Healthy life years statistics*. Available from http://ec.europa.eu/eurostat/statistics-explained/index.php/Healthy_life_years_statistics (accessed September 1, 2018).

68. Madans JH, JD Weeks. A framework for monitoring progress using summary measures of health. *J Aging Health.* 2016;28(7):1299–1314.

69. Institute for Social Research. Past, present, and future trends in population health [Internet]. 2018 [cited September 1, 2018]. Available from https://globalagingandcommunity.files.wordpress.com/2018/06/reves-program-final-4.pdf (accessed May 31, 2019).

70. Bushnik T, Tjepkema M, Martel L. Health-adjusted life expectancy in Canada [Internet]. Canada: Statistics Canada [cited September 1, 2018]. Available from https://www150.statcan.gc.ca/n1/pub/82-003-x/2018004/article/54950-eng.htm (accessed May 31, 2019).

71. The US Burden of Disease Collaborators. The state of US health, 1990–2016: burden of diseases, injuries, and risk factors among US states. *JAMA.* 2018;219(14):1444–1472. DOI: 10.1001/jama.2018.0158.

72. World Health Organization. *Metrics: disability-adjusted life year (DALY)* [Internet]. Geneva: World Health Organization; 2018 [cited September 1, 2018]. Available from http://www.who.int/healthinfo/global_burden_disease/metrics_daly/en/ (accessed May 31, 2019).

73. Wolfson M. Accounting for pain beyond opioids. The Star [newspaper on the Internet]. September 24, 2018 [cited September 30, 2018]; Opinion: about 2 screens]. Available from https://www.thestar.com/opinion/contributors/2018/09/24/accounting-for-pain-beyond-opioids.html (accessed May 31, 2019).

74. Kottke TE, Stiefel M, Pronk NP. "Well-being in all policies": promoting cross-sectoral collaboration to improve people's lives. *Prev Chronic Dis.* 2016;13:160155. DOI: 10.5888/pcd13.160155.

75. OECD (2013). "Overview and recommendations," in OECD Guidelines on Measuring Subjective Well-being. Paris: OECD Publishing, Paris. DOI: 10.1787/9789264191655-3-en.

76. Sharecare, Inc. Well-being index. Available from https://wellbeingindex.sharecare.com/about/ (accessed September 1, 2018).

77. Agency for Healthcare Research and Quality. *CAHPS Measures of Patient Experience*. Available from https://cahps.ahrq.gov/consumer-reporting/measures/CAHPS_FAC_PG_041310.pdf (accessed October 31, 2014).

78. FNX Corporation and Trustees of Dartmouth College. How's Your Health website. Available from http://www.howsyourhealth.org (accessed October 31, 2014).

79. New HEDIS® measures allow purchasers, consumers to compare health plans' resource use in addition to quality [news release]. Washington, DC: National Committee for Quality Assurance; February 22, 2006.

80. The Dartmouth Institute for Health Policy and Clinical Practice. The Dartmouth Atlas of Health Care. Available from http://www.dartmouthatlas.org/ (accessed October 31, 2014).

81. Hornbrook MC, Hurtado AV, Johnson RE. Health care episodes: definition, measurement and use. *Med Care Rev.* 1985;42(2):163–218.

82. Bodenheimer T, Sinsky C. From triple to quadruple aim: Care of patient requires care of the provider. *Ann Fam Med.* 2014;12(6):573–576. DOI: 10.1370/afm.1713.

83. Health.mil. MHS Quadruple Aim. Available from https://www.health.mil/Reference-Center/Glossary-Terms/2013/04/09/MHS-Quadruple-Aim (accessed September 1, 2018).

84. Feeley D. The triple aim or the quadruple aim? Four points to help set your strategy [blog on the Internet]. Boston, MA: Institute for Healthcare Improvement, November 28, 2017 [cited September 1, 2018]. Available from http://www.ihi.org/communities/blogs/the-triple-aim-or-the-quadruple-aim-four-points-to-help-set-your-strategy (accessed May 31, 2019).

85. Corrigan J. *Building a Better Delivery System: A New Engineering/Health Care Partnership.* Washington, DC: National Academies Press; 2005 [September 1, 2018]. Available from https://www.ncbi.nlm.nih.gov/books/NBK22857/ (accessed May 31, 2019).

86. Institute of Medicine. *To err is human: building a safer health system.* Washington, DC: National Academies Press; 2000.

87. The National Academies of Sciences Engineering Medicine. *Unequal treatment: confronting racial and ethnic disparities in health care.* Washington, DC: National Academies Press; 2003.

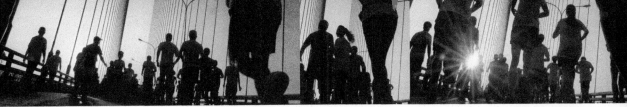

CHAPTER 11

Changing Organizational Culture

Somava Saha

EXECUTIVE SUMMARY

Recognizing the need for change is easy; creating and implementing effective change that leads to equitable and sustainable improvement in population health outcomes are much harder. This chapter reviews common reasons that change efforts fail—failure to build the will for change, failure to generate ideas that lead to effective change, and failure to execute change in a way that makes it readily adoptable and sustainable. It also offers three frameworks for approaching complex adaptive change to drive population health improvement and, using case studies, demonstrates how these frameworks can be applied.

Based on the work of Chip and Dan Heath, the first framework, *Switch*, moves beyond presenting data to motivate people to undertake the change and clarify the path forward. This framework can be applied to create large- and small-scale changes.

A second framework, based on the work of Kate Hilton and Alex Anderson, describes the psychology of change, with a focus on building and sustaining the will to change and shifting culture—a necessary component for the final steps of the third framework.

John Kotter's well-established framework offers an effective eight-step pathway for change, especially one that requires mobilization of large numbers of people. It describes a way to ensure that people are mobilized and that the system itself is changed.

Taken together, these frameworks and case studies offer a set of approaches to the complex, adaptive change that is necessary to achieve sustainable population health improvement.

LEARNING OBJECTIVES

1. Identify the reasons why most change efforts fail.
2. Identify key elements of successful change efforts.
3. Develop an approach to change that is designed to move people and systems together to create sustainable change, building on three frameworks offered here.

▶ Introduction

A receptionist, a medical assistant, a nurse, and a doctor work as a team at a community health center that is part of an integrated health system in Colorado. Their clinic director, Helen, who has just returned from a major conference, tells them with great excitement, "I've just signed us up to be one of the champions of a new model that could improve our care of patients with hepatitis C!" With some trepidation, but also a willingness to try given that they like and trust Helen, the team agrees to pilot the initiative, "Connect for Health, Colorado."

Over the next several months, the team is asked to attend several meetings and perform new tasks, many of which do not seem to directly benefit their patients. Because the system isn't set up for these tasks, they add complexity to the workflow and at least an hour or two to their already long workday. When Helen asks the team about joining a second initiative that builds on the first, the team unanimously votes "no." What went wrong?

This scenario is ubiquitous in health care today. Well-intended **change**, especially at the outset, can make life more difficult for the people who are engaged in it, and often the result is a failure of the initiative to sustain or scale. Improvement initiatives abound, and yet we don't see much real improvement or **organizational transformation**. Some changes, like implementation of electronic health records (EHRs), have brought healthcare professionals to a point of near revolt. High levels of burnout have been reported across the healthcare workforce, and some clinicians are leaving the medical profession, in part because they are losing hope that real change is possible. The Institute for Healthcare Improvement (IHI) grouped "failed change efforts" into three areas: failure of ideas, failure of will, and failure of execution.[1]

Failure of Ideas

Ideas fail when they do not effectively diagnose the problem or generate a set of solutions that would work. Most failures of ideas arise from not having the right people engaged to correctly identify the problem or to create the right portfolio of solutions—that is, those who are most affected by the problem, like patients. Effective codesign and innovation strategies can assure that the right problem is tackled and that a set of realistic solutions can be tested.

Failures of Will

Failures of will occur when everyone, from leadership to front-line staff, lacks the motivation and agency to effectively engage in the process of developing or implementing the solutions. People don't support change when they haven't been invited to provide input about what might work for them. Often, they work around the change if such pathways are possible.

Failure of Execution

A failure of execution occurs when new solutions are not implemented in a way that works. In our experience, most failures of execution arise from not anticipating how the change will affect the human beings involved or from not building systems in which the change becomes the new, **sustainable** norm.

Failures and solutions in these three areas are interrelated and, depending on whether the change is simple and incremental, complex, or transformational, one might combine a set of change strategies that best address the type of change and the context.

Strategies for Success

In this chapter, we will primarily focus on **change management** strategies to create changes that address failure of will and failure of execution. We will introduce three frameworks that have been used by people across industries to create more effective change: one that focuses on improving will (Switch[2]), one that explores the psychology of change[3] with an emphasis on sustaining the will to change and shift culture, and one that is useful in supporting the execution of complex change (Kotter's eight-step change model[4]). In this chapter, we will apply these frameworks to real-world examples of large-scale transformations at Cambridge Health Alliance and in 100 Million Healthier Lives. The chapter will conclude with reflection regarding the responsibilities of change leaders.

▶ Framework 1: Switch

A favorite recent book on creating effective change is *Switch: How to Change When Change Is Hard*,[2] written by brothers Dan and Chip Heath in consultation with hundreds of change makers. Based on sound behavioral science and organizational psychology, it synthesizes a simple yet powerful model for moving humans through the process of change. In the authors' clever analogy, people are like the riders on elephants traveling down a path.

The rider represents the rational brain—the part of us that deals with facts and statistics and consciously decides what to do based on a careful analysis of the facts. The elephant represents our unconscious choices (our limbic system of instantaneous responses that judges within the first moments of meeting someone whether we like them or not) and our emotions and needs (Do we feel safe? Are we hungry? Do we feel loved?). The path reflects our environment, the process of change, and the systems that make life easier or harder.

Most of the time, the elephant is in control. However, when we try to create change, our tendency is to focus messaging on the rider (i.e., using data and statistics to convince people to change through evidence-based practice). If this method were effective, all healthcare professionals would eat healthily, exercise five times a week, and not smoke or drink.

Nearly everyone chooses to make difficult changes during their lives. For instance, getting married and having a baby are complex changes that require us to give up control and resources and take on substantial responsibility. The reason people are willing to make these changes—the "pull" factor—is that the motivation overcomes the negatives. In our analogy, the elephant can be motivated to race down the path to change by sharing stories; using tools to build motivation; making change joyful, meaningful, and easy; and connecting change to purpose.[2]

Switch Framework Case Study 1: Adopting Systemwide Change

Cambridge Health Alliance (CHA), a large integrated safety net academic health system in eastern Massachusetts, was undergoing systemwide transformation to become a patient-centered medical home (PCMH) and accountable care organization (ACO). These complicated, multidimensional concepts were difficult to explain, and the brand names were misleading (for some people, "medical home" connotes "nursing home" or "funeral home").

Switch principles were applied to help people "find the meaning." Rather than present the concept in slides multiple times over the course of a year, the concept was introduced individually to each team and clinic, in the following way:

1. We met people at their home site and invited them to form groups of six. Each of the six group members was asked to take on the role of a patient who might walk through the door (e.g., a 22-year-old single mom with a 2-week-old infant, a 67-year-old Spanish-speaking gentleman with diabetes and an amputation, or a 58-year-old woman caring for her recently widowed 83-year-old mother).

2. Participants in each group were asked to speak from their assigned patient's perspective in answering the question, "What would you want your healthcare system to look like?" The group was given arts and crafts supplies and asked to "play" in building the system together. In

this way, groups rediscovered the principles of the PCMH.

3. After showing a simple, motivating visual about the Switch model, the groups were invited to help build it. Assurance was given regarding the leadership's commitment to changing the business model to align with these principles.

4. To build confidence, data points and stories were shared about other organizations that had made this type of change and achieved significant positive results.

5. Finally, participants were invited to act.

By the end of a year, 93% of all frontline team members understood the vision, rated it 7 out of 10 or higher in importance to them, and felt confident in their roles.[5] Most important, a number of self-proclaimed skeptics had become champions, describing this as one of the most meaningful transformations they had engaged in over their careers. Peer-to-peer spread of ideas was encouraged—and the ideas spread like wildfire.

An often overlooked but highly critical element of creating change is the difficulty or simplicity of the path itself.[2] Whether the path to change is easy or hard to follow makes a huge difference in which way the elephant will go; conscious or unconsciously, it will most often choose the path of least resistance. Complexity, difficulty, and ambiguity can make paths harder. Anything we can do to reshape and simplify the path will make it more likely that people will adopt the change.

There may be very valid reasons why a pathway should be modified for a particular patient. Even Cleveland Clinic, with its strong history of reliably implementing hundreds of evidence-based clinical **pathways,** does not prevent people from choosing to do something that is not consistent with a recommended pathway. But by making the recommended pathway the easiest path to follow in the clinical workflows and EHR, the doctor's administrative burden is lowered, and exceptions are requested only when they are truly indicated. In this way, Cleveland Clinic has shaped the path successfully for *easier* adoption of change.

Switch Framework Case Study 2: Ensuring End-of-Life and Healthcare Proxy Discussions

Promoting change to ensure that conversations occur about healthcare proxies and patients' end-of-life preferences is a complex task. At CHA, where providers are stretched thin, exhorting them to do the right thing was unlikely to work. A family medicine physician facilitated the development of a cross-clinic improvement team that included medical assistants, nurses, physicians, receptionists, and support personnel (e.g., information technology). The team created an elegant workflow for ensuring that healthcare proxy and end-of-life conversations would take place:

1. Work was divided among different roles based on the flow of the patient.
2. The process was integrated seamlessly into the standard flow of team-based care.
3. The process was incorporated into the EHR as a trigger to initiate it.

The following process was put in place:

- A packet with all the forms necessary for a healthcare proxy was prepared.
- A standard flag in the integrated health maintenance section of the EHR prompted the receptionist to give the packet to the patient on arrival.
- The medical assistant answered questions and entered the order for a healthcare proxy into the chart for the clinician to sign.
- The clinician documented patients' preferences about their end-of-life care in the healthcare proxy order with one more click of a button.

Within one year, over 60,000 healthcare proxy orders were entered into patients' charts, and tens of thousands of patients' preferences about their end-of-life choices had been recorded in the EHR. It became the standard of care *without a single physician educational session.* Knowing that physicians already believed in the importance of these conversations, the rest of the team was rallied to shape the path around the process so that the right choice became the easiest one to make. The Switch framework helped focus efforts and built confidence that the change would be good for the people involved.

▶ Framework 2: Psychology of Change

In an approach that dovetails well with Switch, Hilton and Anderson (Psychology of Change Framework to Advance and Sustain Improvement) point out that motivation presents an opportunity to create **agency,** defined as "the ability of an individual or group to choose to act with purpose."[4]

Agency has two key components—power (the *ability* to act with purpose) and courage (the *emotional resources to choose* to act).[3]

Following the initial sessions at CHA (see Switch Framework Case Study 1), we invited people to form a practice improvement team comprised of care team members, patients, and families to select and begin working on a target area. By making it easy to go from motivation to action, we built agency—the power and courage to act.

Framework 3: The Kotter Eight-Step Change Model

The Switch framework applies to many contexts, but when tackling large-scale change, it is sometimes best complemented by the eight-step change model outlined by John P. Kotter, an Emeritus Professor at the Harvard Business School.[4]

Although Kotter's eight steps are often done sequentially, one can reinforce another and also align with Switch strategies (**TABLE 11-1**).

TABLE 11-1 Components of Kotter's 8-Step Change Process

1. Establishing a Sense of Urgency
2. Creating the Guiding Coalition
3. Developing a Vision and Strategy
4. Communicating the Change Vision
5. Empowering Employees for Broad-Based Action
6. Generating Short-Term Wins
7. Consolidating Gains and Producing More Change
8. Anchoring New Approaches in the Culture

Modified from: Kotter, J. P. Leading Change. Boston: Harvard Business School Press, 1996.

1. Create a sense of urgency—elephant
2. Build a guiding coalition—rider, elephant
3. Form strategic vision and initiatives—rider, path
4. Enlist a volunteer army to engage in broad-based action—elephant
5. Enable action by removing barriers—path
6. Generate short-term wins—rider, elephant
7. Sustain acceleration—path
8. Institute or anchor change in culture, systems, and processes—path

Taken together, the Switch and Kotter eight-step frameworks have been applied to create and sustain complex system change. The following two case studies demonstrate the application of a Kotter-Switch approach.

Eight-Step Framework Case Study 1: System Transformation

As described in Switch Framework Case Study 1, CHA cares for 140,000 primary care patients, 75% of whom are on public insurance. Its transformation was precipitated by a funding crisis that occurred when the state's expanded healthcare coverage for Medicaid beneficiaries enrolled nearly four times as many people as expected. The governor informed CHA that $40 million in supplemental funds to cover Medicaid shortfalls would not be paid and that reimbursement for $100 million in Medicaid services delivered for the previous year was questionable. There was no need to create a sense of urgency—there was literally a "burning platform" (*Step 1*).

Rather than panic, the CHA leadership team engaged the organization in envisioning how the organization should look in the year 2015—an approach that proved critical to success.

It was obvious to the leadership that *Vision 2015* should focus on sustainably achieving the organization's mission—*to improve the health of our communities*—rather than on digging out of a financial hole. Three visioning sessions were held with the medical staff:

1. A session where participants considered the principles of an organization they would be proud to be a part of in the year 2015.
2. A session that invited participants to help shape the path to achieving these principles.
3. A session wherein participants assessed care gaps in the current system and made the decision to build a system in which extraordinary care became ordinary—an integrated system that would act seamlessly across primary care, specialties and hospital and community-based services to meet the needs of the community.

Achieving this sustainably would require shifting the business model from *fee for service* to *global payments/ shared savings*—a financial structure that would incentivize the organization to provide what its patients needed (e.g., social care, primary care, or mental health care).

The recommendations from this process became the vision for the organization, and acknowledging the value of these services, the state restored CHA's funding and agreed to support the organization through a change in payment model.

All employees were invited to remain and help build the vision. Over the next several years, new recruits as well as the many who stayed were inspired by the vision and became part of the change.

Step 2 of Kotter's approach was applied by building a Guiding Coalition. The Medical Home Steering Committee (subsequently, the ACO-PCMH Steering Committee) was comprised of a team of senior leaders from across the organization (e.g., Chief Medical Officer, Chief Operating Officer, Chief Administrative Officer for the ACO, Vice President of PCMH Transformation). In the first year, work was informed by five redesign workgroups (including frontline staff and patients); in the second year, ten operating teams made recommendations (e.g., regarding care redesign, collaboration, compensation) that formed the basis of a strategy and operational plan for the transformation (*Kotter Step 3*).

To avoid "spooking the elephant," senior leaders sponsored a Leadership Academy for a critical mass of mid-level leaders and approximately 10% of all physicians to help them own the vision and feel confident in creating change. The senior leaders mentored leadership teams in carrying out projects that aligned with the vision, thereby facilitating broad-based action (*Steps 4 and 5*).

The staff was engaged in envisioning what they would want as patients or community members. Care delivery sites were encouraged to make these improvements, with senior managers removing barriers from their path as needed. Throughout the organization, staff received training in basic design and improvement methods. Innovators and early adopters were invited to enter into learning collaboratives to accelerate transformation and were asked to share their stories at monthly cross-site mid-level leadership meetings, poster sessions, and in the organizational newsletter.

It wasn't easy, but it worked. By aligning the transformation with achieving the mission in a way that made sense for everyone, the collective "elephants" were harnessed, and the path was shaped. As a result, the underlying care model was changed, and, with the engagement of key staff (from CFO to medical assistants) over the next five years, CHA went from 1% to 60% global payments or shared savings.

Within months, dramatic improvements were documented on many levels—from employees' joy in their work, to patient health outcomes, to utilization and costs. These quick wins (*Kotter Step 6*) were useful in refining the care model and spreading it across the organization in waves based on readiness. At two and a half years, a Commonwealth Fund evaluation found that health outcomes had risen to the national 90th percentile at many CHA transformation sites, exceeding their matched controls in the non-transformation CHA sites and of sites across the state. The transformation sites also demonstrated reduced overall utilization and far greater employee joy in work.[6]

Once it was clear that changes were effective, CHA leadership worked with the state to help create a funding glidepath to support CHA's transformation and that of similar hospitals across the state. As CHA shifted its financial arrangements and operational structures to achieve the vision over the five-year period, the changes became anchored in processes and expectations (*Steps 7 and 8*). For example:

- The EHR was redesigned to support teams and integrated care planning.
- Physicians began to share offices with team members to facilitate closer communication and ease of workflow.
- Teams became co-scheduled—which required bringing 18 labor unions on board to support better and more consistent care.
- Business plans were created using new payment model options.
- New data systems and care management processes that crossed payer and delivery systems were created.
- New strategic partnerships with tertiary care and community-based organizations were forged.

With the necessary supports in place to care for the whole person—mental, physical, and social needs in addition to physical health—CHA achieved better outcomes for its patients, its communities, the organization, and its employees. The goals of the transformation were reinforced and became a new norm. The transformation was neither simple nor easy, but it was *meaningful*—and its core message of reshaping the organization to help achieve the mission "to improve the health of our communities" was powerful.

Eight-Step Framework Case Study 2: 100 Million Healthier Lives

When "100 Million Healthier Lives" was launched by IHI, the healthcare field wasn't quite ready for social determinants of health. However, evidence was emerging that the Triple Aim goals[7] of improved

population health, patient experience, and cost—a national imperative—would not be achievable without cross-sector partnerships to address social determinants.[8] Managing costs was essential but had not been achieved in most places.

For decades, the United States had relied on a siloed system of health production without accounting for the substantial interaction between mental, physical, social, and spiritual well-being—despite the World Health Organization definition.[9] Although public health had always operated in a place-based way, the interconnectedness between place and health[10] was not well understood in health care or most other sectors. The business and social service sectors weren't ready to engage in partnership.

A burning platform (*Step 1*) would be necessary to engage a critical mass of change leaders to go on the journey toward change. People had to believe change was possible even without well-developed models or a defined path. Fortunately, a number of major national organizations— Robert Wood Johnson Foundation (RWJF), the Institute for Healthcare Improvement (IHI), the Commonwealth Fund, the American Public Health Association (APHA), Centers for Disease Control and Prevention (CDC), Prevention Institute, Public Health Institute, Communities Joined in Action, Stakeholder Health, the National Academy of Science, Engineering and Medicine, and even the Federal Reserve—were ready to engage. These organizations were not yet working or messaging together, and there was no common playbook or group shaping a common path to make change easier. It was highly unlikely that the elephant would move in the face of this level of complexity.

Using a social networking strategy, a basic community organizing approach of public narrative—for example, "the story of me, the story of us, the story of now"[11]— one-to-one conversations with these organizations and other changemakers yielded recommendations about a common movement that could be built. Stories were shared by people in the system's various silos—stories of people falling through the cracks. Data were shared showing that a reduction in hospitalizations from better primary care would be insufficient to stem the tide of chronic disease or an aging population or to close gaps in equity. With the collective acknowledgment that what different actors were doing separately wouldn't be enough, the decision was made to build a shared movement based on unprecedented collaboration, innovative improvement, and system transformation.

Within three months, over 200 leaders from all walks of life—national organizations to community residents—came together to launch 100 Million Healthier Lives. A leadership team representing more than 30 organizations codesigned a meeting to inspire and to create the confidence to move into uncharted territory. Health was defined as more than the absence of disease. Latino children with Down's syndrome danced their cultural dances; poems and stories of real change were shared. A former member of NASA shared the story of the space race—another far-reaching goal that was set before there was the collaboration, technology, or science to achieve it.

Working groups led by credible leaders across organizations established paths in the 18 areas identified in initial discussions. Conversations focused on assets as well as needs and on what we would do together that we couldn't do alone. At the end of the day and a half meeting, on October 8, 2014, at 2:52 PM, the assembled group committed to an audacious common goal—100 million people living healthier lives by 2020. Changing the way we thought and worked to improve health, well-being, and equity was the highest priority.

Convened by the IHI, the meeting had taken place with 35 partners (potentially reaching 35 million people). One week later, there were over 70 partners (potential reach = 70 million people)—over 100 million people were within reach at three months. Leadership was distributed among the members in the form of collaboration hubs around areas of shared interest. With Robert Wood Johnson Foundation funding, a first national initiative was launched to create SCALE (Spreading Community Accelerators through Learning and Evaluation), the proof points in 24 communities. Highly engaging and trust-building experiences were developed for these communities, focusing on courage and agency to act as well as skills and pathways to make action more likely to be effective. At the end of two years, these communities elected to spread the change to four to ten communities around them, holding over 54 leadership academies with 100+ communities to engage them in the movement and take collective action to advance health, well-being, and equity across sectors.

None of this could have happened without building pathways to make change easier. Major groups in each of the hubs worked together on specific strategic priorities. One of these was the 100 Million Healthier Lives Health Systems Transformation Hub, where groups such as the American Hospital Association, IHI, Network for Regional Healthcare Improvement, Public Health Institute, and Stakeholder Health (with a collective reach of over 10,000 healthcare organizations) joined to build common frameworks and tools to support healthcare organizations on this journey. "Pathways to Population Health: An Invitation to Health Care Change Agents"[12] emerged from this effort. The framework creates a path forward for healthcare organizations to reclaim their mission, purpose, and power to improve health, well-being, and equity. With its supportive tools and graphics, Pathways to Population Health[12] is designed to make a complex journey simpler and easier—and to restore a sense of abundance and possibility for healthcare systems (**FIGURE 11-1**). Hundreds of healthcare organizations joined the effort in its first year, in part because it came from trusted messengers and in part because it made their journey easier.

Together, members of 100 Million Healthier Lives are making the journey easier for one another and demonstrating that real change is possible when assets are brought together across silos. Most important, having become a community of purpose across

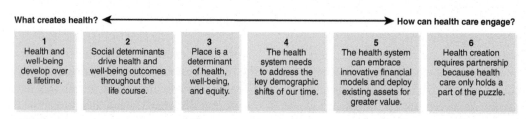

FIGURE 11-1 Foundational Concepts of Population Health Improvement from Pathways to Population Health.

geopolitical and sector boundaries the members have demonstrated that change spreads at the speed of trust. Practices (e.g., partnerships between organizations and people with lived experience of inequity) are spreading along with breakthrough improvements that achieve 50% or better outcomes.

We must sustain the gains, demonstrate that they can scale, and make the necessary changes in systems, processes, and culture the new norm. Fortunately, we are learning that Switch, the Kotter eight-step model, and the Psychology of Change tools and frameworks can apply even at large scale—especially when combined with our best learning about growing networks.

▶ Takeaways for Change Leaders

Poorly designed change processes can add to the burden and complexity of work at best and cause substantial harm at worst—from poor health outcomes to damaged trust with communities. What matters is to plan change well, to quickly identify the pain points, and to actively shape the path to change. Whether the change is small or large, there are methods of creating change that one can learn and apply for far better outcomes. Frameworks like Switch, Kotter's eight-step model, and the Psychology of Change can help to make change easier.

"All improvement will require change, but not all change will result in an improvement."[14] Building in a process of continuous learning and co-design with those who are most affected by the change is crucial. Being both humble and strategic—and always attending to the needs of the people and the process of change itself—can make a profound difference in the well-being of people during and as a result of the journey. Both matter.

Study and Discussion Questions

1. How might Helen have approached her change initiative differently if she had applied Switch or Kotter's eight-step model to her scenario?
2. Where do you see Switch and Kotter's models applied in the 100 Million Healthier Lives case study?
3. Think of a change effort you have been a part of (in work or life) that didn't go well. How might you diagnose what went wrong using Switch and Kotter's eight-step model?
4. Think of a change effort that went wonderfully well. What elements of Switch or Kotter's eight-step model could you identify?

Suggested Readings and Websites

Heath C, Heath D. *Switch: How to Change Things When Change Is Hard*. New York: Crown Business Press.

Kotter's Eight-Step Change Process is outlined in two books:
1. Kotter JP. *Leading Change*. Cambridge, MA: Harvard Business Review Press.
2. Kotter JP. *Accelerate*. Cambridge, MA: Harvard Business Review Press.

Both books may be accessed via https://www.kotterinc.com/8-steps-process-for-leading-change (accessed June 15, 2019).

Hilton K, Anderson A. The Psychology of Change [white paper]. Available at

http://www.ihi.org/resources/Pages
/IHIWhitePapers/IHI-Psychology-of-Change
-Framework.aspx (accessed June 15, 2019).

Synthesis papers on 100 Million Healthier Lives
are available at www.100mlives.org/initiatives
(accessed June 15, 2019).

Pathways to Population Health website is available
at www.pathways2pophealth.org (accessed
June 15, 2019).

References

1. Nolan TW. *Execution of Strategic Improvement Initiatives to Produce System-Level Results.* Cambridge, MA: Institute for Healthcare Improvement; 2007.
2. Heath C, Heath D. *Switch: How to Change When Change Is Hard.* Toronto, Canada: Random House Canada; 2010.
3. Hilton K, Anderson A. *IHI Psychology of Change Framework to Advance and Sustain Improvement.* Boston, MA: Institute for Healthcare Improvement; 2018.
4. Kotter JP. *8 Step Process for Leading Change.* E-book available at https://www.kotterinc.com/8-steps-process-for-leading-change/ (accessed May 3, 2019).
5. Zallman L, et al. *PCMH Workforce Survey.* Cambridge, MA: Cambridge Health Alliance Institute for Community Health; 2011.
6. Hacker K, Mechanic R, Santos P. *Accountable Care in the Safety Net: A Case Study of the Cambridge Health Alliance.* Boston, MA: Commonwealth Fund; 2014.
7. Berwick DM, Nolan TW, Whittington J. The Triple Aim: care, health, and cost. *Health Affs.* 2008;27(3):759–769.
8. Whittington JW, Nolan K, Lewis N, Torres T. Pursuing the Triple Aim: the first 7 years. *The Milbank Q.* 2015;93:263–300.
9. World Health Organization. Constitution of the World Health Organization. [Online] April 7, 1948. Available at https://www.who.int/about/mission/en/ (accessed June 15, 2019).
10. Haley A, Zimmerman E, Woolf S, Evans B. Neighborhood-level determinants of life expectancy in Oakland, California. Center on Human Needs. Richmond, VA: Virginia Commonwealth University; 2012.
11. Ganz M. Public narrative, collective action and power. Chapter 18 in Sina Odugbemi and Taeku Lee (Eds.), *Accountability Through Public Opinion: From Inertia to Public Action.* Washington, DC: The World Bank; 2011: 273–289.
12. Stout S, Loehrer S, Cleary-Fishman M, Johnson K, Chenard R, Gunderson G, et al. *Pathways to Population Health: An Invitation to Health Care Change Agents.* Cambridge, MA: Institute for Healthcare Improvement; 2017.
13. Langley GJ, Moen RD, Nolan KM, Nolan TW, Norman CL, Provost LP. *The Improvement Guide.* San Francisco: Jossey Bass, 1996, p. xxi.

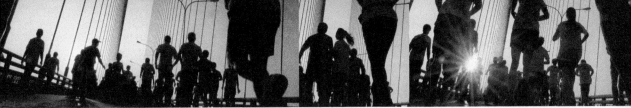

CHAPTER 12

Coordinated Care Delivery Models

Katherine Schneider
Jennifer Puzziferro

EXECUTIVE SUMMARY

Fee-for-service payment for health care in the United States has contributed to creating a non-system of care that is fragmented, costly, and delivers poor outcomes at the population level. Large purchasers of health care, including the Centers for Medicare and Medicaid Services (CMS); large, self-insured employers; and other private payers have begun to shift the mechanism of payment from "volume" (fee for service) to "value" (value-based care) through alternative payment models such as accountable care organizations, bundled payment, and direct payment for coordination of care between visits. Increasingly, hospitals and physicians will not only be rewarded for better population health outcomes but also will bear financial risk for poor outcomes.

Success under a value-based payment paradigm requires providers to significantly reengineer how, where, and by whom care is delivered. Examples of care model transformation include the patient-centered medical home and implementation of team-based care coordination across the continuum.

LEARNING OBJECTIVES

By the end of this chapter, the reader will be able to:

1. Review the context of the shift of payment from volume to value and give examples of alternative payment models.
2. Describe the changes in the use of people, process, and technology required for success under alternative payment models.
3. Identify operational aspects of care coordination across the continuum, and explain how they can be implemented incrementally in a volume-based environment.

▶ Introduction

Rapid and foundational payment reform has been quietly taking place over the past decade in response to the need for a more predictable and sustainable growth rate in healthcare costs in the United States,[1] as well as heightened attention to quality and safety,[2] and geographic variation in all of these metrics.[3,4] Together these represent a shift from payment based on *volume*—that is, fee-for-service—to *value*—that is, "no outcome, no income."[5] While this chapter will highlight specific examples under Medicare, most private payers have followed suit with a commitment to shift the majority of payment to similar value-based models as rapidly as possible.

The Patient Protection and Affordable Care Act of 2010 (ACA),[6] followed by the Medicare Access and CHIP Reauthorization Act of 2015 (MACRA),[7] represent two recent landmark pieces of health-policy legislation. While they are more publicly known for insurance-related issues, they also heralded the most significant payment reforms seen in many decades. The ACA established an innovation center within the Centers for Medicare and Medicaid Services. The Center for Medicare and Medicaid Innovation (CMMI)[8] has unprecedented funding and the authority to pilot new payment and delivery models, including coordination with the private sector. Furthermore, an earlier Medicare demonstration project involving 10 physician groups nationwide[9] was permanently authorized as the Medicare Shared Savings Program (MSSP),[10] a voluntary program for providers who wish to form **Accountable Care Organizations** (ACOs).

Under MACRA, earlier versions of Medicare physician pay-for-performance programs were consolidated into two "voluntary" tracks of a new Quality Payment Program.[11] First, under the Merit-based Incentive Payment System (MIPS), physician groups are scored in four domains: quality, cost efficiency, technology adoption, and clinical practice improvement activities aligned with population health care models. Their fee schedule is then adjusted upward or downward based upon their score, eventually creating a pay gap of 18% or more by 2022. The MIPS track represents traditional pay-for-performance, in which payment for a service is linked to a bonus or penalty for a metric related to that service.[12]

The second track of MACRA drives physician participation in one of an increasing number of Alternative Payment Models (APMs), in particular those that require providers to bear substantial downside financial risk, or "advanced" APMs.[13] These physicians are exempt from reporting on MIPS measures, and instead of variable fee adjustments, they receive a lump sum bonus of 5%. APMs are built upon coordinated care models in which incentives are linked to broader outcomes, especially the total cost of care for people with specific conditions or

TABLE 12-1 Health Care Delivery: Two World Views	
Fee-for-Service (Volume)	**Alternative Payment Models (Value)**
■ Services (visits) generate revenue ■ Code to capture complexity of the service ■ Cost of care is what you are paid for the service ■ Quality is what happens during the service/visit ■ Access to services is driven by provider capacity	■ Visits and services are cost centers ■ Code to capture complexity of the patient (risk) ■ Cost of care is for everything/everywhere (or what you order/control) ■ Quality is what happens to the patient/people daily and year-round ■ The care team is across the continuum, region, country ■ Access to services is driven by patient need

entire populations. Accountability for the total cost of care requires providers to shift their frame of reference 180 degrees, from one that is centered around individual healthcare delivery services, to one that is longitudinal regardless of whether, where, and when services are provided for the target population (**TABLE 12-1**).

Total Cost of Care APM Example: Accountable Care Organizations

An ACO is a group of providers who collaboratively coordinate the care for an "attributed" population, almost always defined according to who receives care from the ACO's primary care physicians (PCPs). Thus, while ACOs *may* include hospitals and specialists, they *must* include PCPs. There are a few exceptions to this rule, where a specialist may be effectively serving in the role of primary care for a unique population—for example, patients receiving dialysis.[14] Despite operating under a similar financial model, ACOs vary widely in structure, scale, and complexity. For example, in the Philadelphia region, there are ACOs covering fewer than 10,000 lives comprised of single, multi-site physician groups as well as

collaboratives of multiple small practices supported by private investors. There are also local "chapters" of a very large national hospital system ACO (Trinity Health), and Delaware Valley ACO (DVACO), which is a joint venture of two regional health systems, Jefferson Health and Main Line Health, and which will be used for further illustrative purposes. DVACO includes a large ambulatory care network with 19 hospitals in the region and roughly 2,000 primary care and specialty physicians (both employed and in private practice). In 2019, DVACO is accountable for roughly 90,000 Medicare beneficiaries through the MSSP, plus 5,000 Medicare Advantage subscribers, 80,000 commercially insured lives, and 60,000 of the health systems' employees and their family members.

ACOs are generally assessed on cost performance through some variation of a "bend the trend" analysis. CMMI's NextGen ACO program operates under a global payment model, which combines aspects of the MSSP with targets set in a manner that is more similar to that for a Medicare Advantage plan (including substantial downside risk).

Because total cost of care includes the entire continuum of services, the ACO's clinical strategy will vary according to what is possible to achieve based upon local care patterns and data. The subacute/post-acute care sector (skilled nursing facilities, home health, physical therapy, and hospice) is a very significant component of the total cost of care, especially for a Medicare population. DVACO combined claims data with publicly reported data, plus care coordination protocols, to develop a preferred regional post-acute network. By concentrating more care in three dozen higher-performing skilled nursing facilities (SNFs), as well as shifting hospital culture to prefer discharge of patients to home when appropriate, post-acute quality improved and cost of SNF care was reduced by 30%. Whether or not specialty and prescription plan pharmaceutical expenses are included should also drive the clinical strategy accordingly—and can make or break an ACO's financial success regardless of ability to keep patients out of the emergency department (ED) and hospital. For example, from 2014 to 2018, DVACO reduced ED visits by 13% and hospital visits by 14%, but the annual cost of specialty drugs increased by 49%!

ACOs also must report on and achieve quality standards to be eligible for financial reward based upon cost management (unlike programs that reward directly for quality). The amount of savings shared with the ACO is often determined by the quality score achieved in multiple domains, including prevention, chronic disease management, care coordination, and patient experience.

The detailed and complex methods for patient attribution to ACOs are generally a thorn in the side of ACO managers and clinicians, since patients very often do not seek care exclusively with a single provider unless their insurance requires it (which is rare). Picture the previously described Philadelphia region, where multiple ACOs and over a half dozen disparate health systems operate, sometimes within yards of one another. Complicating this further, picture a "snowbird" retiree who splits his or her time between two regions. Who is accountable for that individual? In theory, the simplest attribution method is one in which patients actively choose a PCP who participates in the ACO—for example, in a private HMO insurance product. However, this can result in the PCP having accountability for some patients that he or she has never actually seen and therefore having no medical record and limited opportunity to intervene (including for very ill patients cycling in and out of acute care settings). An alternative method is to use administrative data (i.e., claims) to determine which patients have seen the ACO's physicians for a plurality of office visits in the preceding year (i.e., more times with ACO physicians than other physician groups). The ACO can then be assigned responsibility for that population either in that same year (retrospective attribution) or for the following year (prospective attribution). While the former can create frustration about not knowing which patients will end up in the attributed population until the performance year (and opportunities) are long over, the latter makes the ACO responsible for a sizeable number of patients who left the care of the ACO (e.g., those who moved away, switched doctors, or even just had one more visit outside the ACO than in it). To complicate this further, every payer uses a different attribution method—for example, one- versus two-year periods, varying rules for how a specialist can receive attribution, etc. A few simple guidelines can optimize correct attribution and drive more effective coordination of care:

1. Obviously, provide the best possible access and a seamless high-quality care experience so that it is easy for patients to want to stay within the system (also known as the "stickiness" strategy—a win under both volume and value).

2. Ensure that all patients (especially Medicare beneficiaries) see their PCP at least once per calendar year, preferably including a preventive care visit. This is not only good practice but also a fully covered benefit without copay (under ACA rules).

3. Ensure all physicians are listed under the correct specialty in the payer's systems, especially CMS where physicians may have been initially credentialed before they completed specialty training. This issue is irrelevant under fee-for-service but critical in population health/coordinated care models.

Primary Care APM Example: Comprehensive Primary Care (CPC) Program

CPC (2012–2016, in 7 markets) and its successor CPC+ (2017–2021, in 14 markets)[15] is a CMMI-led pilot program designed to provide multipayer alignment in support of primary care transformation. It requires at least one private payer in a market to participate in the program alongside CMS on behalf of fee-for-service Medicare beneficiaries. Primary care practices in the selected markets are chosen from among those who apply and agree to implement care delivery transformations, including integration of behavioral health services, data-driven care management for high-risk segments of the patient panel, enhanced access, enhanced data tracking and reporting capabilities, and establishment of patient and family advisory committees (among other things). CPC builds upon the principles of the patient-centered medical home (PCMH)[16] model for primary care and provides educational and technical support. Primary care physicians are central to the PCMH model and work to create a system that fosters team-based care. All members of the physician-led team have defined roles and functions to support improved care coordination for patients at micro and macro levels, as described in further detail later in this chapter. Participating practices continue to be paid, at least in part, via fee-for-service but can elect to receive part of that as a partially capitated monthly fee. In addition, they receive monthly risk-adjusted care management fees and additional incentives for quality and efficiency (which must be paid back if performance targets are not achieved). Practices are required to invest at least some of these funds in new resources to improve care coordination. As of 2019, Jefferson Health has dozens of primary care practices participating in CPC+ and has invested in additional innovations such as embedding clinical pharmacists in primary care, and centralized outreach teams responsible for keeping preventive and chronic care up-to-date between visits.

Condition-Specific APM Example: Oncology Care Model and the Patient-Centered Specialty Practice

Beginning in 2004, an innovative oncology practice became the first NCQA-recognized non–primary care "medical home" practice in the country,[17] leading to recognition that principles of the PCMH could be applied in specialty care as well; thus came the inception of the Patient-Centered Specialty Practice (PCSP) designation.[18] While formal PCSP recognition has not been widely adopted, the basic tenets are commonly found in descriptions of desirable specialist behavior under coordinated care models—that is, a "medical neighborhood" surrounding the medical home:

- Use of evidence-based guidelines and data to manage, track, and improve outcomes of specific conditions
- Appropriate access to care
- Patient navigation/coordination/ education
- Collaboration and communication with primary care as a virtual team

The concept of the PCSP specific to oncology gained traction in the development of pilot alternative payment models, including with CMMI's Oncology Care Model (OCM).[19] Jefferson oncology practices were selected to participate in the OCM, which is somewhat analogous to the CPC+ primary care model. However, in this case the target population is not 100% of patients and the full year of care, but rather those with specific cancer diagnoses during the 6-month period following the initiation of chemotherapy. The practices receive an up-front care management fee

and are required to redesign care delivery in the practice, including use of patient navigators, after-hours access to a clinician, implementation of patient-centered care plans, and use of data to drive care improvement. The practices are responsible for outcomes including chemotherapy guideline adherence, keeping patients out of the hospital wherever possible by proactively managing side effects, and maximizing quality of life. If quality targets are met, and overall cost of care during the 6 months is lowered, practices can receive additional shared savings payments.

Condition-Specific APM Example: Bundled Payment for Care Improvement

Another way to incentivize coordinated care delivery is in the population experiencing acute events, such as procedures and hospitalizations for specific diagnoses. Episode-based, or "bundled" payments, tie together the cost of all the care that a patient receives in a given period of time, beginning with the hospital admission or a procedure. Some health policy experts feel that bundles are the highest potential alternative payment model for driving value, since care delivery transformation can be highly focused and standardized for a single diagnosis or procedure.[20] Methods for defining and administering bundles vary widely—for example, the length of time, services, and providers included/excluded and whether the payment is actually up front and all-inclusive (and to whom) versus paid in the usual fragmented fee-for-service fashion with an after-the-fact financial reconciliation calculation.

Medicare has been experimenting with bundled payment for decades.[21] The latest CMMI iteration, the Bundled Payment for Care Improvement Initiative–Advanced, or BPCI-A (beginning in 2018 but expanding on an earlier five-year program), targets 29 inpatient medical and surgical diagnoses and three outpatient procedures.[22] Virtually all care that is received during the "index" admission and the subsequent 90-day period is included in the bundle, regardless of its relationship to the bundle diagnosis. For example, following a stroke, typical expected services within 90 days might include the initial hospital stay, inpatient and follow-up ambulatory care from a large team of clinicians (neurology, radiology, hospital medicine, primary care, rehabilitative therapists), a stay in a rehabilitation facility, durable medical equipment (such as mobility aids), a homecare nurse, etc. However, if during the 90 days the patient gets the flu, or breaks a bone, or has care for an unrelated chronic medical condition, those costs are also included. Since the *target* bundle cost is based upon that provider's historical experience with similar patients, if the population size of the program is large enough, these kinds of events would also have occurred historically and may actually be opportunities to optimize care coordination.

Main Line Health System, just outside of Philadelphia, is a new participant in BPCI-A for stroke and sepsis. While already recognized for extremely high quality of care in its five hospitals, participation in BPCI-A is driving significant transformation of the care delivery model to solve challenges. Some examples include:

1. Electronic tools to identify and track stroke and sepsis patients, starting from presentation in the ED and continuing after hospital discharge, whether the patient goes home or to another facility for rehabilitation

2. With data indicating that the 60% of the patients admitted for these two diagnoses are not affiliated with primary care physicians within the system's Clinically Integrated Network, how to best coordinate care once patients return to their own community

3. Systematic methods for ensuring that patients' advance directives and goals of care are available to the care team everywhere

4. Expanded readmission window to 90 days and into any hospital for any reason (as opposed to 30-day window into same hospital for previous pay-for-performance incentives)

Important for system alignment, Main Line's participation in BPCI-A is extremely synergistic with its five-year experience as a member of DVACO as well as dozens of its network's primary care practices also participating in CPC+ since 2017. While the financial accounting becomes extremely complex and challenging when the same patients are in multiple models, if they are managed and governed under a coordinated infrastructure then care delivery transformation can be greatly reinforced. For example, optimized post-acute care for BPCI-A patients leverages the MSSP preferred network and technology. Care coordination in the 90-day period for those in CPC+ and DVACO practices is already in place since CPC+ and MSSP require coordination for 365 days for all conditions (the "mega-bundle"). For those who are not, Main Line Health can expand on these existing resources rather than building a care coordination program from scratch.

It is not a coincidence that so many of the APM acronyms include the letter "C" for Care, because success is driven by care model transformation, whether the changes are on a small (incremental) or large (disruptive) scale. Care models refer to how care is delivered, in addition to what care is delivered (TABLE 12-2). For example, evidence-based clinical guidelines for diabetes include parameters and algorithms for diagnosis, optimal medication use, and monitoring. A full care model for diabetes expands on these and might include (for example):

- How and when a certified diabetes educator (CDE) engages with patients
- A formulary that standardizes a preferred drug within each class of medication
- Level of complexity and urgency for patients who should be escalated from primary care to endocrinology
- How pharmacists should be integrated into the care team
- Adoption of a standard blood glucose monitoring system that uploads real-time results into a centralized monitoring system

TABLE 12-2 Care Models: How We Do It

- Includes value proposition (to all stakeholders)
- Crosses continuum of site of care
  - Now blurring "plan" and "provider"
- Team approach—roles defined
- Defines handoffs
- Risk stratifies (who needs what intensity)
  - Build in primary, secondary, and tertiary prevention
- Includes measurement (triple aim)
- Includes consumer engagement

While clinical guidelines are broadly applicable as medical best practice, care models are likely to be highly local to a health system, community, or population.[23] Care model transformation addresses *people*, *process*, and *technology*:

- Multidisciplinary care teams, both inside and beyond of the traditional four walls of the hospital and office
- Engagement of patients and caregivers as core members of the care team, through self-management skills education, individualized goals of care, and feedback on how to improve the care experience
- Technology beyond just use of a digital health record, such as integration of real-time data exchange (whether across the hall or across the nation), and advanced remote patient monitoring devices and apps
- Advanced analytics that support risk stratification of populations, predictive models identifying patients in whom an intervention today is likely to prevent a bad outcome tomorrow, and performance monitoring/feedback tools for providers
- Innovations in care delivery channels/venues, such as telemedicine and retail-based clinics

The ability to provide care beyond traditional workday hours, (e.g., through virtual visits) for patients who would have otherwise sought care in a more expensive and complicated ED, is both a cost saver and patient satisfier. Access to telehealth for specialty care consults, or care in the home for patients with complex chronic conditions who are otherwise not able to travel to the PCP office, allows for expedited care and provides a level of follow-through and support that has previously not been available. While telemedicine and retail clinics have historically been focused on expanding affordable, convenient access to low-acuity sick patients, they are increasingly being adapted to support chronic disease management. On the other side of the acuity spectrum are "hospital at home" programs that can provide acute illness management at a much higher scope than traditional home health services. However, these models ideally support and supplement access in an organized system context rather than worsening fragmentation with multiple new siloes of care, particularly for high-risk patients.

The recent acquisition of health insurer Aetna by pharmacy and retail giant CVS Health is expected to disrupt multiple aspects of the traditional care delivery model for tens of millions of members/patients through the use of big data and a more consumer-oriented widely distributed network of "HealthHubs."[24]

▶ Care Coordination Operations in Ambulatory Care

Interprofessional Collaboration and Practice Transformation

It is common knowledge by now that change is imminent, and the current system is not sustainable from a cost or quality perspective—so how can the system be transformed into something that is? Unfortunately, there is no standardized playbook for care transformation. Change is contingent upon budget, desire, commitment, and organizational culture.

Strong leadership is required make this journey from volume to value move from theory to practical application.

How much more can we ask physicians to do, and what resources can we provide to facilitate this work? Interprofessional collaboration and practice transformation are foundational. A first step is to establish a care team with clear roles and responsibilities to support business and clinical operations. Key roles include an office supervisor to oversee patient flow, triage patients, facilitate access, and supervise medical assistants (MAs). The supervisor organizes the daily huddle, which is designed to keep team members informed and anticipating the day's work. Sample daily huddle topics include staffing, patient flow, and review of information regarding the care continuum—for example, patients in the hospital, who have had an ED visit, or are in a skilled nursing facility (SNF). The huddle creates a venue to support exchange of information, creates a list of action items and follow-ups, and ensures the most appropriate resource is assigned to each task to ensure all members of the team are practicing to the fullest scope of licensure. In addition to providing lists of high-risk patients to the practices, payers also provide admission, discharge, and transfer information (ADT), all of which inform the practices of patient status across the continuum of care. They may also provide notification of admissions (NOA), which alerts the practice that patients are hospitalized. Rather than passively accepting this information, transformed practices act on it. A first step is socializing this as part of the daily huddle. Patients can be called at the bedside during confinement to schedule follow-up appointments if appropriate, or physicians might consider courtesy visits to the hospital, even if they are not the attending of record. Keeping in close contact with hospitalized patients helps the care team to understand the episode of care and plan for follow-up.

MAs support patient flow by rooming patients; they are often considered the right hand of the physician. They take vital signs, administer injections, and collect information, such as confirming reason for visit, medication changes, and information outlined on patient health questionnaires. In an enhanced care delivery model, MAs reinforce education for certain chronic disease states and can provide chronic care management (CCM) services, which Medicare and some commercial payers offer as a billing incentive opportunity. Regulatory requirements for CCM include a care plan, created with the patient and signed off by the physician, followed by 20 minutes of (documented) coaching in a 30-day period, resulting in a billable encounter. Advanced practice providers (APPs) can support practice flow by managing sick visits and patients with chronic conditions who need to be seen more frequently and require education that would exceed the usual 15-minute physician visit.

Care coordination is the lynchpin to success in a value-based care model. The Case Management Society of America (CMSA) defines the function of care coordinators as supporting a collaborative process of assessment, planning, facilitation, care coordination, evaluation, and advocacy for options and services to meet an individual's and family's comprehensive health needs through communication and available resources to promote quality, cost-effective outcomes.[25] The care coordinator, usually a registered nurse, coordinates care within an interprofessional, collaborative team by linking patients to quality medical care, appropriate community resources, and self-management education to support optimum health. This essential member of the care team identifies and manages patients who are at risk for poor health outcomes by focusing on the social determinants of health (SDOH).

SDOH are defined by the World Health Organization (WHO) as the conditions in which people are born, grow, live, work, and age that affect a wide range of health, functioning, and quality-of-life outcomes and risks.[26] The SDOH are mostly responsible for *health inequities*, the unfair and avoidable differences in health status seen within and among populations of people. Care coordinators engage with the patients and caregivers to facilitate access to community agencies to ensure basic self-care elements are in place, such as access to food, affordable medications, and transportation.

Care coordinator functions include conducting a comprehensive assessment and development and implementation of care plans for high-risk and medically fragile patients in tandem with the patient and care team, facilitating connection to community resources to remove SDOH, and supporting patient self-management through education, motivational interviewing, and increasing patient confidence though self-directed goal achievement. Above all, the care coordinator serves as a patient advocate who helps articulate patient and family goals and focuses the whole care team on working with the patient and family toward those goals.

Care coordinators provide self-management education for patients with chronic conditions, and ensure care is coordinated across the continuum. This adds value for patients and families, team members, and the organization while promoting professional autonomy by supporting clinicians and providing the structure that promotes true team-based care. Utilization of this resource is also a way to succeed in value-based contracting. Assigning a care coordinator to the sickest and most at-risk attributed patients will help to manage total cost of care by ensuring care is delivered in the least restrictive medical setting (ideally the PCP office), thereby avoiding expensive events such as avoidable ED visits and hospitalizations.

Risk stratification is critical in appropriate case finding for care coordinators. Having set criteria, such as patients who have utilized the emergency room more than twice or have had more than two hospital admissions in six months, will help to identify the patients who could potentially benefit from this service. Additionally, care coordinators may have access to claims data from payers, which risk stratifies patients based on predictive models as previously described. Care coordination and transitions are patient-centered medical home (PCMH) philosophies and key to true practice redesign.

Tenets of practice redesign are outlined in the National Committee for Quality Assurance (NCQA) criteria for PCMH. Regardless of whether or not a practice is pursuing PCMH accreditation, these principles align with good medical care and support the Triple Aim. NCQA defines team-based care and practice organization, which creates a system of accountability through definition of roles and functions. Additionally, knowing and managing patients establishes a standard for data collection, medication reconciliation, evidence-based clinical decision support and other activities required to facilitate pay-for-performance or risk-based contracting. Patient-centered access and continuity provides patients with convenient access to appointments and clinical advice. This tenet takes into consideration patient preference and appointment availability during nontraditional hours, such as evenings and weekends. Continuity ensures referrals are managed and that information from required specialists is obtained and available for the care team to review. Finally, performance measurement and quality improvement help practices develop ways to measure performance, set goals, and develop activities that will improve performance.[27] Embedding some or all of these processes into operations provides the opportunity for practices to participate in contracts which pay for performance in quality, also known as closing gaps in care by addressing preventive care measures based on gender and age, and managing chronic conditions more proactively to avoid patient complications, such as testing hemoglobin A1C (HbA1C) quarterly or annual retinal eye exams for diabetic patients.

Coordinating Care Transitions

Real-time knowledge about hospitalizations and confinements to SNFs is a key success factor in risk-based contracts. Receiving information from hospitalists can be challenging and often comes in the form of a discharge summary. Using the huddle to discuss hospitalized patients creates the ability to reserve appointments for post-discharge follow-up and/or potential discussions regarding goals of care, if warranted (see below for description of new codes for these services). It also ensures that your patient will receive care from your practice and not leak into another system of care, which improves patient experience.

As mentioned earlier in the example of DVACO, SNFs are an area worthy of special focus. Many providers feel that these facilities provide ongoing care for patients who have rehabilitation or medical management needs that cannot be performed at home. The truth is that while sometimes medically necessary, these types of facilities have become an epicenter for patients and families with complex care needs, such as end-of-life management. Medicare provides 100 days of SNF benefit to all beneficiaries. Facilities are currently paid by the day, which averages at about $600. Due to the current compensation model, there is no incentive for early discharge. Patients and families are encouraged to use the entire benefit, as long as medical necessity is documented, with the goal of improving or maintaining physical function. In many cases, this care can be futile, and patients are at risk of exhausting the entire benefit which, to be renewed, requires the beneficiary to be community dwelling for 60 days. If the benefit is used in its entirety and patients are re-hospitalized prior to renewal, they are at financial risk upon discharge and are required to pay privately if they cannot return home due to safety concerns or lack of support. If they do not have the financial resources to fund long-term care, patients who meet the eligibility requirements could apply for Medicaid. However, this involves an extensive process

that requires submission of financial documents; waiting for approval could result in a prolonged hospitalization of several weeks or months. There is an opportunity for Medicare to reduce the total cost of care by offering options to patients and families prior to admission to an SNF to ensure there are no suitable alternatives. There truly is no place like home, and with the advent of healthcare reform, it is possible to arrange more robust services to assist people to age in place and die comfortably, bypassing entirely unnecessary confinements in these types of facilities. A tactic that providers can employ is to discuss SNF admissions in the daily huddle and use the care coordinator in the practice to work with patients and families to transition to home as quickly as possible. In his book, *Being Mortal*,[28] Atul Gawande talks in great detail about the use of SNFs and the disconnect providers experience due to their lack of understanding of the care delivered and the absence of clear discharge planning that often occurs in this care setting. He states, "there's this phase of people's lives in which they can't really cope on their own, and we ought to find a way to make it manageable." Using community resources, including social workers, it is possible to implement a plan of care that includes required services in the home based on the patients' individualized needs. Although this is a lofty goal, it is one which the current delivery system should embrace.

How to Manage Change When Providers Are Still Primarily Working on Volume

Managing the change while fee-for-service reimbursement is the primary method of compensation can seem counterintuitive and extremely challenging.

The reimbursement model has not shifted quickly enough to support the investments required for transformation. A way to achieve incremental transformation is to strategically capture all forms of revenue that promote coordinated care (even under fee-for-service) and wherever possible aligning private payer contracts so that practice workflows do not have to differ between payers. Managing quality will generally result in an incentive payment though most important it aligns with good medical care. Furthermore, even outside of the CPC+ pilot program, in recent years CMS has begun to pay (in the regular physician fee schedule) for an "alphabet soup" of newly defined services that are foundational to coordinated care, for example:

The Annual Wellness Visit (AWV), a highly structured preventive care visit that addresses common geriatric risks such as falls, depression, hearing loss, and impaired cognition. The bulk of the AWV can be accomplished by a non-physician member of the care team.

Advance Care Planning (ACP), a detailed discussion and documentation of the patient's goals of care (particularly at the end of life), either as a standalone service or attached to another visit.

Transitions of Care Management (TCM), a single payment for 30 days of monitoring following discharge from a hospital, SNF, or observation stay. This initiative requires outreach to the patient within two business days of discharge and then an in-person visit with 7 or 14 days depending on complexity. Medication reconciliation is a required component of the visit. While an Evaluation and Management (E/M) code can be billed following the visit, the TCM code cannot be billed until post-discharge day 31 after confirming that the patient was not readmitted within the 30-day episode.

Chronic Care Management (CCM), a monthly payment for ongoing telephonic monitoring and care coordination of patients with specific chronic conditions, again primarily a service that can be provided by a care team member other than a physician. Practices in CPC+ are not allowed to bill for this service, since it is an alternative to the monthly care coordination fee in that program.

Telehealth codes, new in 2019, designed to compensate for brief telephonic check-ins with patients or consultations between providers.

▶ Conclusion

The key to sustainability of coordinated care in primary care is panel growth and the ability to take risk—that is, outperform compared to market trends or reduce total medical expense for patients through quality and care coordination. The future care model is sustainable only under alternative payment models and with a commitment to changing people, process, and technology. The highest quality, most cost-effective care must become the easiest path to take for physicians, practice staff, and most important, patients and families. Physician compensation and incentive models must be aligned to facilitate the ability to do the right things with ease while simultaneously achieving value-based contract objectives. Success comes after reaching a tipping point where this becomes the standard care model versus an add-on while also trying to operate under a visit-based fee-for-service model.

Study and Discussion Questions

1. What is driving the rapid move from volume to value in the U.S. healthcare payment system?
2. Give examples of types of care delivery services incentivized by volume-based, fee-for-service payment models, as opposed to value-based, alternative payment models.
3. What are some new skills required of clinicians for success in a future where the bulk of payment may be linked to value?
4. What are some potential benefits and pitfalls of coordinated care models from the perspective of a provider?
5. What are some potential benefits and pitfalls of coordinated care models from the perspective of patients?

Suggested Readings and Websites

Publications on care coordination: https://www .commonwealthfund.org/trending /care-coordination

Primary care transformation (Patient Centered Primary Care Collaborative): https://www .pcpcc.org/

Accountable Care Organizations: https://www .naacos.com/

References

1. Wynne B. May the era of Medicare's Doc fix (1997-2015) rest in peace. Now what? Health Affairs Blog. April 15, 2015. DOI: 10.1377/hblog20150415.046932. Available at https://www.healthaffairs.org/do/10.1377 /hblog20150415.046932/full/ (accessed June 2, 2019).
2. Institute of Medicine. *Crossing the Quality Chasm: A New Health System for the 21st Century*. Washington, DC: National Academies Press; 2001.
3. The Dartmouth Institute. *The Dartmouth Atlas Project*. Available at https://www .dartmouthatlas.org/ (accessed June 2, 2019).
4. Gawande A. The cost conundrum: what a Texas town can teach us about health care. *The New Yorker*. May 25, 2009. Available at https://www.newyorker.com /magazine/2009/06/01/the-cost-conundrum (accessed June 2, 2019).
5. Versel N. Population health expert: health reform as simple as changing incentives. *Forbes*. August 15, 2014. Available at https://www .forbes.com/sites/neilversel/2014/08/15 /population-health-expert-health-reform-as -simple-as-changing-incentives/# d04f9116f039 (accessed June 2, 2019).
6. Rosenbaum S. The Patient Protection and Affordable Care Act: implications for public health policy and practice. *Public Health Rep.* 2011 (Jan-Feb);126(1):130–135.
7. Network for Regional Healthcare Improvement. *What Is MACRA: The Medicare Access and CHIP Reauthorization Act of 2015 (MACRA)*. South Portland, ME: Author; 2019. Available at https:// www.nrhi.org/work/what-is-macra/what -is-macra/ (accessed June 2, 2019).
8. Centers for Medicare and Medicaid Services. The CMS Innovation Center. 2019. Available at https://innovation.cms.gov.
9. Trisolini M, Aggarwal J, Leung M, Pope G, Kautter J. The Medicare physician group practice demonstration: lessons learned on improving quality and efficiency in health care. *Commonwealth Fund* Pub. 1094. Washington, DC: Author; February 2008. Available at https://

www.commonwealthfund.org/publications /fund-reports/2008/feb/medicare-physician -group-practice-demonstration-lessons-learned (accessed June 2, 2019).

10. Centers for Medicare and Medicaid Services. Shared Savings Program. January 24, 2019. Available at https://www.cms.gov/Medicare /Medicare-Fee-for-Service-Payment /sharedsavingsprogram/index.html (accessed June 2, 2019).

11. Centers for Medicare and Medicaid Services. Physician Quality Reporting System. Available at https://www.cms.gov/medicare /quality-initiatives-patient-assessment -instruments/pqrs/downloads/pqrs _overviewfactsheet_2013_08_06.pdf (accessed June 2, 2019).

12. Centers for Medicare and Medicaid Services. MIPS Overview. Quality Payment Program. 2019. Available at https://qpp.cms.gov/mips /overview (accessed June 2, 2019).

13. Centers for Medicare and Medicaid Services. APMs Overview-Quality Payment Program. Available at https://qpp.cms.gov/apms/overview (accessed April 7, 2019).

14. Centers for Medicare and Medicaid Services. Comprehensive End Stage Renal Disease (ESRD) Care Model. ESRD Seamless Care Organizations (ESCOs). Available at https:// innovation.cms.gov/Files/fact-sheet/cec-fs. pdf(accessed June 2, 2019).

15. Centers for Medicare and Medicaid Services. Comprehensive Primacy Care Plus. Available at https://innovation .cms.gov/initiatives/comprehensive -primary-care-plus (accessed April 7, 2019).

16. Agency for Healthcare Research and Quality. Defining the PCMH. Patient-Centered Medical Home Resource Center. Rockville, MD: U.S. Department of Health & Human Services; 2019. Available at https://pcmh.ahrq.gov/page /defining-pcmh (accessed June 2, 2019).

17. Butcher L. Some builders' remorse: the rise and fall of the oncology medical home. *Manag Care*. 2017 (May 1). Available at https://www .managedcaremag.com/archives/2017/5/some -builders-remorse-rise-and-fall-oncology -medical-home (accessed June 2, 2019).

18. NCQA. Patient-Centered Specialty Practice (PCSP) Recognition. Available at https:// www.ncqa.org/programs/health-care -providers-practices/patient-centered-specialty -practice-recognition-pcsp/ (accessed June 2, 2019).

19. Centers for Medicare and Medicaid Services. Oncology Care Model. Available at https:// innovation.cms.gov/initiatives/oncology-care / (accessed April 7, 2019).

20. Porter ME, Lee TH. The strategy that will fix health care. *Harv Bus Rev.* 2013 (Oct);91(10):50–70.

21. Medicare participating heart bypass center demonstration executive summary final report. July 24, 1998.

22. Centers for Medicare and Medicaid Services. Bundle Payment for Care Improvement. Available at https://innovation.cms.gov /initiatives/bundled-payments/ (accessed June 2, 2019).

23. Cranor CW, Bunting BA, Christensen D. The Asheville project: long-term clinical and economic outcomes of a community pharmacy diabetes care program. *J Am Pharmaceut Assoc.* 2003(March/April);43(2):173–184. Available at https://www.aphafoundation.org/sites/default /files/ckeditor/files/TheAshevilleProject -Diabetes-JAPhA-2003-43-173-84.pdf (accessed April 7, 2019).

24. CVSHealth.com. CVS Health testing new HealthHUB store format. Available at https:// cvshealth.com/thought-leadership/cvs-health -testing-new-healthhub-store-format (accessed April 7, 2019).

25. The Case Management Society of America. *Standards of Practice for Case Management, revised 2002*. Little Rock, AR: Author; 2002.

26. World Health Organization. *Social determinants of health*. Available at https://www.who.int/social _determinants/en/ (accessed April 7, 2019).

27. NCQA PCMH standards and guidelines (version 5). Available at: https://www.ncqa.org /programs/health-care-providers-practices /patient-centered-medical-home-pcmh /pcmh-concepts/ (Accessed 8/28/19).

28. Gawande A. *Being Mortal: Medicine and What Matters in the End*. New York: Henry Holt; 2014.

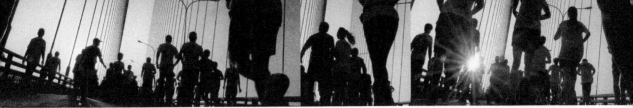

CHAPTER 13

Policy and Advocacy

Vicki Shepard
Michael Park
Brian Lee

EXECUTIVE SUMMARY

The preceding chapters of the book discuss the components of a healthcare system based on population health. This chapter discusses the role that public policy can play in promoting the widespread adoption of population health and how advocacy can be employed to shape policymaking.

In general, policymaking involves the consideration of numerous factors including, but not limited to, politics, budgetary impact, and how the policy would be implemented. There are numerous players in federal policymaking that are relevant to population health, especially in the executive and legislative branches of government. Some of these players, such as legislative branch agencies, play a more supportive role to help inform policy options being explored while other players, such as congressional committees and federal agencies, have the authority to make policy through law or regulation.

There are numerous ways to advance changes in policy or the creation of new policy through both the legislative and executive branches. Advocacy is a key element of advancing policymaking and can be used to advance population health efforts. Lobbying is a common advocacy activity that comes in different forms (e.g., direct lobbying, grassroots lobbying, grasstops lobbying), and advocates often employ multiple lobbying methods. Lobbying can be conducted on the individual or organizational level and also can involve multiple individuals or organizations to band together to form a coalition. Decisions on which lobbying method to employ depend on factors such as preference of the advocate, available resources, and likelihood of success of the lobbying method.

LEARNING OBJECTIVES

By the end of this chapter, the reader will be able to:

1. Understand factors that are considered during the policymaking process.
2. Identify the key players and their roles in federal policymaking for population health.
3. Appreciate population health policymaking in the context of implementing innovative health care and delivery models that promote population health.

▶ Introduction

The preceding chapters of this book discuss the building blocks of the population health ecosystem including organizational structures, reimbursement models, infrastructure, and the workforce needed to support population health. Implementing these building blocks at times requires significant change, and the policymaking process can promote the change needed for the widespread transformation of our healthcare system to one that is based on population health.

The purpose of this chapter is to provide an overview of the policymaking process, including the key players and considerations when making policy. Examples of population health policymaking also will be examined in the context of implementing innovative health care and delivery models that promote population health. Advocacy plays an important role in policymaking, and this especially holds true in the population health field. A discussion of advocacy in both the legislative and executive branches is included.

▶ The Policymaking Process

Public health policymaking can occur at the federal, state, and local levels, with varying scope and scale depending on where and how such policies are developed. As discussed in previous chapters, much of the policymaking related to population health has taken place at the federal level. Federal-level policymaking can drive and incentivize new population health efforts, while also sustaining efforts made by non-governmental stakeholders.

Considerations in Policymaking

Political

Crafting policy brings up numerous political considerations including, but not limited to, the following:

1. Does the policy option have bipartisan support?
2. Who are the supporters and who are the opponents of the policy option?
3. Does the policy option concern an issue that affects the entire population or just a subset?
4. Who will benefit from and who will be adversely impacted by the policy option?
5. Does the policy option address an issue at the nation's forefront?
6. Does the policy option address a controversial issue?
7. Are there data, outcomes, or cost implications that support the policy?

Generally, policy options addressing popular issues that are beneficial nationwide and have bipartisan support are more likely to be implemented than those that are not.

Budgetary

Budgetary issues also arise when considering a policy option. The budgetary impact of a policy option can be significant, especially in the context of federal legislation where "pay as you go" or "PAYGO" budget laws in Congress require that increases in federal program spending or tax cuts must be offset by cuts to federal program spending or tax increases elsewhere. Therefore, under PAYGO, a member of Congress championing a legislative proposal that is estimated to increase federal spending or reduce tax revenues is faced with the task of proposing how to offset these costs. Because they often result in reduced federal spending or tax increases for certain segments of the population or the entire population, offset proposals often produce political ramifications so that the considerations discussed above become more relevant.

Implementation

Implementing a policy option also is a significant consideration that raises questions such as:

1. Does the policy option require the enactment of a law or the promulgation of a regulation?
2. Does the policy option require the creation of a new government program or the creation of a new government agency, or can it instead be implemented within existing programs and agencies?
3. Does the policy option entail a marked change from current policy priorities and require significant culture change?
4. Does the policy option have support from those who will execute the policy, including state, local, or other relevant stakeholder groups?

In such considerations, an analysis is required regarding whether the effort involved in implementation is worth the intended policy goal.

▶ Key Players in Federal Policymaking

Numerous stakeholders affect healthcare policy at the federal, state, and local levels and with key industry groups. The federal government especially plays a significant role in influencing policy and population health directly as one of the largest purchasers of health care and indirectly as an influencer of private sector healthcare purchasing and delivery. As the largest employer and purchaser of healthcare services, the federal government finances and provides coverage to nearly 130 million government employees; the poor, disabled, and elderly; active duty and former military personnel and their dependents; and Native Americans and other populations.[1]

Given this role, federal government purchasing and healthcare delivery policies often can significantly influence other, non-federal health insurance purchasers and providers. For example, independent health plans who participate in federal health programs (e.g., private sector Medicare Advantage plans or Medicaid managed care plans) may impose payment policies on non-government clients similar to those imposed by large, government-managed programs. In other instances, independent health plans that do not participate in federal health programs will rely on federal coverage and reimbursement policy when setting their policies for the commercial market. For example, there have been recent federal developments related to addressing the opioid epidemic. As policies are implemented for federal healthcare programs, independent health plans are likely to implement similar policies for their commercial enrollees.

Private sector purchasers, especially those seeking coverage options for thousands of employees, dependents, or retirees, may seek to negotiate contract rates similar to those paid by government programs, or they may follow the government's lead in directly contracting with newly formed accountable care organizations (ACOs). Clearly, government coverage, payment policies, and ideas regarding system structure extend beyond government-managed programs and can directly affect coverage, payment policies, and contracting for other purchasers, as well as coverage and payment policies for healthcare practitioners.

Policymaking at the federal level mainly is developed in the legislative and executive branches of government. Major players in both of these governmental branches are discussed below.

U.S. Congress

The U.S. Congress plays a key role in establishing healthcare policy and directly influences population health management in the context of broader health policy. Several congressional committees in both the U.S. House of Representatives and the U.S. Senate share jurisdiction over health policy at the federal level. The functions of these committees typically include conducting oversight over federal programs and developing legislation.

In the House, several committees have jurisdiction over health care and make policy decisions that impact both federal health programs and the private sector alike:

- The Committee on Ways and Means (W&M Committee) has jurisdiction over the provision of payments for health care, health delivery systems, or health research. This includes healthcare programs under the Social Security Act, including Medicaid and Medicare, and tax credit and tax deduction provisions related to health insurance premiums and healthcare costs.[2]
- The Committee on Energy and Commerce (E&C Committee) has jurisdiction over health programs under the Public Health Service Act as well as the Social Security Act, which include public health, mental health, and health information technology. The committee also addresses matters related to Medicare and Medicaid, the Children's Health Insurance Program (CHIP), medical research, and food and drug safety.[3]
- The Committee on Education and Labor has primary jurisdiction over matters relating to labor and workforce issues, including employer-sponsored health benefits.[4]

There are two Senate committees with legislative authority over health care:

- The Committee on Finance (Finance Committee) has jurisdiction over health programs under the Social Security Act, including Medicare, Medicaid, CHIP, and other health and human services programs financed by a specific tax or trust fund.[5]
- The Health, Education, Labor and Pensions Committee (HELP Committee) has jurisdiction over health programs under the Public Health Service Act and the Older Americans Act. The committee considers legislation on issues such as public health, biomedical research and development, food and drug safety, access to health care, employer-sponsored

health benefits, aging, and individuals with disabilities.[6]

Also, the Senate Special Committee on Aging (Aging Committee) studies issues impacting older Americans. This committee does not have legislative authority like the Finance Committee and HELP Committee but can "study issues, conduct oversight of programs, and investigate reports of fraud and abuse."[7] The Aging Committee also can submit its findings and recommendations for legislation to the Senate.[7] The Medicare program is a key focus of the Aging Committee.

Furthermore, congressional caucuses play a role in the policymaking process. A caucus is "[a]n informal organization of members of the House or the Senate, or both, that exists to discuss issues of mutual concern and possibly to perform legislative research and policy planning for its members."[8] Caucuses can be based on political affiliation (e.g., House Republican Conference or House Democratic Caucus), region (e.g., House Rural Caucus), ideology (e.g., the Congressional Progressive Caucus or the Blue Dog Coalition), or personal interest (e.g., Congressional Primary Care Caucus or Congressional Public Health Caucus). Caucuses do not have oversight or legislative authority like congressional committees. Instead, caucus members work to advance their shared policy goals through activities that include educating members of Congress and advocating for specific legislation.

Legislative Branch Agencies

Congressional legislative efforts to enact policy changes are informed by numerous sources, including a variety of legislative branch agencies. Among these organizations, the Medicare Payment Advisory Commission (MedPAC), the Medicaid and

CHIP Payment and Access Commission (MACPAC), and the Congressional Budget Office (CBO) play a significant role in advancing the population health agenda.

Medicare Payment Advisory Commission (MedPAC)

MedPAC is a nonpartisan legislative branch agency established by the Balanced Budget Act of 1997.[9] MedPAC has 17 commissioners who bring various expertise in the areas of healthcare administration, delivery, and payment. The U.S. Comptroller General appoints the commissioners to three-year terms, which can be renewed. Several of the commissioners have backgrounds in population health.

MedPAC's purpose is to advise the U.S. Congress on issues related to reimbursement for private Medicare plans (i.e., Medicare Advantage) and traditional fee-for-service (FFS) Medicare. In addition to Medicare payment issues, MedPAC analyzes and provides recommendations on potential changes to the Medicare program related to beneficiary access and quality of care. These recommendations come in the form of two annual reports issued in March and June. MedPAC also submits reports on subjects as requested by Congress and will frequently submit comments on regulations issued by the Department of Health and Human Services (HHS). Further, MedPAC staff, such as the Executive Director, may provide testimony at congressional briefings and hearings.

Following the passage of the Affordable Care Act (ACA), MedPAC accumulated data and evidence related to Medicare's approach to measuring the quality of care for beneficiaries, especially as they relate to traditional Medicare. In its June, 2014 report to the Congress,[10]

MedPAC concluded that the Medicare program relies too heavily on process measures that are weakly correlated to health outcomes. MedPAC concluded that providers are incentivized to focus limited resources on "care processes" that Medicare measures, regardless of whether those measures are significant in terms of ensuring high-quality care is delivered.

The 2014 report highlighted an alternative approach to measuring and reporting on quality of care for FFS Medicare, Medicare Advantage, and Medicare ACOs. Specifically, MedPAC suggested using a set of population-based outcome measures (e.g., potentially preventable hospital admissions, emergency department (ED) visits, and readmissions, mortality, patient experience surveys) to assess the quality of care delivered to Medicare beneficiaries. MedPAC believes that the transition to population health measures is necessary to streamline care delivery and also to improve outcomes. MedPAC continues to explore population health measures, such as the "Healthy Days at Home" (HDAH) outcome measure,[11] which would measure the days during which a beneficiary was neither an inpatient nor had an ED visit.

As MedPAC continues to explore and provide recommendations related to the inefficiencies in the Medicare program, many CMS demonstrations, models, and initiatives have integrated such population health measures as primary or high-priority quality outcomes. For example, preventable admissions, ED visits, and readmissions are now standard metrics in various value-based care arrangements, including the Bundled Payments for Care Improvement Initiative (Original and Advanced demonstrations)

and the Comprehensive Care for Joint Replacement Initiative, and they will likely be included in key metrics in future demonstrations.

Medicaid and CHIP Payment and Access Commission (MACPAC)

MACPAC is a nonpartisan legislative branch agency authorized by the ACA. MACPAC serves as an independent source of information on Medicaid and the State Children's Health Insurance Program (CHIP) and makes recommendations to Congress, the Secretary of HHS, and states on issues affecting Medicaid and CHIP.[12] MACPAC conducts policy and data analysis and disseminates its findings and recommendations in reports that are released in March and June of each year. The U.S. Comptroller General appoints MACPAC's 17 commissioners.

In 2014, MACPAC examined Medicaid's role in promoting population health.[13] In its report, the commission noted that Medicaid enrollees are worse off with respect to social determinants that affect overall health status relative to wealthier and less disabled populations and that this disparity plays a substantial role in the differing health status between Medicaid enrollees and other populations. MACPAC noted that although Medicaid, as primarily a source of health coverage, cannot address all social determinants of health, programs have found ways to address some of these factors, which in turn can avoid costly healthcare services in the future.

MACPAC first identified the various non-treatment-oriented services that Medicaid programs cover. Examples of these services, which advance population health, include (1) screening and preventive services for children and adults; (2) non-medical enabling services ranging from transportation to health education to counseling; and (3) incentive programs to promote healthy behaviors and lifestyles.

The Commission then examined successful partnerships between Medicaid programs and government agencies (other federal and state) and non-governmental organizations such as health plans and providers to promote population health. Examples of these partnerships include working with public health departments to provide preventative services like immunizations, lead abatement and reduction of sexually transmitted diseases. MACPAC also identified challenges in these partnerships, including (1) separate funding streams and other financing challenges, (2) different timeframes for evaluating effectiveness, (3) conflicting eligibility rules and program coordination issues, (4) incompatible data systems, and (5) differences in organization culture or goals.

Finally, the Commission discussed how to monitor population health initiatives in Medicaid in the future as well as what data are available and what data are needed. The Commission noted that there currently are few Medicaid datasets that can provide the information needed to monitor efforts to improve population health. MACPAC did note, however, that work was under way to improve Medicaid data files. The Commission concluded that it "will continue to monitor and to track best practices in Medicaid population health programs, the resources included to promote them, and regulations that may impede or promote their implementation."[13]

Congressional Budget Office (CBO)

The CBO is a legislative branch agency established in 1974 through the Congressional Budget and Impoundment Control Act of 1974.[14] The CBO is the nonpartisan "scorekeeper" for Congressional legislation and provides budget and economic information, especially as it relates to legislation. As part of this role, CBO provides legislators with data, estimates, analyses, and implications of legislative proposals. CBO is required to create estimates of legislative proposals reported out of congressional committees or upon a legislator's request, which must include "discretionary spending" (i.e., budget authority through and controlled by appropriation bills, which set aside federal funds for specific federal departments, agencies, programs, and functions) and "mandatory spending" (i.e., budget authority mandated by law, but not dependent on annual or period appropriation, such as benefits under programs including Social Security, Medicare, and Medicaid).

Currently, CBO is statutorily limited in terms of how far out it can estimate a budgetary impact of specific legislation. Specifically, CBO may only look 10 years to the future when developing cost estimates of how legislation may impact spending and revenues. Because population health comprises changes in long-term health through prevention, wellness, and managing chronic diseases, a 10-year window often does not estimate or include the financial impact of adopting healthy lifestyles or taking steps to better manage chronic conditions. Subsequently, CBO's 10-year forecast does not typically capture the long-term cost savings that result from preventive health. Historically, CBO's scoring methodology has not included financial savings related to prevention or wellness programs.

Despite these limitations, CBO has revised its methodology in light of new evidence, which may improve how CBO estimates the impact of population health measures. For example, in 2012, CBO revised its methodology when estimating the budgetary impact of measures related to prescription drugs.[15] Historically, CBO did not believe there was sufficient evidence related to the "offsetting" effect of prescription drug use on spending for medical services. However, in light of new analyses demonstrating that medication adherence can reduce downstream use of medical services, CBO has synthesized and incorporated such research into its cost estimates for proposals related to prescription drug use by Medicare beneficiaries. This signals that, as new evidence and analyses emerge, CBO may adjust its methodology to capture savings from other population health measures.

In the meantime, members of Congress have attempted to address CBO's limitations through legislation.[16] In 2017, legislation was introduced that would require CBO to determine if a proposed measure would result in reductions in federal spending beyond the 10-year window through the use of preventive health and preventive health services. The legislation would define preventive health as:

An action that focuses on the health of the public, individuals and defined populations in order to protect, promote, and maintain health and wellness and prevent disease, disability, and premature

death that is demonstrated by credible and publicly available evidence from epidemiological projection models, clinical trials, observational studies in humans, longitudinal studies, and meta-analysis.[17]

This legislation would extend the CBO's review period to 20 years for the purposes of scoring preventive health measures in an attempt to capture more of the savings in federal spending associated with these measures. The legislation ultimately was not enacted, but nevertheless shows the interest in addressing this limitation.

Numerous advocacy and industry groups that focus on wellness, prevention, and population health have also addressed the issue of the CBO's scoring period. These efforts will likely continue as these groups advocate for legislation or promote new policies.

U.S. Department of Health and Human Services

Cabinet-level agencies and other offices are also key players in policymaking, with primary responsibility for implementing legislative policy on healthcare issues. Most prominent is the Centers for Medicare & Medicaid Services (CMS), which is an operating division of the Department of Health and Human Services (HHS). Established as a regulatory agency for federal healthcare programs, CMS administers the Medicare program (including covered healthcare services, benefits, eligibility, enrollment, and provider participation), Medicaid, and CHIP (the latter two of which are jointly administered by CMS and individual states). In 2017, almost

138 million individuals were covered under the Medicare, Medicaid, and CHIP programs.[17] As discussed earlier, the federal government has a significant role in the financing and delivery of health care, developing health policy, and managing population health as one of the largest administrators and purchasers of healthcare services. In addition, there are several other divisions within HHS that create policies impacting population health. These divisions include the Centers for Disease Control and Prevention (CDC), the Office of the Assistant Secretary for Planning and Evaluation, the Substance Abuse and Mental Health Services Administration, and the Health Resources & Services Administration. These divisions work on key population health issues including Zika, HIV/AIDS, influenza, childhood obesity, maternal mortality, rural health issues, and substance abuse, including ongoing efforts to combat the opioid epidemic.

The role of HHS in promoting population health management extends beyond the public programs it administers. For example, HHS plays a role in administering regulations related to the use of financial incentives to promote wellness. The Health Insurance Portability and Accountability Act (HIPAA) prohibits private health plans from charging higher premiums or cost sharing for individuals with preexisting conditions, with limited exceptions. The ACA prohibits all insurers from excluding individuals due to their preexisting conditions, charging them higher premiums, or imposing waiting periods for coverage. The population health management industry has pioneered the use of innovative incentive programs to encourage sustained behavior change. After the ACA expanded the

allowable use of wellness-related financial incentives, HHS, the Department of the Treasury, and the Department of Labor collaborated to issue new regulations to enhance and clarify requirements related to the use of nondiscriminatory wellness incentives. Although not part of HHS, the Equal Employment Opportunity Commission (EEOC) also plays a role in regulating the use of wellness incentives and is expected to issue clarifying regulations in the near future.

Additional examples of HHS's expanded role in population health promotion include efforts by the Office of the National Coordinator for Health Information Technology (ONC) and demonstration programs and models implemented by the Center for Medicare & Medicaid Innovation (CMMI or the CMS Innovation Center), which are discussed in more detail below.

Office of the National Coordinator for Health Information Technology

ONC leads the executive branch health information technology (HIT)-related efforts to implement nationwide HIT adoption, use, and interoperability. ONC is the primary federal agency responsible for enhancing HIT infrastructure, supporting HIT adoption, and promoting health information exchange.[18] ONC's mission is to improve the health and well-being of individuals and communities through technology and ensuring health information is accessible.

The National Coordinator position was created through an Executive Order in 2004 and became legislatively mandated in 2009 through the Health Information

Technology for Economic and Clinical Health (HITECH) Act. The HITECH Act provided HHS the authority to establish programs intended to improve healthcare quality, safety, and efficiency through HIT. This included incentivizing the adoption and use of electronic health records (EHR) and secure electronic health information exchange. Originally, HIT was viewed as an important population health management tool, as it could enable providers to improve care coordination, especially for patients with chronic conditions who often see multiple healthcare providers, may take multiple prescription drugs, and require an interdisciplinary care team to effectively manage and treat their conditions.

Through the HITECH Act, which was passed as part of the American Recovery and Reinvestment Act of 2009, HHS invested billions of dollars to incentivize EHR adoption through the "Meaningful Use" program. The Meaningful Use program utilized certified EHR technology (CEHRT) to improve population health management and outcomes. Specifically, the Meaningful Use program had the following objectives:

- Improve quality, safety, and efficiency, and reduce health disparities
- Engage patients and family members
- Improve care coordination, population health, and public health
- Maintain privacy and security of patient health information

In 2015, Congress continued to seek ways to improve population health and passed the Medicare Access and CHIP Reauthorization Act of 2015 (MACRA). MACRA established the Quality Payment Program and its two payment tracks: (1) the Merit-based Incentive Payment System (MIPS) and (2) Advanced Alternative Payment Models (APMs). Through MACRA, the Meaningful Use program and two other CMS quality programs, the Physician Quality Reporting Program and the Value Based Payment Modifier, were transitioned into the MIPS Promoting Interoperability Performance Category. While the Meaningful Use objectives remain the same, the intent was to combine and coordinate physician incentives through a single performance category, which is expected to result in:

- Improved clinical and population health outcomes
- Increased transparency and efficiency
- Empowered patients
- More robust research data on health systems

In addition to consolidating the various physician incentive programs, MACRA required minimum CEHRT use for Advanced APMs. As CMS continues its regulatory process related to the Quality Payment Program, such EHR use and adoption requirements have continued to increase, placing a greater emphasis on the value of HIT in improving patient outcomes and population health.

As technology and EHR vendors entered the market, a new challenge to care coordination and population health management emerged: proprietary EHR systems and networks and subsequent "information blocking." ONC identified this barrier and submitted a Report to Congress on information blocking in 2015.[19] In the report, ONC stated, "Information blocking occurs when persons or entities knowingly or unreasonably interfere with the exchange or use of electronic health information exchange." Information blocking requires three criteria:

1. **Interference**: Some act or course of conduct that interferes with the ability of authorized persons or entities to access, exchange, or use electronic health information.
2. **Knowledge**: A specific decision to engage in information blocking knowing that this is likely to interfere with the exchange or use of electronic health information.
3. **No reasonable justification**: Information blocking should be reserved for conduct that is objectively unreasonable to public policy goals (actions to comply with federal or state privacy requirements would not be unreasonable).

ONC believes that information blocking not only interferes with effective health information exchange but also has adverse impacts on population health, negatively affecting important aspects of health and health care. Patients, especially those with multiple care providers, face barriers in care coordination resulting from information blocking. Further, one of the contributors to the opioid epidemic was a lack of data exchange, which would have illuminated the scope of opioid prescribing for individuals receiving services across multiple providers.

Following the ONC's report, Congress passed the 21st Century Cures Act of 2016 (Cures Act), which included a specific focus on improving the flow and exchange of electronic health information. The Cures Act requires ONC, in collaboration with HHS and other federal agencies, to improve HIT usability and prevent information blocking. ONC is in the rulemaking process to establish regulations related to information blocking, including distinguishing prohibited blocking and permissible information access restrictions. ONC released its proposed rule on February 11, 2019, which is intended to improve interoperability of electronic health information and to prevent information blocking (i.e., impeding the free exchange of patient data across various parts of the healthcare system). As technology advances and HIT infrastructure is further developed, ONC is expected to continue efforts to leverage HIT to improve patient and population health outcomes.

Center for Medicare & Medicaid Innovation (CMMI or the CMS Innovation Center)

The establishment of CMMI within CMS has created opportunities for further development of models that support population health. The CMS Innovation Center funds a broad range of demonstration programs, including alternative payment and delivery models, intended to promote care coordination.[20]

▶ Experimentation Before CMMI

The basis for demonstrations, projects, or other experiments and innovative programs dates back to 1962, when Section

1115 of the Social Security Act was enacted. While this predated the establishment of the Medicare and Medicaid programs, Section 1115 authorized the secretary of what is now HHS to authorize experimental, pilot, or demonstration projects that are likely to assist in promoting the objectives of the programs covered by the Social Security Act. Section 1115 has been used primarily to alter the requirements related to the Medicaid program CHIP, resulting in state-based innovation and demonstrations. The Section 1115 authority is broad and permits states to implement significant changes to Medicaid eligibility, benefits, and how Medicaid services are delivered as long as they support the Medicaid program or CHIP objectives. While not expressly required, Section 1115 waivers are typically budget neutral.

In 1967, Congress passed the Social Security Amendments, which further enabled HHS to undertake and implement various demonstration projects. In 1977, what is now known to be the Centers for Medicare & Medicaid Services (CMS) was established. CMS is where much of today's innovation and reform efforts occur. An example of payment reform during these early phases is the current payment system used to reimburse hospitals for inpatient care—the Medicare Hospital Inpatient Prospective Payment System—that was established through a demonstration project. All redesign efforts pursued under this statutory framework were somewhat limited by statutory requirements and limitations, such as budget neutrality, on the agency.

Originally, Congress would request the demonstration of a particular model and provide funding for CMS to operate demonstrations (or require that the demonstration remain budget neutral). For example, the Medicare Prescription Drug, Improvement, and Modernization Act of 2003 (MMA) required CMS to implement 14 demonstration projects intended to test potential future improvements in Medicare coverage, expenditures, and the quality of care. The results of these programs would then be used to inform and shape future models.

Paradigm Shift: The ACA

The passage of the ACA in 2010 resulted in a major policy shift as the ACA provided new legal authority to CMS. The ACA established CMMI within CMS and provided CMMI with $10.5 billion to design, implement, and evaluate new demonstration models. Essentially, Congress provided CMS with the authority to independently pursue new, alternative, value-based care arrangements. Further, Congress provided CMS with the authority to waive various Medicare and Medicaid requirements, thereby providing CMS with additional flexibility to implement and test models more rapidly without relying on Congress to appropriate funding or provide direction. Prior to the passage of the ACA, approximately 60% of CMS's demonstrations were legislated by Congress.[21]

Congress has not mandated any demonstration projects since the passage of the ACA. Instead, CMMI has actively pursued demonstration models, building off of previously mandated programs and establishing new models. For example, the Medicare Diabetes Prevention Program (MDPP) is an expansion of the Diabetes Prevention Program, a CMMI Health Care Innovation Awardee.

Further, the Bundled Payments for Care Improvement (BPCI) Model is a voluntary demonstration that informed the establishment of the Comprehensive End-Stage Renal Disease (ESRD) Care (CEC), Comprehensive Care for Joint Replacement (CJR), and BPCI Advanced Models. Another example is the Pioneer ACO Model, which was one of the original ACO model types and informed the development of numerous other ACO models (**TABLE 13-2**).

Section 1332 of the ACA also provided an additional avenue for states to pursue innovative strategies and demonstrations through a State Innovation Waiver. As the ACA established new coverage goals and requirements, Section 1332 was intended to provide states with an avenue to experiment with alternative ways to meet these goals. The Section 1332 waivers often work in conjunction with Section 1115 waivers, meaning states now have multiple tracks through which they can innovate and test new models.

▶ Recent Developments

More recently, Congress has passed legislation to expand and build on CMS's demonstration authority, including through the passage of the Bipartisan Budget Act (BBA) of 2018. The BBA of 2018 made significant changes to the MIPS program, but also encouraged and promoted the development of APMs, especially through the Physician Focused Payment Model Technical Advisory Committee (PTAC). There has been criticism regarding the PTAC's process and role. Specifically, the PTAC cannot unilaterally approve new models, leaving it up to the HHS Secretary to decide on whether to implement recommended models. In addition, stakeholders have raised concerns that there is a lack of clarity and direction in the proposal submission and review process. Finally, significant effort, time, and financial resources go into developing a comprehensive proposal. Without any guarantee that the model will be implemented, this has proven to be a significant barrier to the PTAC process. In

---

TABLE 13-1 Categories of CMMI Models

CMMI's models typically fall into one (or more) of the following categories:

- Accountable care

- Episode-based payment initiatives

- Primary care transformation

- Initiatives focused on the Medicaid and chip population

- Initiatives focused on Medicare-Medicaid enrollees

- Initiatives to accelerate the development and testing of new payment and service delivery models

- Initiatives to speed the adoption of best practices

TABLE 13-2 Timeline of Selected Federal Demonstration Projects and Models

Model Name	Description	Start Date
Acute Care Episode (ACE) Demonstration	The ACE Demonstration tested the use of a global payment for an episode of care, which included all Part A and Part B services related to the inpatient stay for a Medicare beneficiary. This Demonstration was intended to better align incentives for hospitals and physicians and lead to greater efficiencies and improved care.	5/1/2009
Medicare Health Care Quality Demonstration	Mandated by the MMA, CMS is using this demonstration to identify, develop, test, and disseminate major and multifaceted improvements to the Medicare program. The goals are to improve safety, enhance quality, increase efficiency, and reduce uncertainty and unwarranted variation in medical practice that result in lower quality and higher costs.	7/1/2009
Medicare Shared Savings Program (MSSP) Accountable Care Organization (ACO) Models	There are multiple MSSP ACO tracks (with staggered start dates), under which participants can assume varying levels of downside risk/shared losses depending on performance. In general, ACOs provide coordinated care and chronic disease management intended to lower costs while maintaining or improving quality of care.	1/1/2012
Pioneer ACO Model	One of the original ACO models, this was designed for ACOs experienced in coordinating care across settings and in coordination with private payers. This model also allowed participants to more rapidly move from a shared savings to a population-based payment model.	1/1/2012
Independence at Home (IAH) Demonstration	The IAH demonstration tests the effectiveness of providing comprehensive primary care services at the beneficiary's home and assesses whether this improves care for beneficiaries with multiple chronic conditions.	6/1/2012
Comprehensive Primary Care (CPC) Initiative	The CPC initiative was a multipayer initiative intended to strengthen primary care. CMS collaborated with commercial and state health insurance plans in seven regions to offer population-based care management fees as well as opportunities for shared savings for participating primary care practices.	10/1/2012
Bundled Payments for Care Improvement (BPCI) Models	The BPCI models link payments for multiple services beneficiaries receive during an episode of care. Participants enter into payment arrangements including accountability for both financial and clinical performance.	10/1/2013

Comprehensive End-Stage Renal Disease (ESRD) Care Model	CEC is designed to identify, test, and evaluate new ways to improve care for Medicare beneficiaries with ESRD. CMS partners with providers and suppliers to test a new service delivery model in providing person-centered, high-quality care.	9/1/2015
Home Health Value-Based Purchasing (HHVBP) Model	The HHVBP model is intended to support improved efficiency and care quality among Medicare-certified home health agencies.	1/1/2016
Next Generation ACO Model	One of several ACO models, this initiative is designed for ACOs more experienced in coordinating patient care. Participants can assume higher levels of financial risk and reward than under other ACO models (e.g., Pioneer and MSSP models).	1/1/2016
Comprehensive Care for Joint Replacement (CJR) Model	CJR built off of the results of the BPCI models and is intended to support improved care for beneficiaries undergoing the most common inpatient surgeries, such as lower extremity joint replacements. This model tests bundled payment and quality measurement for an episode of care for such surgeries.	4/1/2016
Oncology Care Model (OCM)	OCM was developed to test new payment and delivery models to improve the effectiveness and efficiency of oncology care. Under OCM, physician practices enter into payment arrangements (accounting for financial and quality performance) for episodes including chemotherapy administration to cancer patients.	7/1/2016
CPC Plus Model (CPC+)	CPC+ built off of the original CPC Initiative, integrating lessons learned to further strengthen primary care.	1/1/2017
Medicare Diabetes Prevention Program (MDPP) Expanded Model	The MDPP is an expansion of a CMMI Health Care Innovation Award—the Diabetes Prevention Program (DPP). The MDPP is an intervention intended to prevent type 2 diabetes in individuals with an indication of prediabetes.	4/1/2018
BPCI Advanced Model	BPCI Advanced builds off of the BPCI model and is intended to encourage redesigning care delivery through best practice adoption, reducing variation from standards of care, and providing clinically appropriate services for patients throughout a clinical episode.	10/1/2018

response to some of these issues, Congress took steps in the BBA of 2018 to expand the PTAC's work, which was originally defined in MACRA, to facilitate more APM development. The BBA of 2018 provided the PTAC with new authority to provide "initial feedback" to submitters of proposed models. This provides submitters with an opportunity to respond to initial feedback or formally revise and resubmit their proposals.

Following the BBA of 2018, CMS continued to promote care delivery transformation by finalizing regulations to implement the *Medicare Advantage Qualifying Payment Arrangement Incentive (MAQI) Demonstration*. This program will test whether there is an increase in eligible clinician participation in payment arrangements with Medicare Advantage (MA) organizations that CMS determines to be "qualifying payment arrangements," which are similar to Advanced APMs under MACRA. The MAQI demonstration will also test whether participating in Advanced APMs will incentivize care delivery transformation, change utilization patterns, and how these might impact MA plan bids. Most recently, CMS indicated that it will revisit mandatory demonstration models, especially for episode-based payment models.

The agency's statutory authority to implement, eliminate, and expand demonstration models has been well established. Perhaps the biggest challenge related to the future of such models is who controls and leads the agency as well as the associated philosophy and approach to demonstrations. Administration leaders opposed to such activities have the ability to scale back CMMI models while those who are supportive have the ability to expand existing models and create new models.

▶ Advocacy

What Is Lobbying?

In general, advocacy is any action to support a certain cause. There is no limit to the amount of non-lobbying advocacy that an organization or an individual may do. Advocacy in the policymaking process often is accomplished through lobbying, which generally is defined as attempting to influence policymaking

in the legislative or executive branches of government. Essentially, all lobbying is advocacy, but not all advocacy is lobbying. Lobbying often takes the form of "direct" lobbying, which generally entails an individual or group attempting to influence policy through communications to policymakers in the legislative or executive branches of government. There are other types of lobbying in addition to direct lobbying. *Grassroots* lobbying refers to encouraging members of the public to reach out to policymakers in the legislative or executive branches to influence policy. *Grasstops* lobbying refers to encouraging a narrower scope of individuals, usually leaders (e.g., thought leaders, community leaders, organization leaders) to reach out to policymakers in the legislative or executive branches to influence policy. Generally, individuals and entities engaged in lobbying must register and disclose information regarding the lobbying activity, including who was lobbied and on what specific issues.

Advocating for a specific policy option is not limited to one lobbying method. In fact, it is not uncommon for advocates to employ a combination of lobbying methods. The lobbying methods selected largely depend on a number of factors, including (1) advocate's preferences, (2) resources available, and (3) likelihood of success of the lobbying method.

Who Lobbies?

In the United States, lobbying is a protected activity under the First Amendment, which provides the right "to petition the government for a redress of grievances." Lobbying is not limited to individuals and, in fact, often consists of a group of individuals or organizations sharing the same policy objectives. Coalitions, which consist of individuals and organizations with different missions or priorities, but temporarily joining together, often engage in lobbying efforts as well for a shared public policy option. Overall, advocating for policy change and lobbying is a constitutionally protected right with some guardrails.

The vignette discussed in the following section involves a coalition, NashvilleHealth, and its activities, which include advocacy. Non-profit (i.e., 501[c][3]) organizations also are allowed to lobby but are limited in terms of the allowable expenditures on both direct and grassroots lobbying. Subsequently, organizations may lose their tax-exempt status as a result of excessive lobbying.

▶ NashvilleHealth: A Vignette on a Coalition

Nashville, Tennessee, is a thriving, energetic city in the midst of an economic boom. The city has one of the highest rates of employment growth of any large metropolis in the United States, and *U.S. News and World Report* ranked Nashville 13th among their 100 best cities in which to live in 2017. With a $70+ billion healthcare services industry that includes 16 publicly traded health companies, the city is known globally as an innovative healthcare center. Unfortunately, the overall health of the population is poor. This is Nashville's great dichotomy: a thriving "it" city/a city with a dire health problem.

The Honorable William H. Frist, MD, is a Nashville native. He represented Tennessee in the U.S. Senate for 12 years. He was elected majority leader of the Senate in 2003 and served in that role through 2007. As a surgeon, Dr. Frist has performed more than 150 heart and lung transplants, and he is board certified in both general and heart surgery. He is widely considered a leading authority on health, and he joined the Robert Wood Johnson Foundation (RWJF) Board of Trustees in January 2013.

As Frist sat in an RWJF Board meeting in 2014, he learned that the overall health of Tennessee is worse than 41 other states. He also learned that within Tennessee, Nashville/Davidson County fell behind 12 other counties in health rankings. Compared to four peer cities, Nashville ranked fourth for overall health and well-being and demonstrated the worst rates of obesity, children living in poverty, premature and injury deaths, and violent crime of all five cities. Nashville is known worldwide as an emerging, economically grounded, lifestyle-friendly home to creative artists and vanguards of healthcare administration, yet Frist knew that this reputation could not be sustained in a city plagued by poor health.

Frist returned home to Nashville determined to influence city leaders to rally around a clearly defined goal of radically improving the city's health. While recognizing that Nashville already had public health champions going about notable work, he noted that no one organization could possibly be capable of the scale of change needed to reset the trajectory of the population's health. He resolved to form a city-wide collaborative, intent upon leveraging relationships and dollars to attack issues from multiple angles, focus resources on the neediest areas, and ultimately save the city millions of dollars over the next decade.

Frist and a handful of other interested citizens began by investigating other cities' population health initiatives to see what they might adopt. They sought advice from national leaders in the field of regional health transformation. In order to learn about the many existing, but often siloed, efforts under way to address Nashville's health needs, they intensively engaged the local community. In fall 2014, they hosted a town hall to discuss intervention options.

In 2015, Frist established the not-for-profit organization **NashvilleHealth**, with a mission to substantially improve the health and well-being of Nashville residents. Thoroughly steeped in relevant experience and relationships, Caroline Young, former president of the Nashville Health Care Council, stepped into the role of executive director for NashvilleHealth. In just a little over a year, Young and a few volunteers held more than 200 community meetings uncovering issues, interests, challenges, and success stories from a vast array of local entities and national partners. The information gathered informed the course for NashvilleHealth.

NashvilleHealth also partnered with Vanderbilt University's Department of Health Policy (VUHP) to help determine initial activities and to create metrics, a key element in building a sustainable and replicable initiative.

In September 2015, the Nashville-Health and VUHP teams came together to engage in the priority-setting process. NashvilleHealth had a starting goal of targeting three health priorities via pilot projects in Nashville/Davidson County. The teams gathered and assimilated multiple data sets and conducted a comprehensive review of health priorities identified by all local stakeholders. From this process, 14 potential health priorities emerged.

The group then applied nine criteria to narrow the priorities:

1. Is this a real and pressing health issue for Nashville?
2. Is there partner/sponsor interest in this area?
3. Are there successful programs that can be modeled to address this issue?
4. Are measurable, achievable metrics for monitoring and evaluating progress applicable?
5. Is there reliable data about this issue in Nashville?
6. Does it address health equity?
7. Is it novel?
8. Is there a feasible possibility of showing success in a timely manner?
9. Is it scalable?

After extensive discussion and analysis, the working group settled on three initial priority areas: **Tobacco Cessation**, **Hypertension**, and **Child Health** (with a particular focus on infant mortality). They then sought out the most current, evidence-based models to consider for addressing each of the three areas through extensive literature reviews and creation of summary documents of the best practices.

NashvilleHealth applied a two-pronged approach to identify actions for each focus area, as shown in **TABLE 13-3**.

NashvilleHealth had already established a high-level **governing board** and an action-oriented **steering committee**. Armed with the support of those two bodies and the directives established by the working groups, NashvilleHealth was ready to begin implementing the following "prescription" for Nashville (**TABLE 13-4**) as well as amplify the good work already under way.

TABLE 13-3 The NashvilleHealth Two-Pronged Approach

One	Two

Provide a complete environmental and demographic scan of Nashville, including current data and a listing of efforts already under way, to **national panels of scientific experts and distinguished thought leaders for each focus area**, with a directive for them to produce recommendations specific to Nashville.
 	
    Ask them to provide a "prescription" for Nashville after weighing in on a number of evidence-based intervention options within four domains:
 	
1.   health care
2.   community engagement
3.   policy
4.   public awareness
	Create inclusive **local stakeholder working groups for each focus area** and provide them with the recommendations from their area's expert panel with a directive for them to revise and further substantiate those recommendations based on their collective knowledge of local resources and existing work already under way.
	
	    Direct the groups to provide recommended next steps for operationalizing and implementing the "prescription" for each area.

TABLE 13-4 NashvilleHealth's "Prescription" for Nashville

Goal	Make Nashville one of the healthiest places to live in the state and the nation by achieving measurable gains in the health of all residents.
Objectives	1. *Convene* diverse groups of key local stakeholders.
	2. *Identify* specific and measurable community health indicators.
	3. *Develop* a comprehensive and practical health roadmap.
	4. *Leverage* and align Nashville's relevant resources (ongoing).
	5. *Engage* academic partners to measure and monitor outcomes.
	6. *Strengthen* the community-wide integration of health services.
	7. *Scale* evidence-based, countywide success to state and national level.
Measures	1. *Adhere* to the Office of Disease Prevention and Health Promotion's Healthy People 2020 goals, with a 2022 goal date for NashvilleHealth.
	2. *Create* specific equity goals for each area of focus, in order to reduce racial disparities and create a culture of health citywide.
	3. *Consider* process metrics, such as the number of individuals or groups involved in the work, along with media reach.
	4. *Develop* processes for measuring the quantifiable outcomes of each individual program as they are developed for each focus area.

Infant Mortality **Current rate:** 6.8 per 1,000 (TN Dep't of Health 2014) **Broad goal:** 6.0 per 1,000 (HP2020)	• *Established by U.S. Dep't of Health & Human Services Office of Disease Prevention & Health Promotion
Hypertension **Current rate:** 30.5% (BRFSS 2014) **Broad goal:** Prevalence rate: 26.9%	• 10-year national objectives
Tobacco Use **Current rate:** 19.3% (BRFSS 2014) **Broad goal:** Prevalence rate: 12%	• NashvilleHealth timeline = 2017–2022 (with goals achieved as 3-year averages from 2020–2022)

Evaluating NashvilleHealth Interventions Utilizing Healthy People 2020 Goals

Evaluating NashvilleHealth Interventions Utilizing Healthy People 2020 Goals

NashvilleHealth is now actively working to create a culture of health and well-being by serving as the city's principal convener to open dialogue, align resources, and build smart strategic partnerships to forge a dynamic plan to improve the health of all Nashville residents. The power to convene is the key to NashvilleHealth's necessity. Many organizations throughout Nashville are doing good work to improve health outcomes, but it is only through collaboration, alignment, and partnerships among those organizations that substantial improvements in overall well-being and health will be achieved. Examples of initial work within focus areas include the following.

Tobacco Cessation

Nearly 20% of Davidson County, Tennessee, adults smoke, compared to the national rate of 16.8% and the CDC goal rate of 12%. The smoking rate is higher than many of Nashville's peer cities, including Austin and Charlotte. NashvilleHealth supported successful legislative efforts to get Nashville's Ascend Amphitheater to go smoke free, and that is a first step

in passing local control ("preemption") legislation statewide to allow localities to regulate tobacco use in public spaces. The organization also successfully spearheaded efforts, in partnership with Vanderbilt University Medical Center, to secure TennCare's exemption of proven tobacco cessation drugs (pharmacotherapy) from monthly drug limits for enrollees.

Hypertension

More than 30% of Nashville residents self-report as hypertensive, a rate that is worse than peer cities like Austin, Raleigh, Indianapolis, and Denver. In 2013, there were 12 hospitalizations for hypertension per 1,000 citizens. NashvilleHealth worked with the American Heart Association and the American Medical Association to launch "Target BP," a learning collaborative among providers for shared protocols and interventions around hypertension. In just a year's time, more than 16 clinics and hospitals were engaged in the program, with a reach of more than 550,000 hypertensive patients.

Child Health

The infant mortality rate in Nashville is 6.8 infant deaths per 1,000 live births. The African American infant mortality rate is

12 infant deaths per 1,000. With support from Tivity Health, NashvilleHealth began the research phase of a project to create a targeted infant safe sleep awareness campaign. The organization conducted focus groups with African American mothers and mothers-to-be around safe sleep perceptions and reactions to awareness messaging, partnered with Nashville's Metropolitan Public Health Department (MPHD) to take an in-depth look at available data around the issue, and traveled to Cincinnati to learn how an organization there dramatically decreased their city's sleep-related infant deaths through targeted awareness messaging. Moving forward, NashvilleHealth will utilize the information collected to create and disseminate messaging that will resonate with populations deemed high risk for such devastating outcomes.

Data

By design, NashvilleHealth is evidence based and data driven. To that end, NashvilleHealth partnered with MPHD to launch the Nashville Community Health + Wellbeing Survey, a community-wide survey of the health of Nashville residents. Working with a nationally recognized research institute using validated methods and questions from the Centers for Disease Control (CDC), they will survey more than 12,000 residents between October 2018 and January 2019 to more completely understand health-related behaviors, chronic health conditions, and preventive health practices and how environments impact opportunities for well-being. This first-of-a-kind project will provide the critical data to inform and enhance the work being done today and to measurably improve the health of Nashville residents in the future—in a format that will allow for accurate data to track progress over time.

With every newly formed partnership and every newly opened dialogue among diverse groups, NashvilleHealth plays a unique and unprecedented role in Nashville's well-being and future. A city cannot be great without healthy citizens. NashvilleHealth is working to make that state of overall health and well-being for all Nashville residents a reality that can be sustained for decades to come. As for those RWJF county health rankings—Nashville/Davidson County is now ranked sixth out of Tennessee's 95 counties. That's seven steps in the right direction.

▶ Conclusion

Policymaking can take many forms and largely depends on the consideration of numerous factors including the political climate, budgetary impact, and how such policy efforts will be implemented. The policymaking process itself involves numerous players especially in the executive and legislative branches of government. Some of these players play more of a support role to help inform policy options being explored while other players have the authority actually to make policy through law or regulation.

There are numerous ways to advance changes in policy or the creation of new policy through both the legislative and executive branches. Advocacy is a key element of policymaking, which can, and has been, used to advance population health efforts. Lobbying is a common advocacy activity that comes in different forms, and it is not uncommon for advocates to employ multiple lobbying methods. Decisions on which lobbying methods to employ depend on factors such as preference of the advocate, available resources, and likelihood of success of the lobbying method. Overall, while lobbying is a protected right, there are some "guardrails" for this activity. Finally, as noted in the following vignette, involving the key stakeholders in advocacy efforts is also critical to achieving population health goals.

Study and Discussion Questions

1. While the basis for demonstrations, projects, and experiments of innovative programs pre-dates the HHS, how has the authority, pace, and direction changed in the past two decades? What key legislation has impacted federal agency activity? What are the key implications for population health?

2. Federal-level policymaking can drive and incentivize new population health efforts. What are the key considerations in the policymaking process? Who are some of the key governmental players?

3. "Advocacy" can take on many forms, involve a variety of stakeholders, and depend on a number of factors. Describe how to appropriately lobby, including what factors may lead to success, and how lobbying can be used to advance population health priorities.

References

1. Jaffe S. Health policy brief: key issues in health reform. *Health Aff.* August 20, 2009. http://www.healthaffairs.org/healthpolicybriefs/brief.php?brief_id=10. Accessed March 11, 2019.

2. W&M Committee Jurisdiction and Rules. https://waysandmeans.house.gov/about/jurisdiction-and-rules

3. E&C Committee Jurisdiction. https://energycommerce.house.gov/about-ec/jurisdiction

4. Committee on Education and Labor Jurisdiction. https://edlabor.house.gov/about/jurisdiction

5. Finance Committee Jurisdiction. https://www.finance.senate.gov/about/jurisdiction

6. HELP Committee Issues. https://www.help.senate.gov/about/issues/

7. Aging Committee: History. https://www.aging.senate.gov/about/history

8. U.S. Senate Glossary of Terms: Caucus. https://www.senate.gov/reference/glossary_term/caucus.htm

9. About MedPAC. http://www.medpac.gov/-about-medpac-

10. MedPAC Report to the Congress. *Medicare and the Health Care Delivery System.* June 2014. http://www.medpac.gov/docs/default-source/reports/jun14_entirereport.pdf

11. MedPAC Report to the Congress. Chapter 8, Next Steps in Measuring Quality of Care in Medicare. June 2015. http://www.medpac.gov/docs/default-source/reports/chapter-8-next-steps-in-measuring-quality-of-care-in-medicare-june-2015-report-.pdf?sfvrsn=0

12. About MACPAC. https://www.macpac.gov/about-macpac/

13. MACPAC Report to the Congress. *Medicaid and Population Health.* June 2014. https://www.macpac.gov/wp-content/uploads/2015/01/Medicaid_and_Population_Health.pdf

14. About CBO. https://www.cbo.gov/about/overview. An Introduction to the Congressional Budget Office. Accessed at: https://www.cbo.gov/sites/default/files/cbofiles/attachments/2016-IntroToCBO.pdf

15. CBO, *Offsetting Effects of Prescription Drug Use on Medicare's Spending for Medical Services.* November 2012. http://www.cbo.gov/sites/default/files/cbofiles/attachments/43741-MedicalOffsets-11-29-12.pdf

16. H.R. 2953/S. 2164, *A bill to amend the Congressional Budget Act of 1974 respecting the scoring of preventive health savings,* 115th Congress. Available at: https://www.congress.gov/bill/115th-congress/senate-bill/2164/all-info. Accessed August 28, 2019.

17. CMS Fast Facts, Calendar Year 2017 Enrollment Statistics. https://www.cms.gov/Research-Statistics-Data-and-Systems/Statistics-Trends-and-Reports/CMS-Fast-Facts/index.html (accessed February 25, 2019).

18. About ONC. https://www.healthit.gov/topic/about-onc

19. ONC Report to Congress, Report on Health Information Blocking. April 2015. https://www.healthit.gov/sitesdefault/files/reports/info_blocking_040915.pdf

20. About CMMI. https://innovation.cms.gov/About/

21. Congressional Budget Office. Estimating the Budgetary Effects of Legislation Involving the Center for Medicare & Medicaid Innovation. July 30, 2018. https://www.cbo.gov/publication/50692

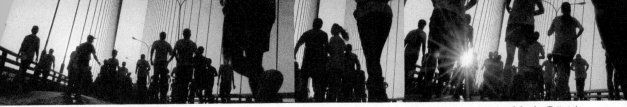

CHAPTER 14

Building Cultures of Health and Wellness Within Organizations

Raymond J. Fabius
Janice L. Clarke

EXECUTIVE SUMMARY

Creating a culture of wellness can sustain population health initiatives within organizations.

Organizations and companies have demonstrated the ability to build a sustainable culture of health and wellness that produces improvements in health status and lowers healthcare costs for a target population (also known as bending the healthcare cost curve). This chapter presents a clear picture of what it takes to create an organizational culture that supports population health.

LEARNING OBJECTIVES

By the end of this chapter, the reader will be able to:

1. Define a culture of health and wellness.
2. Identify benchmark performance measures of a culture of health and wellness.
3. Explain the elements of a road map for creating a culture of health and wellness.
4. Analyze how a culture of health and wellness can contribute to solving the healthcare crisis in America.
5. Explain the connection between a corporate culture of health and their healthcare coverage costs for their workforce and family members.
6. Discuss the connection between health and wealth.

▶ Introduction

The population health movement has been gaining momentum over the past decade, supported by the passage of the Patient Protection and Affordable Care Act (ACA) in 2010 and the subsequent implementation of programs aimed at improving the health of the population. In terms of national statistics, population health remains a daunting challenge; however, some practical applications of its tenets by companies and organizations across the country show great promise. By enveloping population health in an environment that supports its delivery and sustainability, benchmark cultures of health and wellness are appearing throughout the country in large and small companies, in manufacturing and service-oriented organizations, in for-profit and not-for-profit entities, and even in governmental agencies. The population health mandate is now extending its focus on building cultures of health and wellness.

▶ What Is a Culture of Health and Wellness?

A **culture of health and wellness** is defined by its outcomes. Participants in a culture of health and wellness pursue and achieve higher levels of health and wellness than the general population does. The expected outcomes are comparatively better quality of life and reduced incidence of morbidity. Characteristics of cultures of health and wellness include an environment, policies, and cues that lead regularly to healthy choices on both a conscious and unconscious basis.[1] To appreciate the all-encompassing nature of a culture of health and wellness, consider the following attributes:

A culture of health and wellness makes it easier and more rewarding to select lifestyles that foster health. Studies show that eating right, not smoking, exercising regularly, managing stress, and moderate consumption of alcohol can markedly reduce chronic illness over time. In fact, the World Health Organization estimates that 80% of cardiovascular disease and type 2 diabetes, and 40% of cancer could be eliminated by engaging in these activities.[2]

A culture of health and wellness cultivates the appropriate use of healthcare services. Studies by Barbara Starfield et al.[3] at Johns Hopkins University have demonstrated the importance of having a relationship with a trusted primary care provider within a medical home. Despite this, it is estimated that as many as half of all Americans have no satisfactory connection to primary care. In retrospect, the decades- old Healthcare Maintenance Organization (HMO) model that required members to declare an affiliation with a primary care provider was a good policy. An organizational culture focused on health and wellness provides information and education to help its participants become better health consumers.

A culture of health and wellness leverages all population health strategies. The range of available options includes:

- Opportunities for physical activity (e.g., walking trails, intermural competitions, onsite fitness centers, yoga, meditation, sponsored events)
- Policies forbidding the use of tobacco products on the company campus
- Promoting and perhaps subsidizing healthy choices in cafeterias, restaurants, and vending machines
- Enforcing organizational catering policies that ensures healthy foods are served at company events and create safeguards that prevent excessive alcohol consumption

Communication

High-end marketing tactics—including a branded, coordinated campaign—must be deployed to effectively promote healthy choices. For example, General Electric developed the "Health by Numbers 0-5-10-25" program in 2004 as part of its Healthy Worksite initiative. Offered across the globe in eight core languages, this program taught that one should always use 0 tobacco products, eat 5 fruits and vegetables daily, take 10 thousand steps a day (measured by pedometers), and maintain a body mass index (BMI) of 25. All efforts to promote the program were branded with a Health by Numbers logo.[4]

Encouragement and Engagement

A culture of health and wellness provides and tracks the progress of **risk reduction** programs. All participants must know their health risks and develop action plans to mitigate them with the help of health coaches and trusted clinicians. Risks such as high cholesterol or high blood pressure are easily controlled by adherence to a regimen that includes a healthy diet, exercise, and medications. Obesity is a greater challenge, but participants are more likely to tackle it with social encouragement (e.g., Weight Watchers program), and they are more likely to maintain a lower weight in an environment that promotes healthy eating and exercise.

Access

A culture of health and wellness assures that its participants have easy access to healthcare services. Prompt medical treatment for acute illnesses and screening programs to identify chronic and potentially fatal conditions is essential to a culture of health and wellness program (e.g., breast and colon cancer deaths would be much rarer if mammograms and colonoscopies were conducted when recommended in all cases).

Vaccines are arguably our greatest achievement in terms of prevention of disease. Within a culture of health and wellness, all participants receive age- and gender-appropriate immunizations. The availability of influenza and other vaccines at local pharmacies is a great step forward for population health and for promoting health and wellness.

Evidence-Based Practice

A culture of health and wellness fosters the use of evidence-based clinical guidelines. Despite the availability of national guidelines for the treatment of many common chronic illnesses (e.g., heart disease, diabetes, asthma, chronic obstructive pulmonary disease, depression), only half of Americans with these conditions receive recommended care. A culture of health and wellness implements policies and programs that significantly improve the level of individual compliance.

Supportive Environment

A culture of health and wellness promotes health throughout the workplace environment. Social and environmental pressures influence behavior (e.g., a person placed in an environment where the majority of individuals are obese is more likely to become obese). In addition to leveraging **wellness champions** and leaders to promote healthy options, a culture of health and wellness has rituals and places symbols of health promotion throughout the environment (e.g., water bottles, T-shirts, wallet cards, pedometers, tracking bracelets, poster boards). The Internet and social media are utilized as well with messaging on dedicated websites, mobile device applications, video screens, and telemedicine.

Evaluation and Improvement

A culture of health and wellness assesses and improves its programs regularly. Things that are measured can be improved. Today, integrated warehouses of data track medical claims, laboratory values, pharmaceuticals, disability events, workers' compensation cases, durable medical equipment use, and even absence from work or work performance. Regular review and analysis of these data streams can identify healthcare trends and determine whether its population is experiencing better health, less illness, and improved performance.

▶ What Is a Benchmark Organization?

Many corporations, universities, and healthcare systems have been recognized as benchmark examples of cultures of health and wellness, and much can be learned from studying them. One review of benchmark programs identified seven common elements:

1. Employ health and wellness program features and incentives that are consistent with the organization's core mission, goals, operations, and administrative structures
2. Operate at multiple levels, simultaneously addressing individual, environmental, policy, and cultural factors in the organization

3. Target the most important healthcare issues among the employee population
4. Tailor diverse components to the unique needs and concerns of individuals
5. Achieve high rates of engagement and participation, both in the short and long term
6. Achieve successful health outcomes, cost savings, and additional organizational objectives
7. Are evaluated based on clear definitions of success, as reflected in scorecards and metrics agreed upon by all relevant constituencies[5]

Research suggests that benchmark employers have deployed over 200 elements that are available to organizations seeking to build a culture of health and wellness and that a critical mass of these elements (approximately two-thirds) is required for success. It is now possible to measure any organization's pursuit of a culture of health and wellness against these elements and also to generate a score that can be tracked over time. Moreover, this score can correlate to a company's health care cost trend. As the organizational culture of health and wellness improves, the company's medical cost trend moderates and flattens.[6]

Experts suggest that both of the foregoing approaches to measuring a culture of health and wellness are helpful; the former quantifies a reduction of illness over time while the latter provides guidance on narrowing the gaps when compared with benchmark organizations.[7]

The professional literature is a good source of information on benchmark organizations (e.g., peer-reviewed articles, a book by Pitney Bowes about its journey).[8,9] There are industry conferences throughout the year highlighting best practices (e.g., the National Business Group on Health, the National Alliance of Healthcare Purchasing Coalitions, the Institute of Health and Productivity Management, the Population Health Alliance, and the Population Health Colloquium). Among the many award programs recognizing best efforts are the Wellness Council of America, the Health Education Resource Organization, the American College of Occupational and Environmental Medicine, and the National Business Group on Health.[10-14]

Because benchmark cultures of health and wellness demonstrate significant reductions in healthcare expenditures and trends, many employers are pursuing benchmark performance to address their escalating healthcare costs. A benchmark culture of health and wellness documents high screening rates, high compliance with nationally recommended guidelines for care, and low levels of unhealthy lifestyles. For example, after targeting smoking cessation over many years, Johnson & Johnson has decreased the number of smokers in its workforce to 7%,[15] which is less than half the national incidence of over 15%—a remarkable achievement. An IBM initiative encouraging the use of primary care and medical homes has markedly reduced the number of employees who are **medically homeless**.[16]

Research shows that benchmark organizations start with a strong commitment from leadership. The state of Delaware's DelaWELL program has been supported by the governor's declaration.[17] The Dow Chemical Company's benchmark efforts have been led by its CEO.[18] All benchmark organizations have data warehouses, and many have developed scorecards, dashboards, and cockpits to drive improvement at the department, business, national, and organizational levels. Most have physician executives whose jobs are dedicated to promoting health and wellness within the workforce population. Trained in medicine and population health management, these professionals are given adequate resources to identify and address opportunities for improvement on an organizational basis. They monitor and integrate all of the health-related programs from a clinical perspective (e.g., health risk assessments, biometric screenings, disease management services, disability management, and worker's compensation).

As previously mentioned, many benchmark programs have sophisticated branding, marketing, and communication strategies. Most leverage the workplace to create an environment conducive to health and wellness. Some have built comprehensive primary care centers and pharmacies on their campuses.[19] All of these organizations provide health benefits, at least for their workforce and dependents. They have leveraged the science of evidence-based benefit design[20] to foster the appropriate use of health services and healthy lifestyles. A few benchmark employers enable workers to earn higher levels of coverage by taking better care of themselves and family members. Increasingly, they are utilizing **behavioral economics**[21] and, in some cases, reducing their contribution to healthcare coverage when recommendations are not met. All are involved in multiyear strategies and following detailed **road maps** to achieving or maintaining **benchmark performance**.

▶ How Does an Organization Get Started?

There are a number of resources from credible sources that can help to create an organizational road map (e.g., the Change Agent Workgroup,[22] the American Hospital Association,[23] the Centers for Disease Control and Prevention,[24] and the American College of Occupational and Environmental Medicine).[25] The Change Agent Workgroup (a diverse group of experts in this space) published the following seven-step process to achieve a culture of health and wellness:

1. Establish a vision for health
2. Engage senior leadership and align management
3. Develop supporting **workplace environment** changes and implement workplace policies
4. Construct a comprehensive **integrated data warehouse** to analyze what ails the employee population and their families
5. Determine the measurements and goals for success
6. Utilize **value-based benefit design** and behavioral economics
7. Implement broad population health activities[22]

Establish a Vision for Health

Nearly every organization of significant size has developed vision and mission statements, along with related values and objectives. Benchmark organizations embrace a mission and vision that incorporate the value of a healthy workforce. Because these organizations strongly believe that a healthy workforce is a competitive advantage in the marketplace, they require employees to be responsible for maintaining their health as part of the job function. Employees may even be encouraged to assist coworkers in their quests for health and wellness. At the outset of the journey to building a culture of health and wellness, a company's vision, mission, and values statements may need to be amended to clearly state the individual and collective responsibility of all people in the organization to maintain their health and foster well-being among all members of the company.

Engage Senior Leadership and Align Management

Once the vision for health has been established, it must be promoted by the leadership and the management of the organization. Under the best of circumstances, the CEO provides periodic messages to the workforce to reinforce the importance of maintaining health and well-being. One way to communicate this is by videotaping a senior leader "walking the talk" (e.g., exercising) with a tag line such as, "If I can find time to do it, so should you." Many organizations do not actively support taking the time necessary to exercise; stating this as part of every job description goes a long way to building a culture of health and wellness.

A consequence of health benefits being paid through a corporate function is that management is removed from any oversight, understanding, or need to monitor the health of the workforce. Benchmark companies are changing this (e.g., some management compensation and bonuses are being calculated in part by the trend in medical costs and the **health status** of their employee bases).

Develop Supporting Workplace Environmental Changes and Implement Workplace Policies

To establish a foundation for a culture of health and wellness, an organization must provide environmental cues. For instance, most companies have addressed smoking cessation through a series of incremental steps, from designated smoking areas, to policies that do not allow smoking in facilities, to a complete smoking ban on campus. This initiative is often accompanied by expanded health benefits to cover all treatments and services, an unlimited number of times, to support smoking cessation. Some cutting-edge organizations have gone further (i.e., testing new applicants for nicotine in their urine and not hiring smokers).

To promote exercise in the workplace, benchmark organizations ensure that the stairwells are safe and inviting (i.e., clean, carpeted, heated, and air-conditioned, with paintings on the walls and music piped in) to increase their use. Signage at elevators promotes stairwell use as well.

Cafeterias and vending machines in benchmark organizations offer healthy options that are marketed by means of prominent placement and labeling—unhealthy options are discouraged by making them more difficult to find or reach. Entrée choices are identified as being healthy or not. **Best practice** includes subsidizing the healthy choices and taxing the unhealthy ones. Progressive organizations work with nutritionists to eliminate unhealthy options from cafeterias, vending machines, and catering policies.

Construct a Comprehensive Integrated Data Warehouse

Managing the health of a population requires understanding the key health risks, conditions, and diseases. Benchmark organizations integrate medical, pharmacy, disability, and workers' compensation claims along with laboratory values, biometrics, health risk appraisal survey results, and absence data. Highly enlightened companies include presenteeism data in their analyses and use validated tools such as the Work Limitations Questionnaire[26] or the Health and Work Performance Questionnaire.[27] With these integrated inputs, world-class culture of health and wellness organizations can determine the financial effect of specific health risks, conditions, and diseases and prioritize programs and approaches in the best interest of the organization and the employees.[28]

Utilize Value-Based Benefit Design and Behavioral Economics

Companies and organizations whose employees receive compensation and benefits may take advantage of additional methods to promote a healthy culture (i.e., they can manipulate compensation and benefits to reward healthy choices and behaviors). State-of-the-art cultures of health and wellness organizations offer different benefit packages that employees and dependents earn by taking better care of themselves and making healthy choices.

Those that meet a full panel of required healthy activities can earn the highest level of coverage. These companies work closely with consultants and third-party administrators to deliver a health benefit package that is evidence based (i.e., covers proven treatments at a high level and either provides no coverage or charges a steep copayment for unproven or low-value therapies). Benchmark companies understand the nuances of behavioral economics (recognizing that loss avoidance has a three times greater influence on behavior than do rewards; the default choice is most often chosen), and they utilize health savings and health spending accounts to adjust coverage and apply the most influential approaches to rewards and penalties.[29]

Implement Broad Population Health Activities

Whether it be a single company or a national initiative, a benchmark culture of health and wellness must incorporate a comprehensive approach that addresses five key population cohorts across the continuum:

1. Those who are well
2. Those who are at risk
3. The acutely ill
4. The chronically ill
5. Those with catastrophic conditions

Programs must be established to keep well people well using a holistic approach that includes support for social, physical, emotional, career, intellectual, environmental, and spiritual wellness, or SPECIES.[30] People who are "maximally" well have social connections; are physically fit and emotionally stable; have a purposeful, stimulating occupation with potential for advancement; and live in a safe setting that supports physical activity and healthy eating. To keep its population well, a benchmark culture must employ a broad-based, systematic effort to help reduce risks for chronic illness (e.g., attacking obesity, smoking, drug and alcohol abuse, and sedentary lifestyles).[31]

Access to health services must be ensured so that acute illnesses are treated promptly and potentially serious medical issues are addressed early. People with chronic illnesses must be provided condition management support to mitigate potential complications (e.g., people with diabetes must receive an annual eye exam).[32]

Last, a comprehensive population management platform must provide **centers of excellence**[33] and compassionate care for those with catastrophic illness.[34] This most seriously ill population segment benefits greatly from intensive and expensive medical management and coordinated social services. When properly managed, there is a significant return on the dollars spent and great value delivered to the patient and his or her loved ones. With advance directives in place, efforts to eliminate futile care will benefit families and society alike.

▶ Aligning Key Constituencies

Organizations intent on building a culture of health and wellness should leverage constituency partners, with strong consideration given to collaborating with other like-minded organizations in the community through business coalitions and local chambers of commerce. Increasingly, payer organizations, health plans, insurance companies, and consolidated health delivery systems are positioning themselves to be allies in this pursuit. With better **alignment of constituencies** such as among employers, providers, payers, and the citizens, great progress can be made.[35]

▶ Comparison to Benchmarks

Today, there are many benchmark efforts worth studying. Johnson & Johnson and Dow Chemical have published their respective outcomes and presented their successful programs in many forums. The previous leadership at Pitney Bowes published a book on their approach. The state of Delaware's DelaWELL program[36] is an example of an excellent governmental effort directed at state employees. The University of Michigan[37] publishes an annual report on its program. As mentioned earlier, several institutions confer awards on organizations that have built a culture of health and wellness (e.g., the National Business Group on Health, the Health Education Resource Organization, and the American College of Occupational and Environmental Medicine). By studying the scoring systems deployed by these organizations, any organization can determine where it stands in relation to a benchmark performance. To use benchmark program information effectively, an organization should first identify gaps between its efforts and the best culture of health programs. Once identified, the gaps can be prioritized, and the organization can build a multiyear strategic plan to achieve benchmark organization outcomes (i.e., lower healthcare costs and engender greater employee engagement and higher performance).

▶ A Market-Based Solution to the Healthcare Crisis

When a critical mass of organizations in a community or region achieves a culture of health and wellness, the problems of rising healthcare costs and the increasing prevalence of chronic illness are likely to be slowed. Social pressures are likely to shift from consumption of medical resources to promoting wellness. The healthcare industry, especially providers and payers, will begin to direct their attention to economic models that support the elevation of health status rather than primarily delivering more health services to those with illness. Employers will recognize that focusing on the well-being of their workforces is more than a nice thing to do—it is good business.

▶ Justification and Business Case: The Connection Between Health and Wealth

For many years, the prevailing belief was that nations had to attain wealth before they could become healthy. Recent experience in Africa, where the AIDS epidemic has markedly affected the potential workforce, has reshaped our collective thinking on this. Without a healthy working-age population, a country faces insurmountable challenges with respect to productivity and growth in its gross national product. This situation will begin to burden the United States as baby boomers retire and are not replaced by a comparable number of healthy young workers to maintain and advance productivity. When life expectancy is used as a proxy for health, there is a correlation between it and income at the state and national levels. Hans Rosling demonstrated this phenomenon in a powerful short film that looks at 200 countries over a span of 200 years.[38]

The relationship between health and wealth plays out at an individual level. According to a recent estimate from Fidelity Investments, a couple that retired at 65 in 2018 and in average health will need to have saved over $280,000 to pay for their out-of-pocket medical costs. If the couple reaches retirement in poor health, the figure could easily double or triple.[39] Correlating income to health status, health informatics specialists Wendy Lynch and Hank Gardner[40] suggest that higher income earners are more engaged in health and wellness activities. Healthy individuals also are more likely to be higher performers, as demonstrated by the Lamplighter Program at Unilever.[41] Moreover, medical costs are the number one reason for individual bankruptcy. Every discussion of one's savings with a financial advisor should begin with how to maintain maximal health and wellness to preserve your "nest egg."[42]

Published articles also support the notion that companies emphasizing the pursuit of a culture of health and wellness experience less escalation in healthcare costs[43] and outperform in the marketplace.[44-47] Whether one examines the issue from an individual, company, state, national, or global basis, there is compelling evidence confirming the connection between health and wealth.

▶ Conclusion

Studying the achievement of companies and organizations that have successfully built a culture of health and wellness can provide great insights for us as a nation. Replicating these best practices on a broader scale can improve the health status of large populations and enhance the quality of life and performance of individuals at work and at home. Healthier citizens are more productive. The positive outcomes may include more prosperous communities, more involved family members, and more willing civic contributors. As we gradually move toward a national culture of health and wellness, fewer financial resources will be consumed by treating illness, and more can be directed to keeping well people well.

Study and Discussion Questions

1. What is a culture of health and wellness?
2. How can you build a culture of health and wellness?
3. Why does it make sense to pursue a culture of health and wellness?
4. Is there a connection between health and wealth?
5. What does it mean to bend the healthcare cost curve?

Suggested Readings and Websites

Readings

Allen J. *Wellness Leadership: Creating Supportive Environments for Healthier and More Productive Employees.* Burlington, VT: Human Resources Institute; 2011.

Barry R, Murcko AC, Brubaker C. *The Six Sigma Book for Healthcare: Improving Outcomes by Reducing Errors.* Chicago, IL: Health Administration Press; 2002.

Bray I., ed. *Healthy Employees, Healthy Business: Easy Affordable Ways to Promote Workplace Wellness.* Berkeley, CA: Nolo; 2009.

Cascio W, Boudreau J. *Investing in People: Financial Impact of Human Resource Initiatives.* Mahwah, NJ: Pearson Education, Inc.; 2008.

Edington DW. *Zero Trends.* Ann Arbor: University of Michigan Health Management Research Center; 2009.

Edington DW, Pitts, JS. *Shared Values – Shared Results: Positive Organizational Health as a Win-Win Philosophy.* Ann Arbor, MI: Edington Associates; 2016.

Frampton S, Gilpin L, Charmel P. *Putting Patients First: Designing and Practicing Patient-Centered Care.* San Francisco: Jossey-Bass; 2003.

Kaplan RS, Norton DP. *The Balanced Scorecard: Translating Strategy into Action.* Boston: Harvard Business School Press; 1996.

LaPenna M. *Workplace Clinics and Employer Managed Healthcare: A Catalyst for Cost Savings and Improved Productivity.* New York: Productivity Press; 2010.

Lynch W, Gardner H. *Who Survives? How Benefit Costs Are Killing Your Company.* Cheyenne, WY: Health as Human Capital Foundation; 2011.

Pronk NP, ed. *ACSM's Worksite Health Handbook: A Guide to Building Healthy and Productive Companies.* 2nd ed. Indianapolis, IN: American College of Sports Medicine; 2009.

Rath T, Harter J. *Well Being: The Five Essential Elements.* New York: Gallup Press; 2010.

Stephano RM, Edelheit J. *Engaging Wellness: Corporate Wellness Programs That Work.* Palm Beach Gardens, FL: Corporate Health and Wellness Association; 2012.

Websites

National Business Group on Health: https://www
.businessgrouphealth.org/

National Alliance of Healthcare Purchasing Coalitions:
https://www.nationalalliancehealth.org/home

Health Enhancement Research Organization:
https://hero-health.org/

Institute for Health and Productivity Management:
http://www.ihpm.org/

Centers for Disease Control and Prevention: http://
www.cdc.gov/

Integrated Benefits Institute: http://www.ibiweb
.org/

References

1. Fabius R, Frazee S. The culture of health. *Health Productivity Manag.* 2009;7(2):13–15.

2. World Health Organization. Preventing chronic diseases: a vital investment. WHO Global Report; 2005:18. Available at https://www.who.int/chp/chronic_disease_report/en/ (accessed June 6, 2019).

3. Starfield B, Shi L, Macinko J. Contribution of primary care to health systems and health. *Milbank Q.* 2005;83(3):457–502.

4. National Business Group on Health. *An Employer Case Study of General Electric Company: Improving Employee Health Through Prevention.* Washington, DC: National Business Group on Health; April 2009. Available at https://www.businessgrouphealth.org/

5. Goetzel RZ, Shechter D, Ozminkowski RJ, Marmet PF, Tabrizi MJ, Roemer EC. Promising practices in employer health and productivity management efforts: findings from a benchmarking study. *J Occup Environ Med.* 2007;49(20:)111–130.

6. Fabius RJ, Frazee SG, Thayer D, Kirshenbaum D, Reynolds J. The correlation of a corporate culture of health assessment and health care cost trend. *J Occup Environ Med.* 2018;60(6):507–514.

7. National Business Group on Health. C-Suite Reporting Tools and Strategies. WebEx Board Meeting of the Institute on Health, Productivity and Human Capital. Washington, DC: National Business Group on Health; April 24, 2012.

8. Mahoney J, Hom D. *Total Value, Total Return.* Philadelphia, PA: The GlaxoSmithKline Group of Companies; 2006.

9. Flynn JP, Gascon G, Doyle S, Matson Koffman DM, Saringer C, Grossmeier J, et al. Supporting a culture of health in the workplace: a review of evidence-based elements. *Am J Health Promot.* 2018 Nov;32(8):1755–1788.

10. American College of Occupational and Environmental Medicine. Corporate Health Achievement Awards. Available at http://www.chaa.org/ (accessed April 14, 2019).

11. Health Enhancement Resource Organization. C. Everett Koop National Health Awards. Available at http://www.thehealthproject.com/winning-programs/ (accessed April 14, 2019).

12. National Business Group on Health. About *Best Employers: Excellence in Health and Well-Being.* Available at https://www.businessgrouphealth.org/best-employers/about-best-employers/about-best-employers/ (accessed June 6, 2019).

13. American Specialty Health. Healthyroads [website inaugurated 2018]. Available at https://www.healthyroads.com (accessed June 6, 2019).

14. WELCOA. Well Workplace Awards Initiative. http://www.wellworkplaceawards.org/ (accessed April 14, 2019).

15. Henke RM, Goetzel RZ, McHugh J, Isaac F. Recent experience in health promotion at Johnson & Johnson: lower health spending, strong return on investment. *Health Affs.* 2011;30(3):490–499.

16. IBM Institute for Business Value. *Patient-Centered Medical Home: What, Why, and How?* Available at https://www.ebri.org/docs/default-source/policy-forum-documents/67_5grundy-pcmh1210.pdf?sfvrsn=3ba6302f_2 (accessed June 6, 2019).

17. State of Delaware. Governor's "Healthy State Workplace" Page. Available at https://dhr.delaware.gov/benefits/

18. Lindsay GM, for Partnership for Prevention. Leading by Example: Commitment Starts at the Top! International Association for Worksite Health Promotion 2010

Executive Summit [Powerpoint presentation slidedeck]. Available at https://www.acsm-iawhp.org/files/DOCUMENTLIBRARY/Lindsay_executive_Summit.ppt

19. Frost J. Walt Disney World opens on-site health and wellness center for cast members and families. The Disney Blog; October 15, 2008. Available at http://thedisneyblog.com/2008/10/15/walt-disney-world-opens-on-site-health-and-wellness-center-for-cast-members-and-families/ (accessed April 14, 2019).

20. Darling, H. Evidence-Based Benefit Design. Conversations on the Changing Face of Managed Care: Insights from the 2006–2007 Podcast Series. Available at http://citeseerx.ist.psu.edu/viewdoc/download?doi=10.1.1.131.8838&rep=rep1&type=pdf#page=23 (accessed April 14, 2019).

21. Volpp K, Asch D, Galvin R, et al. Redesigning employee health incentives: lessons from behavioral economics. *N Engl J Med.* 2011;365:388–390.

22. Change Agent Work Group. Employer Health Asset Management: A Roadmap for Improving the Health of Your Employees and Your Organization; 2009. Available at http://www.aon.com/attachments/improving_health.pdf (accessed April 14, 2019).

23. American Hospital Association. 2010 Long-Range Policy Committee, John W. Bluford III, chair. A Call to Action: Creating a Culture of Health. Chicago: American Hospital Association, January 2011. Available at https://www.aha.org/system/files/2018-02/call-to-action-creating-a-culture-of-health-2011.pdf (accessed June 6, 2019).

24. Centers for Disease Control and Prevention. Workplace Health Model. Available at http://www.cdc.gov/workplacehealthpromotion/model/index.html (accessed April 14, 2019).

25. Hymel PA, Loeppke RR, Baase CM, Burton WN, Hartenbaum NP, Hudson TW, et al. Workplace health protection and promotion: a new pathway for a healthier—and safer—workforce. *J Occup Environ Med.* 2011;53(6):695–702.

26. Burton WN, Pransky G, Conti DJ, Chen CY, Edington DW. The association of medical conditions and presenteeism. *J Occup Environ Med.* 2004;46:538–545.

27. Kessler RC, Stang PE. *Health and Work Productivity: Making the Business Case for Quality Health Care.* Chicago: University of Chicago Press; 2006.

28. Goetzel RZ, Long SR, Ozminkowski RJ, Hawkins K, Wang S, Lynch W. Health, absence, disability, and presenteeism: cost estimates of certain physical and mental health conditions affecting U.S. employers. *J Occup Environ Med.* 2004;46(4):399–412.

29. Houy M. *Value-Based Benefit Design: A Purchaser's Guide.* National Business Coalition on Health; January 2009. Available at http://www.bailit-health.com/articles/valuebased_apg_bhp.pdf (accessed June 6, 2019).

30. Abbott Solutions Inc. SPECIES—7 Dimensions of Wellness: Survival of the Species. Available at https://abbottsolutionsinc.com/7dimensionsofwellness/ (accessed April 14, 2019).

31. Pronk N, Lowry M, Kottke T, Austin E, Gallagher J, Katz A. Association between optimal lifestyle adherence and short-term incidence of chronic conditions among employees. *Popul Health Manag.* 2010;13(6):289–295.

32. Schoenfeld ER, Greene MJ, Wu SY, Leske MC. Patterns of adherence to diabetes vision care guidelines: baseline findings from the Diabetic Retinopathy Awareness Program. *Ophthalmology.* 2001;108(3):563–571.

33. Coulter CH, Fabius R, Hecksher V, Darling H. Assessing HMO centers of excellence programs: one employer's experience. *Manag Care Q.* 1998;6(1):8–15.

34. Pawlecki JB. End of life: a workplace issue. *Health Aff.* 2010;29(1):141–146.

35. Environmental Scan: Role of Corporate America in Community Health and Wellness. Health Enhancement Resource Organization Research Project Submitted to the Institute of Medicine Roundtable on Population Health Improvement; January 2014. Available at http://nationalacademies.org/hmd/~/media/Files/Activity%20Files/PublicHealth/PopulationHealthImprovementRT/Commissioned%20Papers/PopHealthEnvScan.pdf (accessed June 6, 2019).

36. Louis CJ, Jones, DK. State population health strategies that make a difference: reducing the burden of chronic diseases in Delaware and Iowa. New York: Milbank Memorial Fund;

2017. Available at https://www.milbank.org/wp-content/uploads/2017/10/Reducing-the-Burden-of-Chronic-Diseases-in-Delaware-and-Iowa.pdf (accessed June 6, 2019).

37. University of Michigan Human Resources. MHealthy Annual Report CY2018. Available at https://hr.umich.edu/benefits-wellness/health-well-being/mhealthy/more-mhealthy/about-mhealthy/mhealthys-overview-mission/mhealthy-annual-report.

38. BBC Four. Hans Rosling's 200 Countries, 200 Years, 4 Minutes — The Joy of Stats. Available at www.youtube.com/watch?v=jbkSRLYSojo. (accessed April 14, 2019).

39. Fidelity Investments. A Couple Retiring in 2018 Would Need An Estimated $280,000 to Cover Health Care Costs in Retirement, Analysis Shows. Available at https://www.fidelity.com/about-fidelity/employer-services/a-couple-retiring-in-2018-would-need-estimated-280000 (accessed April 9, 2019).

40. Lynch W, Gardner H. *Who Survives? How Benefit Costs Are Killing Your Company.* Cheyenne, WY: Health as Human Capital Foundation; 2011, Chapter 8.

41. Unilever Lamplighter Program. Report for John Cooper and Dean Patterson. Conference Presentations; 2013. Available at http://www.world-heart-federation.org/

42. Himmelstein, D, Thorne D, Warren E, Woolhandler S. Medical bankruptcy in the United States, 2007: results of a national study. *Am J Med.* 2009;122(8):741–746.

43. Goetzel RZ, Henke RM, Benevent R, Tabrizi MJ, Kent KB, Smith KJ, et al. The predictive validity of the HERO scorecard in determining future health care cost and risk trends. *J Occup Environ Med.* 2014;56(2):136–144.

44. Fabius R, Thayer D. The link between workforce health and safety and the health of the bottom line. *J Occup Environ Med.* 2013;55(9):993–1000.

45. Fabius R, Loeppke R, Hohn T, Fabius D, Eisenberg B, Konicki DL, Larson P. Tracking the market performance of companies that integrate a culture of health and safety: an assessment of corporate health achievement award applicants. *J Occup Environ Med.* 2016;58(1):3–8.

46. Goetzel R, Fabius R, Fabius D, Roemer EC, Thornton N, Kelly RK, Pelletier KR. The stock performance of C. Everett Koop Award winners compared with the Standard & Poor's 500 Index. *J Occup Environ Med.* 2016;58(1):9–15.

47. Grossmeier J, Fabius R, Flynn JP, Noeldner SP, Fabius D, Goetzel RZ, Anderson DR. Linking workplace health promotion best practices and organizational financial performance: tracking market performance of companies with highest scores on the HERO Scorecard. *J Occup Environ Med.* 2016;58(1):16–23.

Appendix I

Case Study: Michigan Primary Care Transformation Project (MiPCT) and the Role of Multipayer Primary Care Initiatives in Achieving Population Health

Marianne Udow-Phillips and Diane L. Bechel Marriott

▶ Overview

In June 2010, the U.S. Department of Health and Human Services released a solicitation for the formation of the Multi-Payer Advanced Primary Care Practice Demonstration. The project was designed to bring Medicare into partnership with health plans and other payers who were experimenting with the implementation of patient-centered medical homes (PCMHs). The demonstration was designed to test whether advanced primary care practices can improve quality, safety, efficiency, and effectiveness of care as well as increase patient involvement in decision making and enhance care in underserved areas. The project is overseen by the Centers for Medicare and Medicaid Innovation. Now, several years into the project, several emerging trends are relevant to the goal of improving population health.

Michigan was one of eight states selected in November 2010 to participate in the demonstration. The Michigan initiative, called the Michigan Primary Care Transformation (MiPCT) Project, has at its core a focus on the effective and extensive use of care managers supported by a common clinical model, rapid-cycle performance feedback, and best practices training and sharing. The care managers are affiliated with one of 35 physician organizations (POs), broad groupings of physician practices throughout the state of Michigan.

To be eligible to participate in the MiPCT, practices were required to demonstrate that they had either National Committee for Quality Assurance (NCQA) level 2 or 3 certification or PCMH designation through the Blue Cross and Blue Shield of Michigan Physician Group Incentive Program (PGIP).[1]

The MiPCT aims to improve overall population health, the value of care, and patient experience through reducing risks for healthy individuals, managing disease and symptoms with self-management support for patients with moderate chronic disease, and coordinating care for patients with complex chronic diseases including end-of-life care. The project is expected to be budget neutral (i.e., the amount spent on care for MiPCT patients will be equal to or less than the amount spent for similar patients not in the demonstration).

The state of Michigan partnered with the University of Michigan to coordinate the statewide project. Coordination support includes learning collaboratives, community governance through multistakeholder committees and advisory groups, organizing opportunities for patient representation on project and practice operations, annual in-person summits to share best practices, a project website, regular communication and educational material, and a data collaborative that provides electronic member lists to identify patients eligible for care management services. The data collaborative also produces PO and practice dashboards that identify performance on key metrics such as:

- Percentage of high-, medium-, and low-risk patients in each practice
- Overall and avoidable (ambulatory or primary care sensitive) emergency room and inpatient visits
- Performance on quality measures for diabetes, well-child, asthma, and other metrics
- Standardized costs

Participating practices are required to have at least one care manager per 2,500 eligible MiPCT patients. Participating payers fund three payment components as follows:

- Care management payment: $3.00 per member per month (PMPM) ($4.50 for Medicare)
- Practice transformation payment: $1.50 PMPM ($2.00 for Medicare)
- Performance incentives: $3.00 PMPM

Although some payers reimbursed practices or POs for practice transformation and incentive components prior to 2012, neither Medicare nor Medicaid reimbursed for these components prior to the demonstration. No payers reimbursed POs or practices for care management prior to the MiPCT; thus, all care management funding was new for all POs and practices.

▶ Magnitude

The MiPCT is the largest PCMH demonstration project in the nation, serving more than 1 million patients (one-tenth of the state of Michigan's population). Seventeen hundred primary care providers in 377 practices statewide partner with more than 400 trained care managers to provide team-based advanced primary care, manage population health, and coordinate care.

Perhaps the most important advantage of the program's large scale is the ability to leverage the influence of five large payers in the state who are aligned on a common approach. This multipayer aspect of the project serves to focus the attention of

POs and practices around the central clinical and financial model. The magnitude of the MiPCT also allows for the cost of project infrastructure to be shared among project funders.

▶ Effect of the MiPCT on Population Health

In 2014, the MiPCT demonstration entered its third year, and final program outcomes from national and state evaluations will not be available until 2016. However, preliminary results suggest that the project has produced quarter-to-quarter improvement in Medicare PMPM payment and hospital admissions compared to a control group. Primary care–sensitive emergency department (ED) visits have also been reduced by almost 4% statewide in the program's first year.

Care manager self-reporting indicates improvement on the extent of physician engagement and championship in identifying and servicing patients most likely to benefit from care management and self-management to reduce health risks, prevent disease, and manage symptoms. This is key to building the infrastructure that will allow population health management to be a focus throughout primary care practices in the state.

Additionally, the MiPCT has expanded the linkages among medical neighborhood partners. In 2013, electronic admission, discharge, and transfer notifications were piloted to provide real-time notification of hospital ED visits and discharges to care managers in primary care practice offices. Work is underway on an electronic directory to allow messaging between MiPCT care managers and care managers in health plans, hospitals, extended care facilities, and specialty offices. The project has enabled the Michigan Department of Community Health to supplement information it provides to primary care practitioners with maternal and child health, mental health and substance use programs, and services information across the state.

▶ Critical Success Factors and Building Blocks

The MiPCT's large statewide reach is unique in its scale and breadth. Although the project continues to evolve, the following factors have been critical to the program's ability to contribute to robust population health management in Michigan:

- POs as partners to practices in program contracting, reporting, and program operations
- Standardized care manager training
- Shared community governance with central project support and coordination
- Multipayer support

Each is described in greater detail in TABLE I-1.

▶ Implications for Population Health

The patient is central to the PCMH and population health. A key article defines PCMH as "focused on improving the health

TABLE I-1 MiPCT Critical Success Factors and Building Blocks

Key Success Factor/ Building Block	Rationale/Example
Physician organizations (POs) as partners to practices in program contracting, reporting, and program operations	Annual participation agreements POs responsible for implementing yearly MiPCT participation agreements and communicating with their practices Program reporting POs help practices collect required self-reported metrics on care management activity and practice infrastructure to support team-based care POs had access to practice and PO dashboards for claims, eligibility, and registry-based measures to facilitate results sharing with practices Program operations Some POs serve as the employers of practice-based care managers, and some organize information sharing with practice team members
Standardized care manager training	To ensure a common approach to implementation of the clinical model, training and continuing education of complex care managers was provided centrally by the MiPCT staff. A select set of available self-management and training programs were approved for moderate care management training.
Shared community governance with central project support and coordination	Stakeholders were encouraged to participate in community project governance to foster achievement of project goals over self-interest. A management team coordinated efforts across stakeholders and facilitated communication via a central e-mail server, a website, webinars, and leadership meetings.
Multipayer support	Payer alignment permits the leveraging of a common voice among participating health plans toward the achievement of common project goals. The greater the alignment of payers, the more likely the achievement of project goals.

of whole people, families, communities and populations, and on increasing the value of healthcare."[2] Thus, patient-centered care serves as a necessary component of an integrated population health infrastructure.

To achieve population health goals, the primary care practice continues to serve as a gateway and foundation, facilitating coordination among the medical neighborhood partners. Multipayer, coordinated programs to build practice capability and spread best practices are essential to achieving population health goals. But, like the promise of population health itself, it will take time and sustained effort to develop and embed the processes that are integral to identifying and effectively addressing risks, symptoms, and conditions and improving the health of individuals and populations.

References

1. Share DA, Mason MH. Michigan's Physician Group Incentive Program offers a regional model for incremental "fee for value" payment reform. *Health Aff.* 2012;31(9):1993-2001.

2. Stange KC, Nutting PA, Miller WL, et al. Defining and measuring the Patient-Centered Medical Home. *J Gen Intern Med.* 2010;25(6):601-12.

Appendix II

Case Study: Assessing Organizational Readiness for Population Health

Keith C. Kosel

▶ Overview

Today, there is widespread agreement that the current structure of health care in the United States is outdated, inefficient, and inequitable and does not optimize the patient experience. When these shortcomings are combined with the fact that the current system's heavy reliance on a fee-for-service payment mechanism is rapidly pushing healthcare to the brink of financial insolvency, it becomes clear that a new focus is required. This new focus is population health. Where our current system focuses on care of the individual, population health widens that lens to include care of populations of individuals. Where our current model emphasizes the delivery of acute care services once an illness or condition presents itself, population health takes a more progressive approach by emphasizing health promotion in the form of preventive and wellness services. By its very design, population health brings with it the potential for meaningful cost management and improved patient outcomes.

Passage of the Patient Protection and Affordable Care Act (ACA) opened the door for organizations to move more aggressively into population health by promoting the concept of accountable care under the Medicare Shared Saving Program (MSSP). Central to the MSSP is the notion of keeping the target population healthy and minimizing the use of inpatient care. Accountable care organizations (ACOs) that are able to do this can share in savings with the Centers for Medicare and Medicaid Services (CMS). As more organizations move into accountable care contracts with CMS or commercial payers, the need to proactively address the health needs of their populations will take center stage and drive much of the transformation of today's health care.

▶ The Challenge

Managing the health of a population of individuals, many of whom are healthy or without discernable disease, is a major challenge for even the most sophisticated healthcare provider systems. For providers without experience in population health or adequate resources, the challenge can be overwhelming. Several factors combine to make the transition to population health a daunting prospect.

- First, population health isn't traditionally taught in medical schools or hospital administration programs. This means that many of today's leaders are learning about population health at the same time they are being tasked with leading population health initiatives for their organizations. Although many nursing programs include elements of community health, most don't include the detailed data analytics and financial considerations (e.g., physician alignment) necessary to seamlessly implement a population health delivery model.
- Second, moving to a population health model requires that the health system redesign its care delivery systems and undertake new models of payment, many of which are risk based. Although simple in concept, these changes are very difficult to bring about, particularly in a short period of time. Development of an integrated medical record across all entities in the network, identifying at-risk individuals, and gaining patients' engagement in their self-care all pose substantial barriers to those embarking on a population health journey.
- Finally, building the necessary network to deliver a wide array of services seamlessly across the care

continuum is a major undertaking. In many cases, the realization that acute care hospitals, physician practices, and postacute community-based provider organizations each have different—and in many cases conflicting—needs and incentives comes only after substantial time and resources have been committed.

What all these challenges have in common is the need for leaders to understand an organization's readiness to undertake a population health model well before implementing it.

▶ Rationale for a Readiness Assessment

A good population health readiness assessment helps leaders to do the following: (1) understand how population health differs for their current practice, (2) identify the critical elements that all population health programs have in common, and (3) identify the organization's current level of preparedness across these critical elements. Although many population health readiness assessments are available,[1-4] it is essential that organizations select one that is both comprehensive in scope and designed to elicit meaningful data to inform the discussion and planning.

In 2012, VHA Inc., a national alliance of more than 1,300 hospitals and some 90,000 postacute provider entities, began working with a small number of member hospitals and health systems that were interested in moving into the population health arena. Preliminary conversations revealed that most of these organizations were unsure about what it would take to become proficient in population health and uncertain that they had the necessary resources and infrastructure in place to succeed. Additional questioning revealed that the first step in the population health journey was to do a critical assessment of organizational preparedness. With that objective in mind, VHA developed the Population Health Organizational Assessment (PHOA), a tool that was easy for hospitals to complete yet provided the level of detail necessary for a reasoned decision about whether to pursue a population health strategy. VHA's organizational approach to population health creates an assessment that pinpoints an organization's strengths and opportunities and enables leaders to gain valuable insights around infrastructure, partnerships, and community collaboration.

In building the PHOA, VHA made use of the lessons learned by developing the Patient Safety Organizational Assessment (PSOA), a tool that proved popular with VHA member institutions and gained the endorsement of the American Hospital Association.

▶ The Nuts and Bolts of Population Health

The PHOA is an easy-to-use tool that assesses six domains that are the recognized building blocks or success factors for population health. These domains include: (1) organization and leadership, (2) care delivery and management, (3) physician integration and alignment, (4) community health promotion,

(5) information technology and informatics, and (6) patient and family involvement. Each of the six domains contains two to four key aspects of population health, which highlight critical strategies required in population health (TABLE II-1).

Within each key aspect are four to seven activities that support the strategic aspects and provide detailed operational requirements. In effect, the PHOA provides a comprehensive look at what is required to be a competitive player in the population health arena.

▶ Talking Together

Although the nature and scope of the information used to fashion the domains, key aspects, and activities are critical to the comprehensiveness of the assessment, how the assessment is administered and how the results are interpreted are of equal importance. Drawing on its past experience in developing organizational assessments, VHA recommended that each organization completing the PHOA create a team of six or seven individuals (including hospital and physician leaders, ambulatory care and postacute services administrators, and internal staff with expertise in risk contracting, epidemiology, and patient experience). It was specified that team members have experience and awareness of the organization's strategic plan and its resources and capabilities as well as market dynamics, competition, and physician relations. Knowledge of population health, while beneficial, was not a prerequisite for participation.

After each member of the team had reviewed and completed the assessment

TABLE II-1 PHOA Domains and Key Aspects of Population Health

Domain	Key Aspect of Population Health
Organization and leadership	Strategic plan Leadership and governance Workforce Financial position and scale
Care delivery and management	Continuum of care Chronic care and disease management programs
Physician integration and alignment	Physician leadership Physician availability and coordination Risk and financial arrangements Physician collaboration
Community health promotion	Coordination with nonclinical community Entities Prevention and screening Educational programs
Information technology and informatics	Electronic health record Data warehouses and clinical registries Analytics and decision support Patient-centric technology
Patient and family involvement	Patient activation and engagement Patient-centric care Self-care/self-management

independently, the team assembled as a group. Each activity was reviewed and scored based on team consensus. Responses were categorized in a hierarchy based on the levels of activity, rated from 1 (low/no readiness) to 5 (fully prepared):

1. There has been no discussion around this activity.
2. This activity is under discussion, but there is no implementation.
3. This activity is under development, but there is no implementation.
4. This activity is partially implemented.
5. This activity is fully implemented.

Final scores, along with demographic information about the organization, were entered into the electronic tool and sent to VHA for processing.

▶ Deployment

Because this was the first time the PHOA would be used in a widespread assessment campaign, a decision was made to deploy the PHOA first to VHA partner and shareholder institutions (i.e., 400 large organizations that form the core controlling membership of VHA). A subset of these partner and shareholder organizations comprises the board that governs VHA's 12 regions. It was decided that the regional board meetings, held quarterly, would provide appropriate opportunities to deploy the PHOA.

The entire assessment process was structured around two board meetings held approximately 12 weeks apart. At the first board meeting, the PHOA was introduced and its intended purpose was discussed. Emphasis was placed on the strategic importance of assessing organizational readiness for population health. After the board meeting, the PHOA was distributed to the chief executive officers with instructions to assemble a team, complete the assessment, and return it to VHA within 4 weeks; most CEOs took between 3 and 7 weeks to complete the instructions. The initial deployment of the PHOA was in five of the 12 regions. Response rates across the five regions varied from a high of nearly 90% to a low of 40%. Once the surveys were returned, VHA analyzed the data using both quantitative and qualitative methods and produced hospital-specific reports for the respondents. At the next board meeting, VHA subject matter experts reviewed the collective responses with the entire board and discussed the implications of findings for individual organizations and the industry.

▶ Findings

Quantitative Findings: Demographics

Analysis of the data provided insights into how well prepared hospitals and health systems were for undertaking population health. As part of the demographic section, respondents were asked two fundamental questions: "How would you rate your organization's commitment to population health?" (Q1) and "How would you rate your organization's ability to provide population health?" (Q2) (TABLE II-2).

Participant responses confirmed that although there is widespread interest in population health and how it can help position an organization for accountable care, most have little strategic or tactical expertise about how to do this.

The demographic questions also shed light on how health systems deliver essential services. TABLE II-3 shows that although most of the essential inpatient and ambulatory care services are already in place, hospitals and health systems generally lack the services typically delivered by community-based, postacute provider

TABLE II-2 Level of Commitment vs. Capability	
Q1: Commitment	**Q2: Ability to Provide**
High—35%	High—4%
Moderate—46%	Moderate—58%
Low—15%	Low—34%
None—4%	None—4%

TABLE II-3 Availability of Key Services			
Service	Owned by Hospital	Provided by Partner	Not Provided
Primary care	60%	35%	5%
Specialty care	56%	37%	7%
Behavioral care	49%	25%	26%
Outpatient imaging	81%	17%	2%
Skilled nursing	25%	31%	44%
Long-term acute care	9%	42%	49%
Home health	49%	30%	21%
Hospice	32%	52%	16%
Outpatient physical rehabilitation	89%	11%	0%
Outpatient cardiac rehabilitation	84%	9%	7%

entities (e.g., long-term acute care, skilled nursing, hospice) and expect to acquire these through a partnership arrangement. Interestingly, the majority of hospitals and health systems reported owning resources related to behavioral health and home health, two components necessary to deliver fully integrated care across the continuum. Long-term acute care and skilled nursing care were the two service areas that were likely to be lacking or not currently available from a partner.

Quantitative Findings: Activities

TABLE II-4 illustrates the overall responses across the six domains along with the range of scores recorded. The grand mean was 3.2 out of 5, indicating that most of the elements assessed were under development but not yet implemented. The domain that received the highest score was community health promotion (3.8), and the lowest, as expected, was patient and family involvement (2.8). We were somewhat surprised to find that the highest scoring domain was community health promotion; it is possible that respondents equated this domain with the community needs assessments that are required in some areas and the associated community outreach services tied to those needs assessments. It is worth noting that the range of scores across the six domains was

TABLE II-4 Respondent Scores by Domain

Domain	National Average	Minimum–Maximum
Organization and leadership	3.0	1.8–4.9
Care delivery and management	3.7	1.7–4.9
Physician integration and alignment	3.3	1.2–4.8
Community health promotion	3.8	1.7–4.8
Information technology and informatics	3.2	1.4–4.9
Patient and family engagement	2.8	1.8–4.6

highly variable from organization to organization. This likely represents a combination of factors including differential level of actual preparedness, misunderstanding of the question, or lack of actual knowledge of one's current resources.

Drilling down from the domains, the key aspects that received the highest scores represented an interesting mix of competencies. The three highest scoring key aspects were (1) delivering services across the continuum (3.8), (2) physician leadership (3.8), and (3) community health promotion (3.8). Although these are not typically considered core competencies for most healthcare systems, substantial progress in advancing these areas has been made by those with an eye on becoming an ACO or undertaking risk-based payer contracts.

At the other end of the spectrum, the key aspects that received the lowest scores were (1) patient engagement (2.5), (2) lack of population health champion (2.7), and (3) patient self-care for chronic conditions. It is interesting that two of the three lowest scoring competencies involve patients. As we have learned from recent studies, patient activation and engagement is central to success with population health and accountable care. As providers become more attuned to the need for partnering with their patients, strong gains are expected in this area. Also telling was the fact that respondents had difficulty identifying universal support for population health and lacked an executive champion. Clearly, an organization must have the support of its key players both within and outside the organization, and it must be able to identify an executive champion to lead this work.

Qualitative Findings

In responding to questions regarding what the CEOs found most helpful about the PHOA, many reported that the most valuable element of the assessment was the process by which their teams completed it.

Specifically, most commented that while they found their individual scores and comparison to the national norms interesting, what added value was the group discussion that preceded the assigning of the final response score. Many realized that they had fewer resources than they initially thought, whereas others were pleasantly surprised to find out that their assets were greater than they believed. Many of the executives commented that having a wide variety of participants helped provide perspective and insight that many of the leaders lacked. Several noted that including frontline staff on the assessment team was instrumental in arriving at a more realistic assessment than would have been possible otherwise. These comments parallel those received from individuals completing the PSOA many years earlier.

▶ Next Steps

Providing the PHOA to approximately 100 VHA hospitals and health systems should not be construed as adequately describing the entire VHA membership, nor the state of the entire healthcare industry. However, the responses generated are likely representative of the vast majority of those organizations that have yet to complete the assessment. To that end, several actions will be taken to further strengthen the PHOA and broaden the insights that can be gleaned from the resulting data.

First, the PHOA will be deployed to all VHA member organizations in the remaining seven regions to increase the sample size and strengthen the reliability of the findings. The focus will be on those organizations that are underrepresented

in terms of demographic characteristics in this first deployment. Second, the questions will be validated through factor analysis and other statistical methods. Third, the breadth and depth of the questions used in the PHOA will be reviewed continually. Questions may be added or removed to make the assessment more comprehensive and meaningful to users. At the same time, efforts will be made to achieve an optimal balance between the total number of questions and the time required to complete the assessment.

Fourth, and most importantly, the findings represented by the PHOA may be subject to intentional or unintentional manipulation. We know with a high degree of certainty that respondents tend to overestimate their experience and capabilities when completing self-assessments. To address this potential shortcoming, review teams will be dispatched to organizations that complete the PHOA with scores of 5 (activity fully implemented) across one or more domains. The teams will review the activities underlying the scores of 5 to determine whether they were accurately assessed. This process will also provide important insights into the correlation between high-scoring organizations and how fully developed their population health programs are. These insights will be especially valuable to organizations beginning the population health journey.

▶ Conclusion

Completing an organizational readiness assessment is a crucial first step for organizations contemplating a population health model. The VHA Population Health Organizational Assessment (PHOA) provides a tool that allows organizations to evaluate their level of preparedness across six foundational areas. Feedback from users confirmed that most organizations are in the early discussion stages of preparing for population health. Further, respondents indicated that the conversations among the group completing the PHOA were by far the most valuable part of the exercise.

References

1. Objective Health, a McKinsey Solution for Healthcare Providers, 2013. http://www.objectivehealth.com/. Accessed November 6, 2014.
2. Population Health Management: Organizational Self-Assessment. Sg2, 2013. https://www.sg2.com/wp-content/uploads/2014/05/PHM_Organizational-Self-Assessment.pdf. Accessed November 6, 2014.
3. Hospital Readiness for Population-Based Accountable Care. Health Research and Educational Trust, Chicago, 2012. http://www.hpoe.org/resources/hpoehretaha-guides/804. Accessed November 6, 2014.
4. Safety Net Accountable Care Organization (ACO) Readiness Assessment Tool. University of California, Berkeley School of Public Health, 2012. http://www.law.berkeley.edu/files/bclbe/Mar6_FINAL_combined.pdf. Accessed November 6, 2014.

Appendix III

Case Study: The Power of Community in Population Health: PowerUp for Kids

Nico Pronk, Marina Canterbury, Thomas E. Kottke, and Donna Zimmerman

▶ Overview

Population health improvement efforts often focus on adults; however, increasing rates of childhood obesity have resulted in a growing emphasis on health improvement efforts for children.[1] The food and physical activity environments have a strong influence on youth behavior and contribute to the sobering prediction that without change, today's children will lead shorter, less healthy lives than the previous generation did.[2] To have a positive effect on children's health, population health improvement efforts must engage the community and address the multiple determinants of health, including medical care; health behaviors; and the physical, social, and economic environments.[3] Involving and engaging the community requires trusted leadership to convene multiple sectors and bring together diverse community stakeholders around the goal of improving children's health.

HealthPartners is a Minnesota-based, consumer-governed, nonprofit, integrated health system serving 1.4 million members. Committed to a population health improvement strategy since the early 1990s, the organization adopted a community health business model to focus on macrosocial determinants of health in 2010. To achieve its mission—"To improve health and well-being in partnership with our members, patients, and community"—health improvement initiatives must reach beyond clinic and hospital walls and include collaboratives with community partners. The case study presented here is one such example of HealthPartners becoming a trusted convener of a multisectoral childhood obesity prevention initiative in the St. Croix River Valley area of western Wisconsin and eastern Minnesota.

▶ PowerUp for Kids

PowerUp is a regional, community-wide initiative with a goal to *make better eating and active living easy, fun, and popular so that youth can reach their full potential.*

PowerUp focuses on children ages 3 to 11 and the adults who influence their food and physical activity choices. This initiative requires a broad approach that goes beyond individual behavior change to encompass the community-level changes necessary to increase access to healthy foods, reduce access to foods of low nutritional value, and develop physical activity–friendly environments.[4,5] PowerUp is designed to work in partnership with community stakeholders in a comprehensive approach to population health improvement for youth. The initiative reflects a 10-year commitment by HealthPartners and Lakeview Health (part of the HealthPartners family of care, located in Stillwater, Minnesota, and including Lakeview Hospital, Lakeview Foundation, and the Stillwater Medical Group) to create community-level change with a focus on childhood obesity prevention.

The PowerUp Health and Wellness Advisory Committee of the Lakeview Foundation comprises representatives from a variety of sectors including businesses, schools, healthcare providers, health plans, nonprofit organizations, community leaders, families, civic leaders, the faith community, and public health organizations. In addition, a PowerUp Steering Committee and numerous work groups help guide the effort. Strong partnerships have formed, and these community advisers support strategy development, set priorities, and hold the initiative accountable for results. Advisers also serve as key agents of change in the community by seeking opportunities to improve the food and physical activity environment for children.

A Focus on Children

Following extensive review and discussion of the evidence pertaining to community health, the need for early prevention, and the importance of positive messaging for childhood obesity, the advisory groups agreed to focus their efforts on children. Obesity and lifestyle issues were identified as a top community health priority in community health assessments performed by local county health departments.[6,7] Local data were considered (e.g., results from the Minnesota Student Survey indicating that the majority of children do not meet recommendations for fruits and vegetables, physical activity, sugar-sweetened beverages, or screen time and that by 8th grade, more than one in five boys and nearly one in seven girls are obese or overweight).[8] The focus on childhood obesity prevention was also supported by the Community Health Needs Assessment (CHNA) completed by Lakeview Hospital, a requirement for all nonprofit hospitals.[9] In essence, PowerUp is a strategy to meet these obligations for Lakeview Hospital and deliver a positive message to the community while working toward achievement of the overall mission of HealthPartners.

A Geographic Focus

The PowerUp initiative serves the St. Croix River Valley, a collection of smaller communities in Minnesota and western Wisconsin that are considered the most rapidly growing section of the Minneapolis and St. Paul metropolitan area. Initially (2013), efforts were concentrated in Stillwater and Mahtomedi, Minnesota, and Somerset, Wisconsin. In 2014, efforts expanded to include another part of the HealthPartners care system (i.e., Hudson and New Richmond, Wisconsin, in partnership with Hudson Hospital and Clinic and Westfields Hospital and Clinic). This local focus is instrumental in developing partnerships and relationships with key stakeholders by drawing on the community's shared values and identity.

▶ Community Initiative Framework

The PowerUp initiative is guided by a multilevel, multistakeholder, community-based framework designed to bring about environment change, community engagement, targeted programs, and clinical interventions. The framework is informed by the socioecological model,

but accepted among all stakeholders as a simplified approach for various audiences. The resulting PowerUp Initiatives Framework Pyramid (**FIGURE III-1**) has five sections. The top two sections represent the greater reach and lower intensity of interventions focused on environment change and community engagement. The bottom two sections represent programs of higher intensity and clinical interventions that reach smaller numbers of children and families. The "engage and transform" zones between the various levels represent the ongoing efforts for relationship and partnership building. Each level of the pyramid is linked to measurement, and reporting objectives and goals of each level are stated as follows:

1. Food and physical activity environment: The community supports and integrates healthy

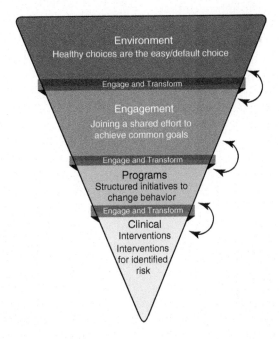

FIGURE III-1 PowerUp initiative framework for multilevel, multisector community change.

food, beverage, and physical activity options.

2. Community engagement: The community joins a shared effort to establish better food, beverage, and activity choices.

3. Programs: The target audience improves food, beverage, and physical activity behaviors.

4. Clinical interventions: The clinic provides resources and referrals to youth and families with identified risk.

5. Engagement and transformation zones between each level of the pyramid illustrate the importance of developing community relationships and partnerships to generate support and create sustainability for the initiative.

All five levels of intervention are necessary for a comprehensive approach that recognizes the vital importance of community involvement, engagement, and adoption for success and sustainability and that requires common goals among all stakeholders to improve children's long-term health and potential. When the community is engaged, change can be contagious—when one restaurant, school, child care facility, or neighborhood makes a change, others see the benefits and are more likely to change themselves.

▶ Communications and Message Strategy

Nutrition and exercise behaviors are rooted in early childhood.[10] A key to the success of the PowerUp initiative is a strong message and communication strategy that includes branding, name, logo, visual look, and main messages. Communications are developed to be relevant to children ages 3 to 11 years, and thus relevant to the adults who influence their food and activity behavior. PowerUp uses positive, simple, and fun messages through multiple channels, including print materials, advertising, a website (http://www.powerup4kids.org), and social media sites (e.g., Facebook, Twitter).

Kid-friendly, PowerUp Countdown messages are consistent, positive, and fun—more like a conversation with a peer rather than a lecture about health (**FIGURE III-2**). The Countdown is also consistent with, and complementary to, the nationally recognized 5-2-1-0 messages for childhood obesity prevention.[11] The Countdown has been well received by adults and children alike. One father reported, "My two girls ask for four colors on their plates at dinner. That means we need to offer more fruits and vegetables, but it's become really fun!"

A PowerUp Superhero

Recognizing that it would have to compete with cartoon characters endorsing sweet treats and advertisements illustrating the power of energy drinks to effectively reach children, PowerUp developed Chomp, a giant carrot superhero. Chomp is an integral part of all PowerUp communications and the Chomp mascot makes personal appearances as well (**FIGURE III-3**). Children strongly identify with Chomp, who receives messages from kids at his own e-mail address.

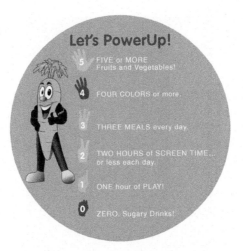

FIGURE III-2 The PowerUp countdown key messages.

▸ Adults Influenced to Change on Behalf of Children

Although focused on change for children, PowerUp expends significant effort engaging and educating adult influencers (e.g., parents, teachers, food service staff, youth leaders, community members) to do what is best for kids. PowerUp encourages adults to consider how to be role models of positive behaviors and how to support the changes necessary for creating a better food and physical activity environment for kids. This call to action for adults has been well received by parents and community leaders in multiple sectors.

▸ Community Outreach

Community outreach has significantly raised the visibility of PowerUp with the target audience. Publically launched with

a community leadership kick-off in the summer of 2012, PowerUp engaged more the 120 community leaders from numerous sectors. On May 4, 2013, PowerUp held a large community-wide launch for families, including an official world record attempt for the most people doing the Cha Cha Slide. More than 750 people attended despite the cold and rainy weather. In keeping with the fun PowerUp brand, the games, food options, and community vendors were consistent with the PowerUp Countdown message. Overall, a strong PowerUp presence at more than 150 community events has reached more than 35,000 families and children with PowerUp resources since mid-2012.

Key PowerUp Programs and Partnerships

As a multilevel intervention, PowerUp works across a wide variety of community sectors. Following are examples of effective partnerships and programs.

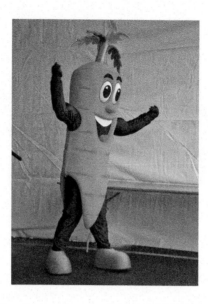

FIGURE III-3 Chomp, the PowerUp superhero mascot, visits with children at an early childhood center.
Courtesy of PowerUp.

PowerUp School Challenge

This 4-week, classroom-based, elementary school program was developed in partnership with the HealthPartners yumPower School Challenge—another community-based program focused on healthy eating and active living (http://www.yumpower.com). The challenge kicks off with a high-energy student assembly featuring Radio Disney to generate excitement about increasing fruit and vegetable intake and physical activity. Students track their fruits and vegetables on weekly trackers. Teachers, parents, and school food service personnel all participate to reinforce lessons and activities. In addition, schools receive incentives for high participation rates in the form of PowerUp bucks, which can be used to purchase wellness-related items for the schools. Data from student trackers and parent and school surveys indicate that students are more interested in fruits and vegetables and are increasing their intake as a result of the challenge.

School Change

The primary local school board issued a PowerUp proclamation in support of PowerUp, and better food and physical activity priorities are incorporated into the districts' 5-year strategic plans. After-school programs have replaced many processed foods with fruits and vegetables, food service offers fruit and veggie snacks, and sugary beverages and foods at school carnivals and concessions have decreased.

Open Gym Events

Open gyms have been a highly successful intervention to increase physical activity. PowerUp partnered with local schools in three communities to provide more than 30 free or low-cost open gyms during cold weather months to give families an opportunity to be active. Hundreds of kids and families attended, with up to 120 people attending a single session, exceeding school district officials' expectations.

Food Shelf Change

In an innovative attempt to reach underserved populations, PowerUp partnered with the local Valley Outreach food shelf. Working collaboratively to revise food lists, inventory, and layout, more fruits and vegetables are now available to clients, at least five a day for each family member for the days food comes from the food shelf. Positive promotion has made fruits, vegetables, and whole grains the easy choice. Food shelves and hunger organizations from across the region have toured Valley Outreach to learn from this model and create change at their own food shelves.

▶ Measuring Progress

PowerUp uses multiple internal and external measures to evaluate progress, including program surveys and data from the clinics, health plans, counties, and school districts. Reporting is summarized in an evaluation dashboard and organized around two types of measures as follows:

- What we are doing: Process measures include outreach and marketing efforts, programs, trainings, and community-sector engagement.
- What difference it makes: Outcome measures include community response; environment or policy change; changes in attitude, awareness, or behavior; long-term health; and body mass index (BMI) trends.

Results are reported at multiple levels of the PowerUp Pyramid Framework, and results to date for key PowerUp activities are summarized in **TABLE III-1**.

TABLE III-1 PowerUp: Intervention Results Summary: 2013–Q1 2014		
PowerUp Key Intervention/ Resource	**Reach (January 2013– First Quarter of 2014)**	**Results**
Community Outreach Activities, games, and information at local community fairs and events	More than 35,000 people reached at more than 150 events	Majority of target audience aware and value PowerUp after 1 year of outreach. Requests for PowerUp at events is growing rapidly.
Open Gyms Offered in partnership with three school districts as an alternative for family physical activity in cold-weather months	30 open gyms in three communities; attendance ranges from 45–120	Surveys indicate great appreciation by families for low-cost physical play options. Attendance continues to grow.

(continues)

TABLE III-1 PowerUp: Intervention Results Summary: 2013–Q1 2014   *(continued)*

PowerUp Key Intervention/ Resource	Reach (January 2013– First Quarter of 2014)	Results
PowerUp Kids Cooking Classes Offered for two age groups in partnership with local cooking school and hospital dietitians	18 classes with a total of 325 attendees	75% of attendees indicate that they will make a specific food behavior change as a result of the class
The PowerUp Pledge A call to action for a family, a person, or an organization to PowerUp (http://www.powerup4kids.org /pledge)	Pledge included at events and website	700 have taken the pledge
PowerUp Food Coach Training Training food service and child care staff on methods to increase and positively promote fruits and vegetables offered	205 staff trained	More than 9,000 children are exposed to positive messages about fruits and vegetables.
PowerUp Sports Nutrition Playbook Developed at request of local coach to provide athletes and parents with information about better food and beverage choices for athletes	300 athletes, coaches, and parents reached	Sports teams no longer provide sugar-sweetened sports drinks to athletes but rather provide and encourage water. Parent volunteers lead changes in concessions at school events to reduce sugary foods and beverages and provide better choices.
PowerUp School Challenge A 4-week, classroom-based, elementary school program with an assembly to generate excitement about fruits and vegetables. Students track fruits and vegetables daily. Teachers, parents, and school food service personnel participate with lessons and activities.	2013: 5,300 students, two school districts, three other schools 2014: 8,200 students, four school districts, four other schools	Data from student trackers and parent and school surveys indicate that students are more interested in fruits and vegetables and are increasing intake as a result of the challenge.
Website and Social Media Powerup4kids.org (https://www.facebook.com/#!/ PowerUpKids)	14,762 unique website visitors; 813 Facebook and 75 Pinterest followers	Community response on website and social media grows consistently. Popular content includes recipes, "Veggie Voting," and letters to Chomp.

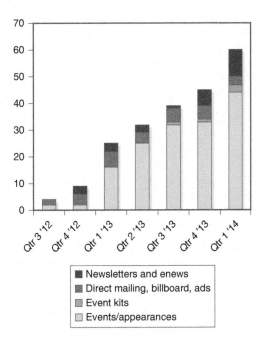

FIGURE III-4 PowerUp community outreach by quarter, Q3 2012–Q1 2014.

The consistent growth of community outreach is illustrated in **FIGURE III-4**. The evaluation approach also includes a family survey tool that measures child and family behaviors, attitudes, and awareness. Households with young children were randomly selected to receive the survey in five communities in January 2014. The survey will be repeated at 2-year intervals over the course of the intervention to measure progress. Early survey results indicate very high awareness and perceived value of the initiative, with three out of four being aware of PowerUp and 95% indicating that the initiative is important or very important. Responses related to intake of fruits, vegetables, and sugar-sweetened beverages; screen time; and physical activity are being analyzed and will be compared over time.

The PowerUp initiative is an excellent example of engaging the local community to affect a large population and working collaboratively toward sustainable change and improved population health. The initiative also demonstrates how a health system can work in partnership with the community as a trusted convener of multiple stakeholders—a role that is paramount for successful community initiatives. Importantly, this initiative targets both individual behavior change and the relevant social, physical, and economic environments, thus changing the social norms that affect overall health.

References

1. Centers for Disease Control and Prevention. Childhood obesity in the United States, 2010. http://www.cdc.gov/about/grand-rounds/archives/2010/download/GR-062010.pdf. Accessed May 30, 2014.

2. Olshansky SJ, Passaro DJ, Hershow RC, et al. A potential decline in life expectancy in the United States in the 21st century. *N Engl J Med.* 2005;352:1138-45.

3. Isham G, Zimmerman D, Kindig D, et al. HealthPartners adopts community business model to deepen focus on nonclinical factors of health outcomes. *Health Aff.* 2013;32(8):1446-52.

4. Glickman D, Parker L, Sim L, et al., eds. *Accelerating Progress in Obesity Prevention: Solving the Weight of the Nation.* Committee on Accelerating Progress in Obesity Prevention, Food and Nutrition Board. Institute of Medicine. Washington, DC: National Academies Press; 2012.

5. Keener D, Goodman K, Lowry A, et al. *Recommended Community Strategies and Measurements to Prevent Obesity in the United States: Implementation and Measurement Guide.* U.S. Department of Health and Human Services. Centers for Disease Control and Prevention; 2009. http://www.cdc.gov/obesity/downloads/community_strategies_guide.pdf. Accessed November 7, 2014.

6. Washington County, Minnesota, Community Health Board. *Washington County 2008 Community Health Assessment: Community Health Improvement Plan 2009–2014.* http://www.co.washington.mn.us/DocumentCenter/View/6. Accessed November 7, 2014.

7. Healthier Together—St. Croix County: Community Health Improvement Plan, 2009–2014. http://www.co.saint-croix.wi.us/vertical/Sites/%7BBC2127FC-9D61-44F6-A557-17F280990A45%7D/uploads/Healthier_Together_-_St__Croix_County_Plan_FINAL_6-15-11.pdf. Accessed November 7, 2014.

8. 2010 Minnesota Student Survey. Washington County Tables. http://www.health.state.mn.us/divs/chs/mss/countytables/washington10.pdf. Accessed November 7, 2014.

9. Minnesota Hospital Association. Community health needs assessment. http://www.mnhospitals.org/policy-advocacy/priority-issues/community-benefitactivities/communityhealth-needs-assessment. Accessed November 7, 2014.

10. Cunningham SA, Kramer MR, Venkat Narayan KM. Incidence of childhood obesity in the United States. *N Engl J Med.* 2014;370:403-11.

11. Childhood Obesity Action Network: Expert committee recommendations on the assessment, prevention and treatment of child and adolescent overweight and obesity, 2007. http://obesity.nichq.org/resources/expert%20committee%20recommendation%20implementation%20guide. Accessed June 1, 2014.

Glossary

Accountable care organizations (ACOs) Integrated groups of providers that include hospitals, physicians, and post-discharge care delivery organizations that work together to deliver coordinated care that is focused on quality, efficiency, and value.

Administrative services only An insurance model in which the employer directly bears the risk for the costs of the benefits.

Advocacy Efforts to enlist support to a particular cause; lobbying.

Agency The ability of an individual or group to choose to act with purpose.

Alignment of constituencies Coordination of the priorities of different stakeholders in order to achieve a particular overarching goal that they have in common.

Allostatic load The cumulative wear and tear on the body's systems owing to repeated adaptation to stressors.

Alternative payment models Payment models that offer incentives to physicians to provide more focused care as a way of saving patients and insurers the cost of care with less optimal outcomes.

Analytic epidemiology Epidemiological research focused on searching for the determinants of diseases.

Analytics The science of utilizing systematic analysis of data to identify and predict trends.

Attribution Methods to identify which patient is in the care of which provider for billing purposes.

Autonomy Lack of dependence on another for managing decisions and life activities.

Behavioral economics The study of the psychological, cognitive, emotional, cultural, and social factors affecting financial or economic decisions made by individuals and institutions.

Behavioral intervention A plan of action designed to help a patient alter his or her behavior to improve health.

Behavioral psychology The study of the psychological underpinnings of human behavior.

Benchmark performance The level of performance that sets the standard for quality.

Best practice Methods shown by evidence to provide the best options.

Big data Analysis of large sets of structured and unstructured data to enable the prediction of trends.

Bipartisan policy or law that has support from members of the two major political parties.

Bundled payment Reimbursement for services based on the expected costs of a clinically defined episode of care.

Capitation A payment model in which the provider is paid a set amount per patient regardless of whether the patient seeks care.

Care coordination Steps taken to ensure that care provided by different providers works in tandem to improve patient health, rather than at cross-purposes or in isolation.

Care management Steps taken to provide support to the patient in managing chronic or long-term conditions such that outcomes are improved (e.g., coaching or training for diabetes management or wound care).

Care model The basic framework that determines how care is provided, coordinated, and billed, developed with an eye toward improving cost effectiveness and outcomes.

Care transformation A process of altering the structures and delivery methods of health care within an organization.

Caucus A group of political leaders who work in concert to achieve specific goals or agendas on behalf of a subgroup they represent or to which they belong.

Centers of excellence Healthcare systems or institutions that offer high-quality evidence-based care for a specific disease condition or population.

Change The process of altering prior behaviors or structures.

Change management Management processes intended to guide organizational or personal change.

Children's Health Insurance Program (CHIP) A health insurance program designed to provide insurance for children whose parents do not qualify for Medicaid but are unable to afford commercial insurance.

Choice architecture The organization of the context in which people make decisions.

Chronic care management Care coordination across the many settings where care is delivered that uses evidence-based clinical management and effective self-management such that treatment decisions are made jointly by the patient and the provider.

Cohort A group of people assembled or observed by researchers in order to learn about the extent or causes of health problems. Cohorts have similar demographic, risk factor, or health outcome characteristics.

Collaboration A cooperative effort by various stakeholders to achieve a specific goal.

Commercial insurance Health insurance policies sold on the open market to companies so they can cover their employees' healthcare needs.

Community health workers Lay volunteer or paid advisors who offer interpretation and translation services; provide culturally tailored health education; and help community members connect with needed resources inside and outside of the health system.

Comparative effectiveness research (CER) Research that seeks evidence comparing the benefits and harms of alternative methods to prevent, diagnose, treat, and monitor a clinical condition or to improve the delivery of care so that consumers, clinicians, purchasers, and policy makers can make informed decisions about what will improve health care at both the individual and population levels.

Competencies The combination of knowledge, skills, and behaviors a person must demonstrate to be successful in a defined position.

Competency model A framework that defines the skills and knowledge required for a specific job.

Compression of morbidity The research finding that the longer one can maintain good health, the shorter the period of significant illness before one dies.

Congressional Budget Office (CBO) A nonpartisan agency mandated to provide Congress with unbiased assessments of the costs and benefits of a particular policy initiative or law.

Cost effectiveness Assessment as to whether the value of an intervention is in alignment with its monetary cost; that is, whether outcomes are sufficiently positive to warrant the expense of obtaining them.

Critical roles The roles with the most significant impact on outcomes.

Cultural competency A set of congruent behaviors, attitudes, and policies that come together in a system or agency or among professionals and enable that system, agency, or those professions to work effectively in cross-cultural situations.

Culture of health and wellness Policies developed to encourage people to choose healthy behaviors that help prevent poor health and avoid unhealthy behaviors that promote health problems.

Data governance A system of decision rights and accountabilities for information-related processes, executed according to agreed-upon models that describe in detail the circumstances, methods, actions, timing, information and responsibile parties involved.

Data science The science of developing algorithms and analytics to generate insights from a dataset.

Delivery The components that influence whether a patient receives appropriate and necessary care within the healthcare system, including access, cost controls, quality improvements, prevention, workforce development, revenue, and administrative billing and costs.

Demand The buyer's willingness to acquire a product or service at a given price.

Descriptive epidemiology Epidemiological investigations summarizing the impact and extent of health-related events among particular groups.

Determinants The varied factors that affect the health of individuals, ranging from aspects of the social and economic environment to the physical environment and individual characteristics or behaviors; a definable entity that causes, is associated with, or induces a health outcome, such as death or disease.

Disease surveillance Routine collection of data to identify the prevalence and distribution of a given health condition over time.

Distribution Variation in the frequency of disease and mortality from disease among different demographic groups.

Downside risk A situation in which an ACO that is reimbursed by capitation assumes responsibility for the difference between the premium and the cost of care provided.

Driver diagram A visual tool that organizes the theory of improvement for a specific project, visually connecting the outcome or aim, key drivers, design changes, and measures.

Ecological model of health behavior A model focused on the influence of the totality of the environment on human behavior that delineates the elements of that environment and theorizes ways in which those components complement or oppose each other in shaping an individual's decision making.

Effectiveness A pragmatic assessment of whether an intervention works in routine clinical care.

Efficacy An assessment regarding whether an intervention can work under ideal conditions.

Efficiency Measurement of the amount of effort or resources needed to obtain positive outcomes or results.

Electronic health record (EHR) A database containing routinely updated patient records.

Epidemic The occurrence of cases of an illness, health-related behavior, or other health-related event at a higher rate than expected within a population and derived from a common source.

Experimental studies Research studies in which the investigator manipulates both the study factor (drug, treatment, or intervention) and randomly assigns subjects to the exposed and non-exposed groups.

Fee-for-service (FFS) An insurance model in which healthcare providers are reimbursed for every service they perform regardless of outcome.

Financing The system through which healthcare services are reimbursed.

Federally Qualified Health Centers (FQHCs) Community-based healthcare providers that receive funds from the HRSA Health Center Program to provide primary care services in underserved areas.

Grassroots Lobbying efforts that encourage members of the public to reach out to policymakers in the legislative or executive branches to influence policy.

Grasstops Lobbying efforts that encourage a narrower scope of individuals, usually leaders (e.g., thought leaders, community leaders, organization leaders) to reach out to policymakers in the legislative or executive branches to influence policy.

Health behavior theory Concepts of how health behaviors impact health and what strategies help in changing health behaviors that draw upon various disciplines such as psychology, sociology, anthropology, consumer behavior, and marketing.

Health behaviors Behavioral factors that have strong effects on health, including smoking, poor diet, physical inactivity, and alcohol consumption.

Health disparities Preventable differences in the burden of disease, injury, violence or opportunities to achieve optimal health that are experienced by socially disadvantaged populations.

Health ecosystem The collection of diverse yet interdependent sectors with a shared interest in improving health outcomes and quality of life.

Health equity The absence of avoidable, unfair, or remediable differences in health among groups of people, regardless of the way these groups are defined (socially, economically, demographically, geographically, etc).

Health information exchanges Organizations that manage and enable the exchange of health data for a particular region or state.

Health information technology (HIT) Computer systems and networks enabling the collection, analysis, and maintenance of health data by healthcare organizations.

Health policy Policies and laws that identify health priorities and support and promote public health initiatives.

Health promotion The process of enabling people to improve their health.

Health status An assessment of the overall health of a population including identification of specific priorities to be addressed.

Healthcare exchange Government-regulated and standardized health care plans offered by the insurers participating in the exchange, which can be a national exchange (Healthcare.gov) or a state-run exchange.

Healthcare policy Legislative and public policy initiatives intended to improve healthcare access and quality for the majority of people in the society.

Healthcare quality An assessment of the systems and processes implemented to make health care safer, more efficient, more cost effective, and better in overall outcome.

Healthy life expectancy A metric that combines the ultimate outcome measures for population health (i.e., length and quality of life) to identify the amount of time the majority of the population lives in a state of good health.

Healthy People 2030 The most recent update to the federal *Healthy People* policy priorities agenda that confirms that achieving health and well-being requires eliminating health disparities, attaining health literacy, and achieving health equity.

HHS The U.S. Department of Health and Human Services, the federal agency tasked with executing health and social service policies and laws passed by Congress.

Incidence The rate of development of new cases of disease among people in a group over a certain time period.

Influencers Individuals or organizations that have the ability to convince others in society to behave in specific ways.

Informatics The science of data processing; information science.

Insurance An agreement in which a participant pays a set fee to an insurer to offset risk; the company receiving the fee agrees to reimburse expenses covered by the agreement should they occur.

Integrated data warehouse An IT system that allows different components of the healthcare system to access data about a specific patient.

IT system The network of computers, servers, and software used to obtain and store health information.

Learning approaches and modalities Different techniques used to define a range of development approaches, including training, which matches the identified development needs.

Lobbying A formalized method of public policy advocacy. *See also* **Advocacy**.

Meaningful Use A standard for electronic health record implementation set by the Affordable Care Act.

Medicaid A public healthcare insurance option intended for individuals who live in poverty created by a 1965 amendment to the Social Security Act.

The Medicaid and CHIP Payment and Access Commission (MACPAC) A nonpartisan legislative branch agency authorized by the ACA. MACPAC serves as an independent source of information on Medicaid and the State Children's Health Insurance Program (CHIP) and makes recommendations to Congress, the Secretary of HHS, and states on issues affecting Medicaid and CHIP.

Medical-legal partnerships Formal collaborations between attorneys and healthcare systems to address those social determinants of health for which there are civil law remedies.

Medically homeless An individual who lacks a connection to a healthcare organization and must seek care on an uncoordinated, piecemeal basis.

Medicare A public healthcare insurance option intended for elderly individuals (those age 65 and older,) or those with disabilities, created by a 1965 amendment to the Social Security Act.

Medicare Payment Advisory Commission (MedPAC) A nonpartisan legislative branch agency established by the Balanced Budget Act of 1997 to advise the U.S. Congress on issues related to reimbursement for private Medicare plans (i.e., Medicare Advantage) and traditional fee-for-service Medicare.

Model for Improvement A change management tool that combines basic problem-solving techniques—identify the problem and what constitutes success—with continual plan, do, study, act (PDSA) cycles to test and implement changes in real-world settings.

Morbidity A measurement of ill health.

Mortality The measure of the number of deaths in a particular population.

National Priorities Partnership A collaborative venture convened by the National Quality Forum in 2008 to address four major healthcare challenges that affect all Americans: eliminating harm, eradicating disparities, reducing disease burden, and removing waste.

Nudges Information intended to remind or encourage patients to move toward healthier behaviors.

Observational study A study in which researchers do not intervene to impose an exposure on subjects or randomize study subjects. Instead, epidemiologists "observe" the natural exposure categories or disease diagnoses that characterize people and assign them to groups based on these characteristics (e.g., case-control studies and cohort studies). These types of studies measure patterns of exposure in populations to draw inferences about cause and effect.

Organizational culture How organizations make decisions and characterizes the behaviors that are consistently demonstrated and reinforced within an organization.

Organizational transformation A change management process that seeks to restructure an organization to achieve a new set of goals or priorities.

Pandemic An epidemic affecting populations of an extensive region, country, or continent.

Pathway A sequence of choices or decisions that leads to a specific outcome or destination.

Patient navigator An individual who helps guide patients through the healthcare system and works to overcome obstacles that are in the way of the patient receiving the required care and treatment.

Patient Protection and Affordable Care Act A comprehensive healthcare reform law passed in 2010 under the Obama administration.

Patient safety A set of standards that outline what constitutes reasonable versus unacceptable risks to a patient's health or well-being.

Patient-centered medical home A model of care in which the patient's disparate healthcare needs are assessed, coordinated, and managed through a single organization.

Payment The reimbursement of a healthcare provider for services or treatment provided.

Payer The organization (insurance company, Medicare, etc.) that pays for services rendered by healthcare providers.

Plan, do, study, act (PDSA) cycle A time-tested framework for generating and testing ideas for improvement. The *plan* step involves developing objectives, predictions, and plans to carry out the cycle. The *do* step involves carrying out the plan and documenting data and observations. The *study* step involves analyzing the data, comparing results to predictions, and summarizing what was learned. The *act* step involves determining the changes to be made in the next cycle, after which the cycle repeats.

Population health The distribution of health outcomes within a population, the health determinants that influence distribution, and the policies and interventions that affect those determinants.

Population health management The combination of information gathered to define problems and build awareness and the strategies to Address Population Health Needs.

Population health management (PHM) systems Systems to support population health initiatives by coordinating care based on the level of risk in a cohort. These systems include data aggregation, data analysis and risk stratification, and care management and coordination.

Predictive analytics Data analytics that are used to identify trends with the goal of anticipating future developments.

Prevalence The number of existing cases of a disease or health issue at some designated time.

Private sector Nongovernment entities and organizations.

Program evaluation The systematic collection, analysis, and use of information to answer questions about effectiveness and efficacy of healthcare projects, policies, and programs.

Program planning Development of processes and activities that may be used to improve public health.

Public health The science of protecting and improving the health of people and their communities by promoting healthy lifestyles, disease and injury prevention, and preventing/responding to infectious diseases.

Qualitative research A scientific method of observation in social sciences to gather non-numerical data that can complement quantitative data by providing richer context and background.

Quality-adjusted life-years (QALYs) A year of life lived in less-than-perfect health compared to a year of life in perfect health.

Return on investment (ROI) An assessment of the value received for inputs of time or resources.

Risk reduction Mechanisms to lower a patient's likelihood of developing a disease or slow the progression of an illness or condition.

Risk stratification Identification of high-risk populations versus lower-risk populations.

Road map A plan or outline of steps to take a person or an organization to a desired outcome.

Run chart A basic data analytics tool consisting of a trend graph that includes a median line.

Shared savings Reimbursement models in which any savings obtained by accountable care organizations are split between the payer and the healthcare provider.

Social determinants of health (SDOH) The conditions in which people are born, grow, live, work, and age. These circumstances are shaped by the distribution of money, power, and resources at the global, national, and local levels.

Social media Online platforms and publishing apps that enable rapid information exchange.

Sponsorship Efforts by leaders to promote a particular project or workforce development effort.

Stakeholders Individuals and organizations within the healthcare system who have a vested interest, skill sets, and networks associated with the delivery of services.

Stigma The co-occurrence of labeling, stereotyping, separation, status loss, and discrimination in a context in which power is exercised.

Strategy The decisions made for how organizations will use resources to create value for customers and achieve their objectives.

Structural racism The totality of ways in which societies foster racial discrimination through mutually reinforcing systems of housing, education, employment, earning, benefits, credit, media, health care, and criminal justice. These patterns and practices in turn reinforce discriminatory beliefs, values, and distribution of resources, which all potentially impact health. Structural racism has resulted in reduced access to care; lower-quality care; denial of services (including recommended diagnostic tests and treatments); fewer referrals to clinical research programs; and delivery of unneeded and harmful interventions.

Structure The organization of different components that interact in healthcare delivery.

Success profile A tool that categorizes the competencies needed for success.

Supply The seller's willingness to offer the good to the buyer at an agreed-upon price.

Sustainable A process or structure that can be maintained in the long term without the addition of new or extra resources.

Systems A collection of components that work together in an organized way, such as a group of hospitals and clinics that provide care for patients.

Telemedicine The exchange of medical information from one site to another through electronic communications to evaluate, diagnose and treat patients in remote locations.

Triple Aim The goals of health care, as defined by the Institute for Healthcare Improvement, consisting of (1) improving the individual experience of care, (2) improving the health of populations, and (3) reducing the per capita costs of care for populations.

Upside risk A reimbursement model that allows healthcare providers in an ACO to share in the healthcare savings if the cost of the services provided are less than projected.

Value The amount an individual would be willing to pay for health care in monetary terms or give up in terms of other resources or time to receive it.

Value equation The relationship between the outcomes of healthcare delivery and the cost of healthcare delivery, such that value is equal to outcomes divided by cost.

Value-based benefit design An insurance model that offers benefits based on what options will offer the most beneficial outcomes for the most reasonable cost.

Wearables Electronic devices worn on the body that collect data related to health status.

Weathering A hypothesis developed by Arline Geronimus and her coauthors that posits that black Americans' health deteriorates more rapidly than that of other groups because they bear a heavier allostatic load.

Wellness The process of becoming aware of and consciously selecting habits and behaviors that improve or maintain good health.

Wellness champions Individuals designated or self-selected to promote wellness to their peers.

Workforce development plan A plan that defines a range of development approaches, including training, that matches the organization's identified development needs.

Workplace environment The physical, social, and organizational culture environment in which a person works.

Index

Note: Page numbers followed by *b, f,* or *t* indicate material in boxes, figures, or tables, respectively.